Remedies and Rituals

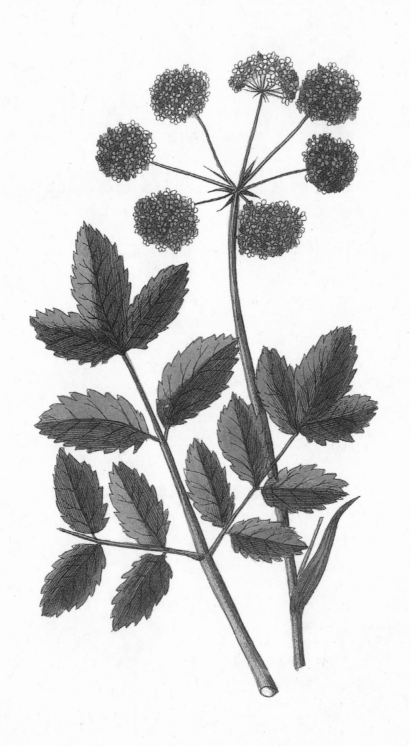

Remedies and Rituals

FOLK MEDICINE IN NORWAY AND THE NEW LAND

Kathleen Stokker

 MINNESOTA HISTORICAL SOCIETY PRESS

www.mhspress.org
The Minnesota Historical Society Press is a member of the Association of American University Presses.

Manufactured in the United States of America

10 9 8 7 6 5 4 3 2 1

♾ The paper used in this publication meets the minimum requirements of the American National Standard for Information Sciences—Permanence for Printed Library Materials, ANSI Z39.48–1984.

International Standard Book Number
ISBN 13: 978–0–87351–576–4 (cloth)
ISBN 10: 0–87351–576–5 (cloth)

Library of Congress Cataloging-in-Publication Data

Stokker, Kathleen, 1946–
    Remedies and rituals : folk medicine in Norway and the New Land / Kathleen Stokker.
        p. ; cm.
    Includes bibliographical references and index.
    ISBN-13: 978–0-87351–576–4 (cloth : alk. paper)
    ISBN-10: 0–87351–576–5 (cloth : alk. paper)
    1. Alternative medicine—Norway—History.   2. Traditional medicine—Norway—History. I. Title.
[DNLM: 1. Medicine, Traditional—history—Norway. 2. Medicine, Traditional—history—United States. 3. History, 19th Century—Norway. 4. History, 19th Century—United States. 5. Magic—history—Norway. 6. Magic—history—United States. 7. Phytotherapy—history—Norway. 8. Phytotherapy—history—United States. WZ 309 S864r 2007]
    R733.S76 2007
    615.8'809481—dc22

2006027948

To the memory of T. U. ("Tiny") Fretheim, Evelyn Thykeson Fretheim, and "Bami."

To Liv Dahl, Jane Jakoubek, Deb Miller, Ann Regan, and E. S., midwives of the manuscript.

To the self-trained healers who filled the void.

Contents

Preface

ALL THE STOKKER COUSINS knew the story of Grandpa. We often reviewed its horrifying details—the fall from a skittish horse that dragged the young husband and father over rough ground until his head hit a tree stump. They had laid him out on the counter of the grocery store he managed in Hayward, Minnesota, though by then he was beyond help. The "popular Otilia Gulbrandsen," as one newspaper dubbed our grandmother, had been his bride only four years earlier. Now a widow with two young daughters, she left the apartment above the store, returned to her parents' farm, and, one month later, gave birth to my father. As tradition decreed, she named him George for the father he would never know.

Of course, we all knew this story; it had transformed our parents' lives. Strangely, the story of another ancestor who had touched many more lives went untold. Only far into research for this book did I learn that my mother's great-grandmother had been a self-trained caregiver. She apparently never said much about it to her family, and her work would have been entirely forgotten had she not lived to be one hundred years old. To celebrate this milestone, an *Albert Lea (Minnesota) Tribune* journalist interviewed her in December 1927. The Sunday rotogravure section of the *Minneapolis Tribune* published a picture of her, wearing a lovely lace cap and satin gown and holding a Bible in her lap, with the caption: "Reads without spectacles at 100."

Though I recall seeing this photo proudly displayed in my mother's childhood home, the story of her great-grandmother's "doctoring" never became part of family lore. If the newspaper reporter had not included these details, this aspect of her life would now be unknown. "Handy at nursing, she was called often to the bedside of a neighbor, where she took the place of a doctor in times of need," says the old clipping. Born on December 1, 1827, at Leikanger in Sogn, Norway, Mari Samson married Nels Simonson in 1855 and emigrated with him and their two daughters in 1865. The family stopped in Dane County, Wisconsin, for a year before settling in the Riceland Township of Freeborn County, Minnesota.

In the interview, Mari Simonson told about a night in 1868 when she was busy making a pair of overalls for her husband. Neighbor Ole Wangen rushed to her house to ask for assistance with his wife, who was in labor and very ill. At first Mari refused because she needed to finish the overalls for her husband, who would leave early the next day to walk more than forty miles to Rochester for harvest work. When Wangen pleaded, Mari relented and returned with the worried neighbor.

Later that night, when the mother and new baby were comfortable, Mari started back in the dark. The mile-and-a-half distance would have seemed short in daylight, but the road was difficult to follow at night, and she became lost in a marsh. Confused, she wandered until the first gray streaks of dawn finally guided her home, just in time to finish the overalls for her husband to leave as planned.

Many readers of this book, whether they know it or not, have someone like Mari Simonson in their own family. Every settlement had at least one self-trained "healer" who cared for neighbors' ills, but most of their stories have been lost. Little has been written about the everyday medicine practiced in a time when most Norwegians lacked access to the country's few professionally trained doctors.

Since standard histories have left this story untold, I turned to the family histories written in recent years by amateur genealogists and found in the libraries of the Norwegian colleges, the Minnesota Historical Society, the Norwegian American Historical Association, and Vesterheim Museum. Diaries, letters, memoirs, church histories, personal interviews, and newspaper accounts were also primary sources for my research.

Some of the contemporary medical details have come from "doctor books," or popular health manuals. Included are C. E. Mangor's *Lande-apothek* (Country apothecary), published in Copenhagen in 1803; *Lægebog for hvermand* (Doctor book for everyone [Chicago, 1879]); *Huslægen* (The house doctor), a portion of *Husvennen* (The home companion [La Crosse, 1883]); and *Før doktoren kommer* (Until the doctor arrives [Decorah, 1892]). Except for Mangor, these publications were issued by Norwegian American newspapers as premiums for their subscribers. Also consulted was *People's Home Medical Book*, by T. J. Ritter, the first third of the black-bound, thousand-page *People's Home Library*, published in 1915.

Another source, *The Diary of Elisabeth Koren, 1853–1855*, revealed the medical role of the pastor's family, and the classic midwifery text by F. C. Faye (Christiania, 1844) granted unparalleled glimpses of nineteenth-century obstetrical practice. The so-called black-book formulas (most notably published as *Norske Hexeformularer* in 1901 by A. C. Bang) detailed the magical medicine that lived on in both the Old Country and the New Land.

Among secondary sources, I would especially mention Olav Bø's *Folkemedisin og lærd medisin* (Folk medicine and professional medicine [1986]), for its overview of legal actions and court cases endured by several self-trained healers, and Per Holck's *Norsk Folkemedisin*, for its general look at Norwegian folk medicine. My chapter on childbirth relies heavily on Lily Weiser-Aall's *Svangerskap og fødsel i moderne norsk trasisjon* (Pregnancy and childbirth in modern Norwegian tradition [1968]) and Kristina Kjærheim's history of midwifery, *Mellom kloke koner og kvitkledde menn* (Between magical folk healers and white-coated men [1987]). Two works by Norway's incomparable scholar of folk medicine, Injald Reichborn-Kjennerud—*Våre norske lægeurter* (Our healing herbs [1922]) and his extended article about old Scandinavian doctor books—have been indispensable resources throughout this project.

Travel has been essential to my research. Visiting the old neighborhoods where Mor Sæther and Anne Brandfjeld tended their patients when Oslo was still Christiania; searching for Olene Solberg, who "cupped" her neighbors in Arkdale, Wisconsin; tracing Trondheim emigrant Olava (Yttervik) Wick, whose renown as Doctor Gamla (the old lady doctor) reached far beyond her home in Dalton, Minnesota; and finding the drugstore in Cooperstown, North Dakota, owned by Severin Almklov, whose Itch Specific cured untold thousands with scabies—each journey added new and otherwise unattainable insights.

Much of the success of these expeditions depended on helpful guides, including Ragnhild Slette, who drove me through the green hills of Dovre, Gudbrandsdal, to fill in the background of Ole Toftelien and his black book; Lorraine Becken, who told me the lore associated with Toftelien's daughter in Hanska, Minnesota; Gloria Gransberg, who led me to Valborg Skåret's account of nineteenth-century childbirth and showed me where Valborg had lived in Trysil; and Kari Grønningsæter, who scouted persons and places associated with Valborg Valand, introducing me to them as we made our way along Norway's idyllic southern coast from Kristiansand to Mandal.

Museums have also played a major role in this project. Having Vesterheim Norwegian-American Museum so close to my home in Decorah, Iowa, is a gift beyond measure that has influenced my work in countless ways.

I have also appreciated my association with the Sogn Folkemuseum in Kaupanger, where curator Aud Ross Solberg mounted an exhibit on traditional Norwegian healing practices in the 1990s. Realizing our shared interest in folk medicine, she arranged for the two of us to interview thirteen elderly residents of Vik, Balestrand, Fortun, Fjærland, and Sogndal about the home remedies used by their families.

To gain a better understanding of botany, once the most important of the medical sciences, I visited the herbal gardens in Hamar, the Esrum Cloister and Steno Museum in Denmark, and the apothecary garden of the Folk Museum in Oslo. At the Hatton-Eielsen Museum in Hatton, North Dakota, one of Aagot Raaen's former pupils vividly recounted Raaen's work as an inspiring teacher, then took me to the neighborhood where the Raaens had lived and the Goose River churchyard where they are buried.

For financial assistance in making these journeys and in traveling to research libraries at Norway's Rikshospital in Oslo, the National Institutes of Health in Bethesda, Maryland, the Academy of Medicine in New York City, the Library of Congress, the New York Public Library, and the University of Wisconsin at Madison medical school, I am sincerely grateful for travel grants from the Norwegian Ministry of Foreign Affairs and faculty research funds from Luther College. I am also indebted to the constant and consistently gracious help of Preus Library's Kathy Buzza and Eddie Attwell and the staff of the college print shop.

Deb Miller's invitation to use the McKnight Research Suite at the Minnesota Historical Society in St. Paul, Minnesota, enabled me to derive maximum benefit from my 2002–03 sabbatical leave from Luther College. Developmental readings of early versions of the text provided by Jane Jakoubek, Ann Regan, and the ever elusive E. S. proved crucial to the ultimate completion of this project.

In the following pages are the names of others who generously shared their ancestors' stories. Added to these are the many unlisted helpers who have in letters, conversations after lectures, personal visits, or other ways vitally assisted my understanding of this extremely complex subject. Aware of having barely scratched the surface, I am nevertheless deeply grateful for this help. Without it, this book would simply not exist.

Remedies and Rituals

A note about spelling

I have used the nineteenth-century spelling of the word *"almuen"* (term for the "common classes" used by the elite, or *kondisjonerte*, class), although in modern Norwegian the word is spelled *"allmuen."* Conversely, I have used the more modern spelling *"svekk"* (instead of the nineteenth-century *"svek"*) for the disease now known as rickets, because it better suggests its pronunciation with a short "e."

The name and spelling of Norway's capital city has changed several times. At its founding around the year 1050, it was called "Oslo." In 1624 the city adopted the name "Christiania" to honor King Christian IV, who suggested rebuilding with brick instead of wood after a catastrophic fire. The spelling changed to "Kristiania" in 1877, and in 1925 the city once again became "Oslo."

·1

Healing the People

"People weren't so quick to go to the doctor in the old days."

Thor Økland (born 1885 in Tysnes, Hordaland)

NOTHING SHAPED THE LIVES of nineteenth-century Norwegians more than their health, but historical accounts remain vexingly silent on the subject. Though some sources mention doctors, nurses, and hospitals, they completely overlook the meaningful medicine practiced by mothers and neighbors, by pastors and pastors' wives. These "folk healers," trained only through hands-on experience, bridged the yawning gap in people's health care, often providing remedies that equaled and even surpassed those favored by Norway's few doctors. Not until acceptance of the germ theory of disease near the end of the nineteenth century did professional medicine meaningfully diverge from folk medicine and begin to offer technologically superior treatment.

Once science had revolutionized medicine, self-trained caregivers were quickly forgotten. Even at the height of their popularity, they were often dismissed as quacks or feared as witches. Though some deserved their questionable reputations, many self-trained caregivers tended their patients with sincere dedication and rational means. These folk healers, who merit recognition for their intelligence and resourcefulness, provided most of the health care available to Norwegians on both sides of the Atlantic Ocean.

Unearthing these healers' stories is no easy task, in part because nineteenth-century Norway's strong class divisions obscure the healers' accomplishments. The nation's few professionally trained physicians—less than three hundred in 1850—belonged to the elite (*kondisjonerte*) class, which included clergy, civil officials, wealthy merchants, shipbuilders and sea captains, mine and mill operators, and large landowners. Politically powerful, the elite amounted to no more than 2 percent of Norway's citizenry at the beginning of the 1800s.[1] The remaining population fell almost equally into the middle class, consisting of small landowners, craftsmen, and small businessmen, and the lower class, made up of servants, day laborers, cotters, and paupers. The *almue* or "common folk" differed in every way from the cosmopolitan kondisjonerte, not least in their lack of access to formal education for the professions.

While the kondisjonerte congregated in towns and cities, more than 90 percent of Norway's population in 1800 lived in rural areas, where people labored as farmers, foresters, and fishermen. Norway's cities initially remained small: the largest, Bergen, had only 17,000 inhabitants, while the capital, Christiania (now Oslo), had less than 11,000 until rapid development after 1814 brought its population to 30,000 by 1830.

A decline in mortality sparked by the introduction of a potato crop and vaccination against smallpox doubled the country's population between 1815 and 1865. This growth brought increasing impoverishment, because modernization could not match the exploding demand for employment. Rising taxes forced small landowners and other members of the middle class to slide into the lower class. Farm foreclosures doubled the number of day laborers and cotters (*husmenn*), a rural class between independent farm owners and destitute paupers. Cotters, the fastest growing group in nineteenth-century Norway, sometimes owned land, but most worked on someone else's property.

Threatened with impoverishment, middle-class family groups began emigrating in large numbers to the United States in the late 1840s, but cotters and day laborers soon dominated the emigrant surge. By 1850, some 18,200 Norwegians had departed Norway for America, and the number increased to 70,000 by 1860. The transition from sailing ships to steamships made possible three great waves of Norwegian emigration—from 1866 to 1873, 1880 to 1893, and 1900 to 1910.

By 1925, more than 850,000 Norwegians had left fjord districts such as Hardanger and Sogn and mountain valleys like Hallingdal, Numedal, Valdres, and Setesdal. Most people settled in the upper Midwest's Wisconsin, Iowa, Minnesota, and North Dakota. Newcomers wanted to improve their economic prospects, but many also sought to preserve a way of life no longer possible in a rapidly changing Norway.

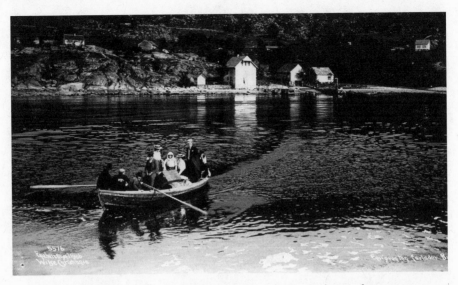

Norwegian emigrants beginning their journey from the country's rugged west coast. (*Photo by Wilse*)

Whether by choice or necessity, many immigrants retained traditional patterns from home, not least in their health-care choices. As in the Old Country, distance and poverty enhanced the settlers' wariness of doctors and perpetuated reliance on self-trained healers. The fact that most doctors in the New Land spoke English raised an additional barrier between the immigrants and professional caregivers.

Although self-trained healers provided most nineteenth-century health care, interested historians have been forced to rely on the written records left by doctors who served the tiny elite class. Annual reports filed by Norway's rural "district doctors" occupy a prominent place in the historical record. While these documents offer valuable insights into medical practices, they prove far less reliable in portraying the people whom these doctors served. The gap in life experience and worldview between the elite class, to which the doctors belonged, and Norway's commoners resulted in an overwhelmingly negative view of both rural dwellers and the self-trained healers they consulted. Accordingly, the district doctors' reports need to be balanced by the voices of the people who provided and who received everyday medical care. It is from their observations that historians can work to construct the remarkable account of how most Norwegians secured their health care.

Folk medicine and science

Folk medicine—human knowledge and experience about illnesses, medicine, and treatment through time—may have first developed by observing animals' healing instincts, such as a deer licking a wound after chewing leaves of sage or a sparrow applying pine resin to a sore foot.[2] Folk medicine's first written sources are medical papyri from the ancient Egyptians that date to about 1500 BC. Passed down by a myriad of folk healers, who added their own trial-and-error experiences, the lore lived on in both oral and written form for thousands of years before being tapped by nineteenth-century healers.

Folk medicine has always coexisted with regular medicine—as it does today—because it meets health needs not fully addressed by professional caregivers. Nineteenth-century folk healers followed a combination of rational remedies and magical medicine. While their rational remedies differed little from those used by doctors of the time, the healers' magical medicine aimed to cure more mysterious ailments, caused by the witches and *huldre-folk* (hidden people) that preindustrial Norwegians believed shared their world. Curing supernatural ailments required supernatural means such as those found in the so-called "black books." These compendiums of magical procedures and incantations allegedly granted the power necessary to ward off hidden spirits and evil persons who caused diseases.[3] Sometimes these magical formulas were used to enhance the potency of a rational remedy, most commonly an herb.

Herbs for medicinal use also characterized medicine during the Viking era, roughly 800–1000 AD. Medieval sagas and eddas tell of using elderberry, juniper, plantain, angelica, gentian, and onion. With the arrival of Christianity in Norway around 1000 AD, foreign monks brought new herbs to Norway and cultivated them in their cloister gardens. From such a monastic setting came Scandinavia's first medical book, *Liber Herbarum* (Book of herbs), written in the thirteenth century by Danish cleric Henrik Harpestreng (died 1244 in Roskilde). The treatise contained plant lore as it existed before the voyages of discovery to the New World added a wealth of new medicinal herbs to European folk medicine.[4]

Folk medicine relied on the same materials as conventional medicine but was more conservative. While eighteenth- and nineteenth-century medical research sought to find the effective ingredients of herbs and developed synthetic drugs, folk healers continued to use the herbs themselves. Their choices were often influenced by the so-called "doctrine of signatures." Originally promoted by the influential Swiss physician and alchemist Paracelsus (Theophrast von Hohenheim, 1493–1541), this doctrine held that a plant's physical appearance signaled its medicinal effects. While the theory encouraged positive experimentation, not simply slavish reliance on the herbs recommended by ancient practitioners, it also led to frivolous treatments, such as plants with heart-shaped leaves for heart ailments and yellow flowers for jaundice.[5]

In whatever ways nineteenth-century folk healers chose their herbs, they usually extracted the active herbal ingredients with alcohol and concentrated them into tinctures known as *"dråper,"* or "drops." Despite the growing strength of temperance movements, alcohol, whether as herb-flavored tinctures, patent medicines, or straight spirits, remained an essential medication among Norwegians on both sides of the Atlantic.

Minerals such as gold, silver, mercury, copper, iron, pewter, and lead had also played a vital role in medicine since ancient times, and during the 1600s the element antimony became the popular "philosopher's stone" thought capable of curing all illness. By causing both vomiting and violent diarrhea, it supposedly eliminated harmful substances responsible for disease. In the nineteenth century, both physicians and self-trained healers continued purging therapy by means of the antimony-based, poisonous "tartar emetic."[6]

Bloodletting also persisted in nineteenth-century medicine, practiced not only by professionals and folk healers, but by people who bled themselves as an invigorating pick-me-up. Blistering, another ancient therapy involving application of highly irritating "plasters" to the skin and cutting open the resulting blisters to release supposed disease toxins, also continued. Together, these three purging treatments constituted state-of-the-art medicine on both sides of the Atlantic around 1870.[7]

Printed "doctor books" (*legebøker*) describing these therapies became mainstays for many folk healers, including the pastors and pastors' wives who provided much of the health care for rural Norwegians in the first half of the 1800s. As the century progressed and literacy levels improved, people increasingly read and interpreted doctor books for themselves.

Early druggists depended on doctor books, too. Norway's first apothecary shop appeared in 1595 (Svaneapotek, in Bergen), and several others soon followed (in Kristiania in 1628, Kristiansand in 1651, and Trondheim in 1661). Apothecaries were an urban development, however, leaving rural areas without access to medicine. Ministers often filled this void by obtaining medicines to distribute among their parishioners.

As late as 1750, Norway had only five officially appointed public doctors and an equal number in private practice. All of them lived in towns and cities. Though the number of doctors grew to ninety-nine by 1816 and to 120 by 1827, most served only urban areas. An 1810 law divided rural Norway into districts, each to be served by a "district doctor." These posts were assigned slowly, however, and when a district doctor finally assumed his position, he was often the only formally trained physician within a radius of a hundred miles or more. Filling out the ranks of doctors available to rural people were a few military officers, who had served as battalion surgeons during the Napoleonic War years (1807–14). Though they lacked a full medical education, many received authorization to continue in private practice.[8]

By the 1850s, the number of district doctors had begun to grow, but their territories remained large, requiring too much travel for most rural dwellers. In addition, doctors frequently dispensed lectures instead of care. "The Halling farmer wears highly decorative clothing," disdained the district doctor of Ål and Hol in late 1800s, "but underneath most strikingly we meet the opposite, for washing the body, with the exception of face and hands in the faucet, occurs seldom, and for many, never." For struggling Norwegian peasants, however, carrying and heating sufficient water was itself a significant challenge; access to soap, washcloths, and towels was limited. Traditional beliefs also held rural dwellers hostage, and many regarded bathing as unhealthy or a ritual only for special times of the year. Normally sleeping on beds of straw, they seldom aired their sheepskin bed coverings, thereby encouraging body lice and scabies. While district doctors tried to change these practices, their judgmental attitudes stymied reform and instead fueled simmering class conflicts.[9]

Ministers, though members of the elite kondisjonerte class, often possessed better psychological skills and insights that won their parishioners' confidence in medical matters. Moreover, many ministers had studied medicine while at the university. Some would have chosen a medical career had not the ministry offered a more secure living.

With or without medical training, self-trained ministers seem remarkably to have escaped the harassment regularly endured by folk healers. Thus, while authorities frequently sued folk healers for breaking kvaksalver (quack) laws, ministers escaped similar legal reprisals. Popular legend reflected this reality, portraying ministers as using the magical black book with impunity, while other users of the black book sacrificed their souls.

The term *kvaksalver* (literally, one who "cheats with salves") suggests illegal medical activity. When the term is applied to self-trained healers, as most standard histories do, it impugns the healers with bad motives. Economic and political factors, along with social factors, however, often prevented the professional class from seeing or acknowledging the aptitude, dedication, and sense of calling that many self-trained healers brought to their work.

Some folk healers treated patients in their homes, often over an extended period of time. Though modern hospitals came into being during the late 1800s, most Norwegians feared them as places only for dying. Mothers who delivered in hospitals did more frequently die than those who gave birth at home, in many cases because doctors did not wash their hands between seeing patients, operating, and doing autopsies. Among the first who vehemently criticized the practice was a Hungarian doctor, Ignác Semmelweis (1815–65). In 1848, he ordered physicians under his jurisdiction to wash their hands with calcium carbonate before inserting them into the birth canal during childbirth. The death rate subsequently fell to zero, but Semmelweis's abrasive personality and the general ignorance about bacteria—whose existence was not proven until six years later by Louis Pasteur—kept this crucial discovery from being implemented for several decades.[10]

In any case, most nineteenth-century Norwegian women delivered babies at home. Although the 1810 law dividing the country into medical districts also stipulated the appointment of a professionally trained midwife for each district, decades passed before these positions were filled. Even after they became available, only women of the elite class used them. Commoners continued their traditional practice of delivering each other's babies.

By the nineteenth century's end, germ theory had explained childbed fever, and antiseptic procedures radically reduced its incidence. Doctors could at last reliably cure simple infections that often had led to gangrene and amputation. But one childhood killer, rickets, remained a mystery. Doctors had no cure, so Norwegian parents of all classes consulted folk healers when their children showed telltale signs of the disease. This gave folk healers substantial experience and enabled them to understand the benefits of outdoor exercise and cod-liver oil long before investigators learned that lack of Vitamin D produced the soft bones of rickets.

Prior to the discovery of germ theory, many folk healers similarly learned effective treatments for infected wounds, using alcohol, pine tar, tobacco, camphor, and other substances now recognized as antibacterials. In this sense, folk healers really did possess two magical qualities that most doctors lacked—experience and trust. As long as doctors remained inaccessible to common people, folk healers saw more patients and had a better opportunity to evaluate which treatments worked. Perhaps most importantly of all, they had their patients' faith that their homegrown methods of healing would work.

Stories of healing

"It was hard for us to get hold of a doctor, for he lived over nine miles away," writes Jens Stubseid (born 1882 in Askvoll, Sogn). Yet, the nine-year-old and his twelve-year-old brother made an arduous journey to fetch medicine for their ailing mother. "We set out at five in the morning and first had to row over the fjord a good three miles, then walk equally far and borrow a boat to cross yet another fjord. When we finally got there, the doctor was taking his after-dinner nap. So we had to wait outside on a little hillock, where in the fine weather we almost fell asleep ourselves. At last my brother went into the doctor's house and almost immediately came back out again with a small bottle of castor oil."[11]

The difficulty of traveling to a doctor who might be unavailable or away, and who often had nothing better to offer than a home remedy, was a familiar story. Though some doctors provided dedicated and effective assistance, a letter in the widely circulated capital-city newspaper *Morgenbladet* on April 4, 1852, confirms that good medical care could not be taken for granted: "Twice we've had doctors up here. One of them we owe special thanks. The other we would rather forget. He had the strange custom of pointing out the harshness of the winter weather in Tydal, as though we had not already noticed. A woman who came to him complaining of chest pains, especially when she went up hill, received the laconic reply, 'Well, then, you'd better turn and go back down hill.' Not the most helpful advice!" No wonder most nineteenth-century Norwegians preferred to consult local, self-trained caregivers.

They continued this preference in America, where their letters, diaries, and memoirs reflect a persistent preoccupation with good health. "Except for the three weeks when I was seasick," wrote immigrant Johanne Svenningsdatter Sogne on July 16, 1854, "I have been healthy the whole time, and I must thank Him who oversees all that He has preserved both my life and health since many of the Norwegian immigrants have died this year of cholera." Johanne's contemporaries would have shared her belief that God determined the state of their health. "Yes, here at home we are all in good health, which we can also thank God for," wrote E. T. Rogne from Austin, Minnesota, on December 9, 1895, to his brother and parents. "Ingeborg has in this past summer been healthier than she has been for a long time, and that can also be useful because she has many things to do all the time." Because immigrants recognized that good health was fundamental to their success in the New Land, many ranked it important above all else: "First and foremost I want to say that I am well, which is the best news," wrote Ragna, a Norwegian housemaid, on October 5, 1910, shortly after her arrival in America, and on January 26, 1911, she repeated: "First I want to tell you that I am well, which is the best of all."[12]

The importance of good health to immigrants' success is obvious, but the nature of the health care that immigrants received has largely gone unexplored. "The general conditions of health, the prevalence of diseases, and the nature of medical practice among the early Norwegian settlers in this country have received so scant attention," observed physician Ludvig Hektoen and historian Knut Gjerset in 1926, "that this side of pioneer life is known only imperfectly." Detailing the diseases—malaria, cholera, and typhoid fever—that most often plagued the immigrants, Hektoen and Gjerset emphasized the lack of Norwegian doctors to treat them: "As there was no field for remunerative medical practice among the first pioneers and no physicians from Norway accompanied the early immigrants, medical assistance was therefore often limited to questionable remedies recommended by 'wise' women, superstitious old men or unscrupulous quacks."[13]

Rather than researching the nature of the care and "questionable remedies" that immigrants received from self-trained caregivers, Hektoen and Gjerset dismissed them out of hand, an attitude as typical of their time as it is now regrettable. Their skepticism kept them from learning firsthand about the remedies actually used by immigrants. As a result, historians today spend long hours piecing together fragments of half-forgotten lore that frequently end in frustration. The scarcity of detailed stories makes the few accounts that remain all the more valuable.

Folk medicine: valued or reviled?

Immigrants to the New World suffered their afflictions thousands of miles from home, after a long, arduous, and often disease-plagued journey that most could neither afford nor bear to repeat. Typhoid fever, cholera, and measles impaired health and claimed lives on many immigrant ships, and even after passengers arrived safely on solid ground, illness often struck again to sap their strength just when it was most needed. "Practically all the Norwegians have been sick," observed immigrant Munch Raeder from Muskego, Wisconsin, in 1847, "some of them as much as a year at a time."[14]

Poor health kept settlers from making a living and sapped meager financial resources. Worse yet, it threatened to break their spirit—as Gunder Torgersen Mandt could attest. He had left Telemark in 1843, intending to make his home in the well-known Koshkonong settlement in Wisconsin's Dane County, but he found the inhabitants too impoverished to pay for his carpentry skills. This problem Mandt solved by walking seventy miles back to Milwaukee, where he readily found employment. Two weeks later, however, he was "visited by the new-comer's most dangerous enemy—climate fever [malaria], which in those days seldom passed anyone." Abandoned "among utter strangers" and unacquainted with the language, Mandt became "a prisoner of the sickbed. . . . Added to the pain of feeling forsaken was the longing for friends and homeland. In

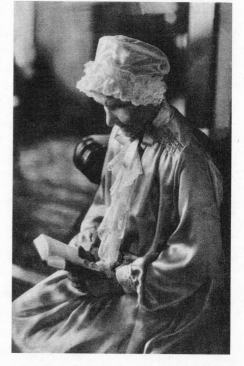

Healer Mari Simonson, photographed on her one-hundredth birthday in Minnesota's Freeborn County. She tended neighbors' illnesses and births, but her calling, like that of many folk healers, was forgotten by her family. (*Minneapolis Tribune*, Dec. 15, 1927)

various shapes, memories of the happy days of youth were conjured up before my mind's eye and around the melancholy feeling called homesickness."
Aided by "the kind treatment of neighbors," Mandt eventually "regained so
much strength that I could strike out west for Koshkonong." There, according to the Norwegian American journalist Sven Nilssen, this "once poverty-
stricken newcomer" eventually became "one of the most prosperous and best
informed individuals in the township, despite barely being able to write his
name when he arrived in America."[15]

The people who provided the "kind treatment" that put Mandt back
on his feet had no medical degrees; they were simply helping a neighbor in
need. Sven Nilssen chronicled Mandt's trials and triumphs in the February
5, 1870, issue of his *Billed-Magazin* (Picture magazine), but all too typically
he included no details of the medical care Mandt received.

The memoir of another immigrant, Ole Løkensgaard, is more helpful,
providing at least a few facts. His account (serialized through several issues
of *Hallingen* from 1917 to 1921), however, displays the doubtful disdain toward folk medicine common during the first half of the twentieth century.[16]

Løkensgaard's parents and three children emigrated in 1857 from Ål in
Hallingdal. They initially settled in the Nerstrand Woods near Northfield,
Minnesota, but subsequently moved farther west. During the summer of
1863, they built a twelve-by-fourteen-foot cabin on an eighty-acre homestead
in Nicollet County's Lake Prairie Township (now known as Norseland).
The new cabin had an attic, accessed by an almost vertical ladder through
a hole in the ceiling, and it was to this attic that Helga Løkensgaard sent
the nine-year-old Ole to fetch the washboard one morning. Fifty-six years
later, Ole Løkensgaard vividly recalled what happened next: "I took off up
the ladder with brother Mikkel on my heels trying to beat me. When we
reached the top of the ladder, he tried to get there first by grabbing the attic
floor and swinging himself up. But he lost hold and fell straight down, tip-
ping over on himself a copper kettle full of water boiling on the wood stove."
Helga tore the scalding clothing off her son, and as she removed the stock-
ing from his right foot, skin and muscle tissue followed. "Screams followed,"
too, wrote Løkensgaard, "the likes of which I've heard neither before nor
since. I sometimes think I hear them still."

Løkensgaard continued, "There was no talk of a doctor in those days,
but every woman who came had a new remedy, all said to be 'Godt probat'
(well proven). So every one of them was tried." He later reflected, "I have

no doubt these women were intelligent, but some of their remedies didn't seem very sensible. I was sent hither and yon to fetch the most unlikely things: sugar and salt, milk, and rainwater, salted butter and unsalted butter, *makkemjøl* ["worm flour," produced by insect larvae as they gnaw through log-cabin walls], goose grease, and more items, both mentionable and not."

Mikkel's burns kept him in bed for eighteen weeks. "That his foot wasn't completely destroyed was not the fault of these many wonder cures," wrote the doubting Løkensgaard. "At last, Mikkel's strong and healthy nature won out."

While Mikkel's strong constitution significantly aided his recovery, the remedies Løkensgaard so readily rejects probably saved his life. Though we do not know how Mikkel's mother applied them, accounts by other nineteenth-century caregivers suggest that she probably used the milk and rain water to soothe and cleanse the wound, the makkemjøl to remove excess moisture, and the butter and goose grease to exclude air, an essential objective for treating burns. Most significantly, the sugar and salt prevented infection, the greatest threat to life and limb as long as the existence of bacteria remained a mystery.

Helga's Home Remedies

Milk, makkemjøl, sugar, and salt have deep roots in Norwegian and international folk medicine. "Milk just seems to help health," says Ester Hegg (born 1913), whose Valdres ancestors "used boiled milk for any sickness." To this day, Norwegians drink more milk per capita than any other nationality, perhaps as a legacy from the Vikings who believed milk warded off evil powers. Well into the nineteenth century, Norwegian mothers customarily squirted breast milk into the eyes of their newborns to protect them from blindness.[17]

For centuries Norwegians have used milk to soothe wounds and treat infections, making *grautomslag,* or poultices (literally, "porridge wraps") from clotted milk and flour, spreading this mixture on cloths, and placing them on the wound to be healed. Helga Løkensgaard probably applied many such poultices to Mikkel's foot during the eighteen weeks it took to heal.

Makkemjøl, the yellow dust produced by insect larvae (*mark* or *makk*) that gnaw through the walls of pine or spruce log cabins, served as baby powder for generations of Norwegians. Soothing the damp, irritated skin of infants when their wet swaddling clothes were changed, it would similarly have removed moisture from Mikkel's wound, reducing the risk of further infection.[18]

Sugar provided the most potent protection of all. For centuries, folk healers around the world have used sugar to reduce the danger of infection in wounds and sores. Why it worked remained a mystery until the 1950s, when bacteriologists showed that sugar and salt prevent infection the same way they preserve food: by osmosis, the tendency for solutions on two sides of a membrane to achieve equal concentrations. When a cell is surrounded by a highly concentrated solution, water rushes out of the cell to dilute it. Filling a sore with sugar or salt causes the bacteria in the wound to lose water rapidly, making them shrivel and die.

Hjalmar Lie experienced this dramatic effect as a child in 1893, when his mother packed a deep gash on his leg with crushed loaf sugar. Eight years earlier their neighbor had died when gangrene set into a similar wound, but thanks to the sugar, Hjalmar believed, he made a full recovery. In a similar way, the sugar Helga Løkensgaard used on the advice of her neighbors may have saved Mikkel's life.[19]

Though Løkensgaard disparaged these "medications," he performed an invaluable service by recording them. Handed down orally in the midst of other pressing concerns, Norwegian-immigrant home remedies seldom found their way onto paper and have largely been lost to history. Yet, the few examples cited here suggest their time-tested worth. Even "cures" that provided no clear physiological benefit often helped psychologically by allowing patients and caregivers an active role in the healing process and sustaining their hope of a favorable outcome.

Løkensgaard's account further reveals the extensive repertoire of remedies possessed by a random group of neighbors when he writes that "every woman" who came to the house seemed to have a cure. The now-derogatory term "kjerringråd" (old wives' remedies) accurately reflects the role wives and mothers took as the family's principal providers of health care. Diagnosing illnesses and determining, preparing, and administering appropriate medicines was largely a female task in nineteenth-century Norway.

Men sometimes took an active role in folk medicine, especially when injuries happened while working. Their Old Country experience as farmers, foresters, and fishermen had taught them that their survival, especially when they were away from home, could depend on this lore.

The ability to apply traditional remedies proved no less crucial in the New Land, where winter blizzards were frequently followed by spring floods, summer farming in snake-infested fields, and fall prairie fires, all threats to crops, homes, and lives. To meet these challenges, immigrants supplemented the remedies brought from home with some gleaned from their new surroundings. In the Nerstrand Woods, where Løkensgaard's family first settled, for example, Ole benefited from an Indian remedy. In 1858, while four-year-old Ole was helping his seven-year-old sister Sigri shorten sticks on a chopping block, he suffered an axe blow intended for the sticks. Ole's blood-curdling screams brought their mother running, and her urgent calls quickly summoned men from the nearby forest. One of these men, Christofer Lockrem, bandaged Ole's hand. According to Ole, "Tendon and bone were exposed, but Christofer knew how to treat an injury. He bandaged it so well that within a few weeks' time it had healed, and I have never been troubled by it since, though I can still see the scar." To help the wound heal, Christofer's father, Ivar, made a dressing by "cooking roots he found in the woods. He had learned how to make it from the Indians, so we called it *Indi Plaster*. It certainly did the trick."[20]

While Norwegian settlers surely learned other remedies from Native Americans, written diaries, letters, and memoirs yield very few examples. Yet, intuition insists that such exchanges occurred with some frequency. Immigrants were thoroughly familiar with herbal remedies from their homeland and must have been eager to learn how to use the unfamiliar plants in their new surroundings. Though mutual wariness and even open hostility characterized some encounters between Norwegians and Indians, historical sources also depict friendlier exchanges of food and assistance. Moreover, Indian ways of viewing illness resembled those of the Norwegians. Both believed in the spiritual component of health, for example, and the necessity of identifying the supernatural powers that caused the malady before proper treatment could be determined.[21]

The missing accounts of exchanged medical lore remain a mystery that may be explained by the hard work and physical challenges of settling the land, the belief that remedies were too commonplace to write down, and the subsequent discrediting of this lore as medicine modernized. That these factors conspired to leave unrecorded the exchanges that actually did occur, Løkensgaard indirectly confirms. He, too, fails to identify the plant used to make the "Indi plaster" despite his satisfaction that it "certainly did the trick."

From folk medicine to professional care

Despite settlers' positive experiences with folk remedies, they quickly fell from favor as health care became increasingly professionalized. Stella Kirby (born 1897) told of a childhood incident that illustrates this transition. Raised by grandparents on a farm near Decorah, Iowa, Kirby was frequently ill as a child and at age seven contracted "double pneumonia," or severe pneumonia in both lungs.

> Grandpa didn't know what to do, so he went into town and got the doctor. Now, this doctor was a licensed Norwegian-American physician. He looked at me and said that he didn't know of any professional medical remedy or therapy that would cure me. He did, however, say that he knew some folk medicine that might work if they could try and keep it quiet, because as a licensed doctor he was not supposed to do this. He told my grandmother to cut up onions and mix it together with honey and bake it. Then put it in soft cloth rags and place one on my chest and one on my back. I don't understand how it worked, but by morning I was so sick, coughing up large amounts of green mucus. After I got all of that out of my lungs, I felt so much better and was cured.[22]

This doctor, who had "learned this cure from his parents in Norway," hesitated to use it for fear that someone might find out. His nervousness makes sense in the context of strides made by the American Medical Association, founded in 1847, to bar all nonorthodox treatments as a way of addressing "the disorganized state of the profession in the wake of the country's rapid westward expansion."

Specifically, the association aimed to remedy the absence of legal regulations, lowered educational standards, and ruthless commercialism that had resulted. Hundreds of "proprietary schools" had sprung into being and become a powerful educational and political force after legislation declared the diploma for one of these short courses of study to be equivalent to licenses granted by county and state medical societies. These "schools" soon filled the country with medical practitioners whose education depended less on literacy, prior academic achievement, and good moral standing, than on the applicants' ability to pay their fees.[23]

"Believe me, it is a frightful, often sinful business that is carried on here with the medical arts," wrote recent immigrant Caja Munch on February 23, 1857, from Wiota, Wisconsin. "A man may one day be a farmer, the next day he has bought himself an American drugstore, where liquor actually is the most important article, and after having carried on this for about a month, he sets himself up as a doctor and takes some of his medicines in a satchel on his back and drives around to the poor sick ones, who in their distress take what help is offered." The previous year she had written on January 22, "There are two doctors here, of whom the best one used to be a grocer, but all of a sudden he sold the whole lot, disappeared for three months, and returned as a doctor, has now a large practice and earns money." Summing the situation up in her later letter, Caja declared: "There is hardly a doctor here who can be compared with our skillful Norwegian physicians; if some of them would like to come over, they would quite certainly make good business because here you pay an extraordinary amount to *have your life ruined*." Many people who found these conditions deplorable abandoned official medicine to follow so-called sects such as "botanics," which urged the use of herbs, or "hydropathists," who embraced dietary change and water treatments. Orthodox medicine suffered a great crisis of confidence.[24]

To counter these alternative methods, the American Medical Association introduced a code of medical ethics that forbade regular physicians from consulting sectarian practitioners, treating any patient under a nonorthodox doctor's care, or using nonorthodox practices themselves.[25] In this context, Stella Kirby's physician felt it necessary to be very careful about recommending a folk remedy although it might, in fact, work.

Pharmacist Severin Almklov (1850–1938)

On the spectrum of healers, somewhere between Kirby's licensed physician and the self-trained caregivers, stands another kind of healer personified by the ethnic pharmacist Severin Almklov. Born in 1850 at Vanylven in Sunnmøre, Almklov had already received an exceptionally advanced education when he graduated from Tromsø Seminary in 1871. His rural contemporaries rarely went beyond *omgangsskole* (ambulatory school, conducted by itinerant teachers for a few weeks on local farms) and "reading for the minister" in preparation for the Lutheran Church's rite of confirmation around the age of fourteen.[26]

After graduation, Almklov became a private children's tutor in the home of the district doctor on Senja, a large island about a hundred miles from the city of Tromsø. Almklov worked afternoons in the doctor's office, helping to compound various medicines. "No ready-made pills, capsules, tablets, or elixirs were then available in Senja," he writes in a 1931 memoir, "and the nearest pharmacy was on the mainland in Tromsø."

Almklov credits the district doctor with "making everything interesting as well as instructive." When a scabies epidemic raged among the district's fishermen and farmers, however, the doctor showed considerably less insight. Blaming the malady on the almue's lack of cleanliness, he echoed the careless diagnosis of other district doctors. "Farmers are not happy unless they have the pleasure of constantly scratching and clawing themselves," wrote the doctor at Seljord in the 1840s, Hans Angell Krabbe.[27] "Taking an occasional bath or washing their underwear once a week might help," Almklov's employer observed with no less sarcasm.

The doctor's judgmental attitude rankled Almklov. In retaliation, he liked to tell about the burly fisherman who came for advice about "itching so bad that he couldn't sleep." When the district doctor "commenced his usual diatribe," the fisherman retorted that he "hadn't come to be lectured." In response, the physician furiously pounded the table with his fist and shouted, "I'm the doctor and I prescribe." But the fisherman just laughed. "I've sailed the seven seas, and have seen far worse storms than this little tempest in a tea cup. If I pounded my fist on that table, it would break in two." The doctor then gave the fisherman mercury tablets to take four times a day.

Noticing that the doctor's prescription for scabies often did more harm than good, Almklov began reading about skin diseases and finally came upon a dissertation by the eminent German dermatologist Paul Gerson Unna (1850–1924), who invented skin peeling. Unna explained that the itching of scabies was caused by parasites that laid eggs under the skin.

Almklov experimented with chemicals that could penetrate the skin and ultimately developed a salve that killed parasites and healed the broken skin in a week's time.

In 1874, Almklov visited America and enrolled at Augsburg Theological Seminary in Minneapolis on the invitation of a family friend and the school's dean, A. Weenaas. Three years later Almklov graduated with a degree in theology and married Hansine Wadel, a merchant's daughter from Tromsø. The couple settled in Benson, Minnesota, where Almklov had accepted the call to minister to a large parish covering Kandiyohi, Pope, Swift, and Chippewa counties in west-central Minnesota.

Many of the area's impoverished settlers lived in sod huts and suffered the same skin disease that had plagued the fishermen of northern Norway. This observation revived Almklov's interest in dermatology, but it took a family tragedy to change the course of his career. When Almklov's sister and only blood relative in America, Anne Reite, died in childbirth and left five small children, Almklov, who at age four had lost his own mother to tuberculosis, promised to take care of them in lieu of their alcoholic father. With four small children of his own, as well, he realized he could not support two families on a pastor's income and decided to study pharmacy. In 1888, degree in hand, he took over a small, woodframe drugstore on the main street of Cooperstown, Dakota Territory. He did so with relief, for his brother-in-law was far from the only parishioner who frequented Benson's many saloons and ignored Almklov's plea for temperance.

As a pharmacist, Almklov again observed the scourge of scabies. Harvest hands and workers from logging camps, mines, and factories brought "the itch" to town, where it quickly spread to settlers on far-flung homesteads. Almklov then mixed up a batch of the salve he had invented in Norway, which seemed to clear up the condition in a matter of days. This was sensational news that traveled fast. Harvest hands and other itinerant workers talked about Almklov's salve when they returned home, and soon mail orders began to come to his pharmacy from around the country.

Almklov's "Itch Specific," a salve consisting of "Sulfur, Pine Tar, and Oil of Pine," came in a flat tin resembling a can of shoe polish. "Take a good bath first, dry the body well, and rub the salve in well all over body every night for six days," directed its bright orange label. "Bathe seventh night and change underwear and sheets."

In addition to his sister's five sons and their own children, the Almklovs

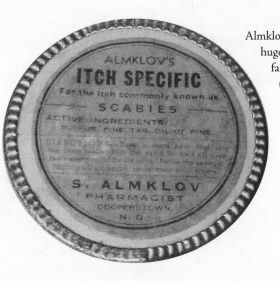

Almklov's Itch Specific ointment,
hugely popular among settlers,
farmers, and ranch hands on
the American prairie

raised their grandson, Norman Hoel, after Almklov's oldest daughter died
in 1918. Hoel became "the same kind of pharmacist his grandfather was,"
writes his daughter Erlys Haerter from Williston, North Dakota. "He enjoyed making the compounds to prevent pain and suffering."[28]

As a child, Erlys watched her father "take powdered chemicals from the
tall apothecary jars, grind them with mortar and pestle, and precisely measure them in one pan of his small scale against the weights standing in the
other pan." At the counter with its "multitude of small drawers filled with
all sizes of medicine bottles and pill boxes," Norman worked with his uncle,
Dr. Leif Almklov, to devise new remedies.

By then Severin Almklov had developed an entire line of products to
treat skin ailments, along with a reputation for curing them as no one else
could. For many years Norman continued to make and distribute one of
these salves, mixing it in a large boiler in the basement and packing it into
tins with a palette knife. "By the time I was in the 6th, 7th and 8th grade,"
Haerter writes, "Dad would let me help fill cans or pack tins into cardboard
cartons to be mailed all over the U.S. or shipped to Norway, Sweden and
Denmark." Even during Almklov's lifetime, mail orders arrived from "every
state in the Union, every province in Canada and from Alaska, as well as
from South America, England, Norway, Sweden, Finland and Denmark." A
few regular orders even came from missionaries in China and India.[29] Then,
however, "the federal government started getting pretty tough on what the

label and list of ingredients required. Things just went from bad to worse with rules as to what was required of the room where the salve was made." Finally, says Haerter, her father "just stopped making it," and the "formula went to the grave with his passing" in 1933 at age eighty-five.

Gone now, too, were the druggist's never-ending workdays. "Growing up with Dad was difficult for me in the early years," Haerter writes, "because he was not able to be home very much." The drugstore was open Friday and Saturday nights until midnight and on weeknights until 10 o'clock. "I felt bad when Dad would have to leave the house during a holiday dinner or a Sunday evening supper to go fill a prescription for a customer and even have to deliver it to the home."

Able to speak the language of the immigrant, ethnic pharmacists like Almklov often found themselves in greater demand than local doctors. "Winter was the worst," writes Haerter, who, with her mother and brother, would "put all the lights on in the house facing East and South in hopes Dad could see them as he walked the three blocks home in snow storms and blizzards." The nearest hospital was in Fargo, one hundred miles away, and her father sometimes had to drive patients there for surgery or other medical attention, using a hearse to transport patients who needed to lie down. Her father and uncle ran the town's funeral business, Severin Almklov having bought the town's coffin supply when he took over the drugstore. His descendants inherited the business, along with the neighbors' jokes about having "everyone covered from cradle to grave."[30]

•2

Folk Healers and Folk Cures

Filling the void

> "Everyone knew something about medicine in those days. Children learned simple remedies for common ailments just as surely as they learned Luther's catechism. Each community had its specialists, too, and people had great faith in them."
>
> *Anne Marie Djupdalen (1841–1945), describing Vågå, Gudbrandsdal*

EVERY NEIGHBORHOOD IN NINETEENTH-CENTURY Norway had at least one folk healer. Helping others, often at the risk of their own well-being and good name, hundreds of healers provided badly needed and otherwise unavailable health care. Though their names are mostly lost, some have stories that can be pieced together.

Three Norwegian healers, Mor Sæther (1793–1851), Anne Brandfjeld (1810–1905), and Valborg Valand (1812–93), developed national reputations, an unusual feat for women of their time. Mor Sæther ran a boardinghouse where Henrik Ibsen briefly stayed before he became the world-famous dramatist; she also treated the renowned poet and patriot Henrik Wergeland, who made her the subject of a poem. A generation later Anne Brandfjeld also became a literary subject, the title character of a novel. In another arena, Valborg Valand gained fame when public criticism of court cases decided against her eventually led to changes in Norwegian law.

Mor Sæther (1793–1851)

When did Anne Johannesdotter Wiger, as she was baptized in 1793, leave her birthplace at Grue in Solør for the capital city some fifty miles away?

Sources do not say. By 1820, Anne, the oldest of seven children born to Johan Eriksen Wiger, had arrived in Christiania (now Oslo), married, and become a widow though still only twenty-seven years in age. Her first husband, whose family name, Sæther, she kept for the rest of her life, worked as a caretaker in the anatomy department at Royal Frederick University (now Universitetet i Oslo, Norway's first university, founded in 1811).[1]

Anne came to the capital city with a strong interest in medicinal herbs, an interest likely stimulated by the veterinarian Martin Noer, who lived next to the Wigers' farm in Grue. Noer introduced several new plants to the area, using them to make his own medicines. A letter written in Mor Sæther's defense during an 1842 court case against her refers to her thirty years of experience, suggesting that Anne may have been treating patients before she left home.

During her first seven years in Oslo, Anne learned more about medicine by working as an assistant in the anatomy department. For three of those years she also did light housekeeping for the military surgeon Jens Essendrop Knopf in exchange for medical instruction and the opportunity to borrow medical books and observe operations.

It was as the wife of her second husband, Lars Bastian Nielsen (whom she married in 1825, at age thirty-two), that Anne briefly became Ibsen's landlady in 1850. Nielsen bought the three-story building at Vinkelgate 17, near the fjord in Pipervika where Oslo's City Hall now stands. The couple kept cattle on the land now occupied by Studenterlunden, a large park in downtown Oslo across the street from the parliament building, and ran a farm supporting twenty well-tended cows that grazed each summer at Frognersæteren in Nordmarka, the forested recreation area north of the downtown.[2] With a good reputation for her animal husbandry, Mor, or "Mother," Sæther supplied butter and cream to the Oslo bishop and the royal household when the Swedish king Karl XIX Johan resided in Oslo.

Mor Sæther's reputation as a folk healer proved considerably more controversial. She was summoned to court on three occasions—in 1834, 1840, and 1842—for breaking Norway's "quack law" (kvaksalverlov). Formally known as the Ordinance of September 5, 1794, this law sought to punish quack healers, or kloke menn og kloke kvinner ("wise men and wise women," the common term for self-trained healers, especially those thought to use witchcraft). The law targeted healers "who take upon themselves, despite their lack of professional training, the treatment of illnesses among the common classes." *Kvaksalvere* (quacks), the law stipulated, should be fined twenty dollars for the first offense or "jailed on bread and water for eight days." Second offenses brought six months in jail, with the punishment doubling for subsequent offenses.[3]

Sæther's 1834 trial featured three cases. The first concerned a minor official's wife, who testified that Mor Sæther had successfully treated her for a serious illness after a prominent physician, Dr. Christen Heiberg (1799–1872), had failed. Her "hopes awakened," said the woman, upon hearing of Mor Sæther, who, once persuaded to take the case, listened carefully to her symptoms, diagnosed the condition as "cramping in the chest and back" (a diffuse diagnosis typical of the time), and gave her some "drops," probably the tincture of valerian Sæther favored. The mild sedative addressed only the symptoms, but the patient's "hope" no doubt did its part, too. Two weeks later the woman resumed her employment as a housekeeper and had enjoyed good health ever since. Sæther had asked no payment, but the woman insisted on paying Sæther "against her will."[4]

The 1834 trial continued with testimony from a group of women whom Mor Sæther had successfully treated for stomach pains using aloe drops, a tincture of *aloe ferox* commonly used as a cathartic. The last witness, an employee of the local jail, testified that Mor Sæther's "drops and salve" had healed his eleven-year-old daughter's sores, which the prison physician could not do, and again she asked no payment. The court ultimately determined that Mor Sæther had done no harm in any of these cases, but it nevertheless fined her in accordance with the quack law.

The 1840 trial, instigated by Dr. Heiberg, concerned Mor Sæther's treatment of a customs agent for indigestion and constipation. When the court ordered her to submit the "drops" she had used, Mor Sæther presented two bottles, one containing a plant extract she produced by boiling various herbs in water, known as a "decoction," and then adding aloe and turpentine, a common ingredient in nineteenth-century medicine. The other contained a decoction of valerian and other herbs. While the patient had recovered and the court admitted that no harm had been done, by the terms of the quack law, Sæther was sentenced to six months in jail and assessed with the court costs. She appealed the sentence to the supreme court, and the case remained unresolved until 1842, when her punishment was reduced by royal decree to a fine.

The positive resolution of this case reflects the good relationship Mor

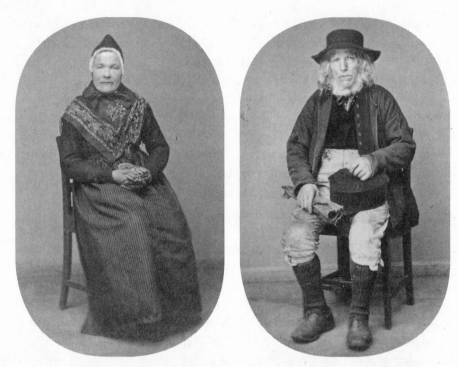

A woman from Jølster and a man from Østerfjorden, photographed wearing local *bunad* (traditional clothing) in Bergen, Norway, about 1870 (*Photo by K. Knudsen*)

Sæther enjoyed with a number of the capital city's most prominent individuals. Some she had helped personally, others had friends and acquaintances who had sought her services. Though the court cases involved middle-class patients, Sæther also treated people from the lower classes, as evidenced by an August 24, 1841, document signed by the Poverty Commission at Eidsvoll. The town had enlisted Mor Sæther to treat their destitute in order to "save some doctor bills and other expenses," official scruples over quackery apparently being overcome by the bottom line. "People came from all over, about 140 of them," the document continued, and Mor Sæther gave them medicine at no charge. "Everyone was satisfied with her treatments," and those of better means who had also come "wanted to pay her more than she could be persuaded to take." The document's signatories therefore hoped "that Madame Sæther may soon receive royal permission to practice her form of medicine" because of her "great benefit to the common classes and especially the poor, to whom she not only gives free care but also money to support their travel back home and never demands specific payment."

Sæther may have requested this document as part of a plan to expand the scope of her work, but before she could act, she found herself back in court. Records from the 1842 trial instigated by Dr. Johan Hjort (1798–1873) reveal a great deal about the relationship between self-trained healers and the medical establishment.

The case concerned a local official's son, who had fallen during fencing practice and suddenly gone lame. Feeling such terrible leg pain that he could neither walk nor stand upright, he sought the services of Dr. Hjort, then a brigade doctor, but a director at the National Hospital (*Rikshospitalet*) by the time of the trial.

On October 11, 1842, the patient's father, the "distinguished judge" S. Sørensen, submitted the following testimony: "At the request of Anne Johannesdatter Sæther, I certify that during the past summer she successfully treated my eldest son for a paralysis he acquired in both legs. It is to be noted that only after having told the tending physician, who had already taken care of the patient for some time, did I decide to seek the help of Mor Sæther, since so much time had passed under his care without any noticeable improvement." Sæther then confirmed that she had treated the patient only after the judge had received Dr. Hjort's approval. Why, then, did Hjort bring a case against her?[5]

Hjort's motives emerge in a letter he wrote to Sørensen. First, he cast doubt on Mor Sæther's diagnosis: "You term your son's sickness a 'paralysis in both legs,' a conclusion you have probably reached based on his inability to stand or walk. But rather than paralysis, it was merely a sprain of one knee joint, and there was nothing wrong with the right leg." He then explained his own treatment. "The first objective in his care was to bring down the considerable swelling and to deaden the initial extremely sharp pain. My treatment succeeded in completely ridding the limb of swelling; the leg subsequently had its normal shape and could be moved by me in every natural direction. Once the swelling has gone down, it is of the greatest importance in this condition to see that the stretched muscles and tendons receive rest so they can heal, though the healing time can then be significantly shortened by the use of stimulating massage." Hjort had barely begun massage therapy, he asserted, when Mor Sæther took over, and she merely continued the regimen he had already begun.

In a written reply, Sørensen acknowledged the correctness of Dr. Hjort's words. The paralysis only appeared to affect both legs because the boy couldn't stand up and because Mor Sæther massaged both legs. He realized now that only the left leg had been injured and recalled that his son had remarked that the swelling was going down even before Mor Sæther began her treatments. Still, the boy was in pain and thought it would continue for a long time. Going to someone like Mor Sæther had not been easy, Sørensen admitted, and he readily conceded that Dr. Hjort's treatment could well have contributed to the quick recovery for which Sæther had gotten credit.

"The writer of the testimonial has told me that Anne Sæther herself identified the illness as a paralysis in both legs," Dr. Hjort testified in court. "By massaging also the right leg with alcohol, she led the family to believe the illness was more serious so they would regard her cure as miraculous." Seeing Sæther massage both legs probably did lead the family to assume the "paralysis" involved both limbs, but had she purposely misled them as Hjort accused? If so, was it greed that motivated her, or her desire—based on the healing power of hope—that they have faith in the efficacy of her treatment? While the doctor appears willing to rush to judgment, he did have good reason to resent Mor Sæther. Struggling to make a living at a profession that had not yet become established, he, like other doctors, no doubt saw much of his business lured away by folk healers and quacks. "This woman has for years shamefully played on the public's gullibility," wrote one of Hjort's colleagues in the 1842 medical publication *Ugeskrift for Medicin and Pharmacie* (Weekly magazine for medicine and pharmacy). Despite being sued in court, the letter continued, she persisted in the same illegal activity "while an unsuspecting public deliberately shields their eyes from the truth and eagerly continues to seek her assistance as if they had ten lives to lose instead of only one." The author, who signed himself "Philaletos," declared that he had come to regard his own professional training "more a liability than benefit" because knowledge "repulsed" a public that "preferred to believe in miracles." He continued that the more unlikely a quack is to have the slightest bit of medical knowledge and the more unreasonable the methods she uses, the more strongly the public believes in her power, while a person who has actually studied medicine has no chance of winning renown. "Only blacksmiths, unlettered farmers, and old crones of the lowest sort, known to be 'uninfected' by academic knowledge, can do so," because their wisdom is credited as divinely inspired and therefore infallible. "If the quack in addition has the guile to express herself with a certain degree of imperial decisiveness," the writer concludes with obvious reference to Mor Sæther, "she will succeed in arousing in many a patient the confidence which in itself can work wonders."[6]

Frustrations on both sides of the case emerge in the ensuing court testimony. Hjort's charge that Mor Sæther's cure had been no miracle since she merely followed the course of treatment he had begun reveals a greater concern with his own reputation than the patient's well-being. Though Mor Sæther did submit her medicine, as the court ordered, identifying it as "spirits to which a decoction of fifteen types of herbs had been added," this time she refused to specify the herbs and told the doctors instead to figure this out. The fact that they could not identify the herbs, of course, indicates the state of nineteenth-century science.

Sæther's trial finally concluded on September 16, 1843, with her being sentenced to jail as required by the quack law for a third offense. Once again she appealed to the supreme court, which found that since Dr. Hjort had been informed of her intent to take over the boy's care, and inasmuch as she had used essentially the same treatment as the doctor, she had not endangered the patient. They therefore reduced her punishment to twenty days in prison on bread and water.[7]

Even as the case was pending, Mor Sæther implemented her plan, having "the unmitigated gall," as Philatetos wrote in 1842, to apply for royal dispensation to treat patients from all over the country for "external injuries, cancerous lesions, eye diseases, rheumatism, paralysis, colic, convulsions, tumors, and similar complaints" (a list that reflects the era's vague differentiation among diseases). For the next three years, Mor Sæther waited as her application moved from office to office in the city bureaucracy. Despite strong objections from health officials and the university's medical faculty, she finally received in 1845 the permission she sought. "She persists in giving help to anyone who seeks it," the granting document noted, and "her reputation for successful treatments grows daily." The "widespread desire among people both within and far beyond Christiania [Oslo] that the applicant be permitted to practice" was, moreover, demonstrated by the "over one hundred signatures that accompanied the application." Though she lacked the requisite education, the applicant "seemed to possess an unusual competence in healing certain illnesses.... Denying permission would, in any case, fail to have the intended effect, for it would not keep people from coming to her for help, something she seems unable to refuse regardless of the persecution she thereby incurs."[8]

Mor Sæther's Medicines

Aloe (*Aloe ferox*)—Unlike aloe vera, the familiar colorless gel used to treat irritated skin, Mor Sæther's dark-brown, glistening aloe was a strong laxative, and its active principle (aloin) was once a component of most laxative pills, including Carter's Little Liver Pills. Effectively stimulating the lower bowel within twelve to eighteen hours, it also caused cramping, nausea, vomiting, diarrhea, and kidney inflammation. When less irritating materials became available, they quickly replaced aloe. Combining aloe with antispasmodics such as valerian or hops, as Mor Sæther seems to have done, would have counteracted these gripping tendencies.[9]

Valerian (*Valeriana officinalis*)—Deriving its name from *valere*, or "be well" in Latin, valerian supposedly cured diseases ranging from tuberculosis to gout. Modern research shows it has a mild tranquilizing effect. Medieval monks cultivated valerian in monastary gardens and used it medicinally, as *officinalis* in its Latin name suggests. European apothecaries still sell valerian for insomnia, excitability, and exhaustion, probably the very symptoms Mor Sæther treated with *baldrian dråper* (valerian drops), as she called her frequently used tincture of valerian. Administered by dribbling a specified number of drops on a lump of sugar for the patient to ingest, valerian is also known in Norwegian as *vendelrot*, since it is the root that holds the plant's medically active ingredients.[10]

Hops (*Humulus lupulus*)—Known in Nowegian as *humle*, this vine can grow as much as fifteen to eighteen feet in a summer, faster than any other plant in Norway. A mild sedative, hops entered Norway with the Christian monks, and it was often used with valerian. Bitter in taste, it has long been used to preserve beer. The herb's sedative effect became known in the Middle Ages when hops pickers were observed to tire easily. The bitter acids located in the conelike "strobile" are believed to cause this effect.[11]

Turpentine—Produced by distilling pine sap, this volatile oil played a prominent role in nineteenth-century medicine. Norwegians applied cloths soaked in turpentine to soothe rheumatism (*gikt*) aches, added a few drops to milk or coffee to treat coughs, and applied cloths rubbed with turpentine and sheep tallow to their chests to cure congestion due to colds. Turpentine also added significant antiseptic action to the warm porridge poultices (*grautomslag*) commonly used to treat wounds.[12]

Henrik Wergeland: Impressive patriot, impossible patient

In the same year, 1845, that Mor Sæther's application was approved, she treated her most famous patient: the beloved poet and patriot Henrik Wergeland (1808–45). Best remembered for initiating the annual celebration of Norway's national day, *Syttende mai* (17th of May), Wergeland worked tirelessly for many other worthy causes. Social commitment ran in the family. Henrik's father, Nicolai Wergeland, served as one of the 112 influential men convened in 1814 to draft Norway's Constitution, signed on May 17 at Eidsvold, where Nicolai subsequently served as parish pastor.[13]

Despite his privileged background, Henrik Wergeland had a strained relationship with the "cultured class" and fought tirelessly for the less comfortable almue. He initiated numerous projects to advance popular enlightenment and wrote a pamphlet in 1831 about the medicinal herbs of the Norwegian countryside, *Den norske Bondes nyttige Kundskab om de Læge-, Farve, Garve, samt Gift-Planter, der voxe paa hans Jord* (Useful knowledge for the Norwegian farmer about the healing, dying, tanning, and poisonous plants that grow on his land). The restless and energetic Wergeland also studied medicine from 1834 to 1836 and started several public libraries, including one in his own home.

Most famously, Wergeland campaigned against Article 2 of the otherwise liberal Constitution that banned Jews, Jesuits, and members of monastic orders from admission to Norway. (The article was finally repealed in 1851, six years after Wergeland's death, largely due to his efforts.)[14] Wergeland also opposed Norway's union with Sweden, begun shortly after Norway gained freedom from Denmark in 1814 and lasting until 1905, and he wrote a profusion of patriotic speeches and poems to arouse public sentiment for Norwegian independence.

Appointed national archivist by King Carl Johan in 1840, Wergeland would later blame his chilly office at the medieval Akershus Fortress with its "six foot thick" walls for inducing the lung disease that on May 2, 1844, sent him to bed for the rest of his short life. Through the first two weeks of May, he nursed his sore throat and "desperate cough," but on May 17, as he wrote in a November 30, 1844, letter, he "simply had to see the procession." Doctors reluctantly gave their permission. In the excitement, Wergeland forgot he was sick, ran across town to the home of friends, and collapsed. Racked with a violent cough, the formerly towering and robust young poet watched the parade hunched in tears.[15]

The next day he knew he had "broken" his health. Doctors diagnosed the condition as pneumonia, "whose consequences I still suffer," his November 30 letter continued. "I have not been dressed as much as an hour during all this time, but my mind has been active, and against doctors' orders, I have written with great industry." It was on his deathbed that Wergeland wrote his most beloved poems.

Wergeland's ultimately fatal disease, usually identified as tuberculosis, was reassessed in 1995 by Per Holck of the University of Oslo's Anatomy Department as pulmonary cancer. Wergeland had made the same diagnosis himself, calling it a "hardening," *forhærdelse,* of the lung, as this cancer was then known, and declaring in the same November letter that "the victim knows best from which illness he suffers."[16]

Regardless of the malady's actual identity, it provided Wergeland with ample opportunity to display his long-standing skepticism of doctors and hospitals. "The duration of my illness and the enormous waste of medicine has done nothing to increase my respect for physicians," he grumbled in the November letter, and on February 4, 1845, he proclaimed, "I am tired of this experimentation. No more prescriptions will be written for me!"[17]

Somewhat more patiently, Wergeland had submitted himself to familiar folk remedies. In August 1844, he told of a "Spanish fly plaster as big as a wall map" being applied to his "already raw back." (Spanish beetles known as cantharides were dried to produce a highly corrosive substance used in blistering.) In January 1845, Wergeland wrote that he had spent his "worst night ever," coughing "every minute" and relieved only when the housemaid made him an øl-ost (a drink made with two parts milk and one part beer, heated separately, and then mixed), which finally brought him some much welcomed sleep.[18]

Financial woes worsened Wergeland's plight and forced him to sell his beloved home, Grotten ("the grotto"), still situated on the split in a rock outcropping just north of the Royal Palace. In April 1845 he moved to the nearby but considerably smaller Hjerterum ("heartroom") in rural Pilestredet. Wergeland called Hjerterum a "husmannsstue" (cotter's cabin) and looked forward to its quiet surroundings, but the new house was cold and damp, and the constant hammering of carpenters completing it hardly suited a convalescing patient. His wife, Amalie, insisted he would be better off in the hospital, but Henrik adamantly refused, wrote Wilhelm Lassen, who witnessed the couple's quarrel. At last Henrik relented on the stipulation that the hospitalization last no longer than eight days (it lasted ten) and that he be allowed to bring his canary.[19]

Though the official records of the Rikshospital mention no canary, they do show Wergeland being admitted on April 20, 1845, to a single room with the "better care" appropriate to his class and station. Lassen visited him a few days later in the hospital's main building (located between Akersgaten and Grubbegaten, now occupied by the government office building). He found Wergeland "more dissatisfied than sick," complaining that the "echo chamber" produced by the long corridor outside his room amplified beyond endurance the "hysterical screams" of the patient in the room next door. Wergeland groused about the service, too, and wondered "if he was receiving such poor service, how bad must it be for those less favorably situated?" A painful earache magnified Wergeland's discomfort, and it was on this ailment the doctors focused their treatments.

On April 21, the physicians administered quinine for agitation and chills, along with anise drops to clear his lungs. They also massaged his ear with cod-liver oil. The next day they sprayed lukewarm water into the ear, followed by a continual drip of lead acetate, commonly used to soothe bruises and sores. Wergeland's physicians repeated this procedure on April 23, substituting a soap solution, and later that day they applied a poultice of kavring grøt (bread-rusk porridge) to Wergeland's ear, that evening adding some powdered *hundetunge* (hound's tongue, *Cynoglossen officinalis*), a calming, astringent herb used on difficult wounds. On April 29, the doctors administered Griffith's mixture, a solution containing iron to address the bleeding in Wergeland's lungs. Finally, on April 30, they released him as "uncured."[20]

Wergeland then contacted Mor Sæther, who had also visited him at the hospital. "This much is certain," he wrote to his father on May 13, "after coming home and putting myself in Mor Sæther's care, my appetite, healthful appearance, and vigor have returned." She also apparently restored his will to write. "For over a month the thought of books and writing has sickened me, but now I can not only read but am also writing my 'Life Sketches'—with, I presume, a good measure of dry humor."[21]

In gratitude, Wergeland wrote one of his last poems "*til ære for gamle Moer Sæther og hendes Phioles Kraft*" (in honor of Mor Sæther and the power of her herbs). Titled "*Mulig Forvæxling*" (Possible confusion), the poem compares the folk healer's comforting presence to the watchful eye of the moon shining through his hospital-room window and to a cat keeping silent vigil on the ground below. It also credits Mor Sæther's medicine for granting him the strength to write.

> *Thi Draaber tre jeg smagte, og deraf Følgen blev*
> *de tre Minutters Helse, hvori jeg dette skrev.*

> (For the three medicinal drops I tasted
> gave three minutes of health, not wasted,
> but transformed to the present verse.)

In response, Mor Sæther sent Wergeland oranges, apples, and breads made of peas and oats, along with a delicious *pultost* (a soft, sharp cheese) and hand-churned butter with chives, appetizing and nutritious food that may have helped Wergeland as much as her "drops." It certainly brought him greater enjoyment. As Wergeland complained to his father, her medicine (a tincture of valerian called "baldrian drops") "stinks so bad that I stopped using it this morning, giving myself over to the pain, which bothers me tremendously."[22]

Wergeland died on July 12, 1845, at age thirty-seven, by no means mistaken about the pungency of *vendelrot* (valerian). (Peasants believed its repulsive odor could protect livestock from evil spirits and hung bunches of the plant from barn ceilings.) Mor Sæther chose valerian to induce relaxation and sleep. Mixing its dried rhizome and roots with mildly sedative hops, she also made a soothing salve subsequently endorsed by such prominent university medical professors as Ernst Ferdinand Lochmann and Joachim Andreas Voss. Through the 1980s her salve continued to be offered for sale at Norwegian apothecaries as *"Mor Sæther's gikt smørelse"* (Mor Sæther's rheumatism salve).[23]

Mor Sæther treated patients outside the capital city, too, attracting attention wherever she went. "Our town is currently being visited by a highly remarkable personality, the miracle woman, Mor Sæther from Christiania," reported the April 18, 1843, Bratsberg *Amtstidende* (County times) when she visited Skien. "Far wiser than all the medical professionals combined, as everyone knows, she has many testimonials from the most learned, well-born, and highly respected individuals proclaiming her cures of many patients declared incurable by the most respected, best-educated doctors. Clearly more than a mere mortal . . . she is certainly attracting an enormous crowd of townspeople who stream to the wonder woman as she somehow manages to find remedies for them all."[24]

Faced with sarcasm, controversy, and court cases, what kept Mor Sæther going? Most likely she regarded her work as a calling and felt compelled to learn all that she could about medicine and help others. Confirming the healer's thirst for knowledge, her niece (born 1841) reported in 1908 that during an 1851 operation performed on Mor Sæther by Doctors de Besche, Conradi, and Faye for a stomach tumor, "she insisted on watching the entire procedure in a hand mirror."[25]

Confirming her equally strong desire to help others, the inscription on her tombstone declared:

Hun var de Syges Hjælper og de Armes Pleier,
Ved Herrens Gaver styrked Hun de Svage.

(Caretaker of the poor and healer of the sick,
with God-given gifts, she gave strength to the weak.)

The headstone, placed by Pastor Wexels and several of Mor Sæther's friends, stood for decades after her death on April 30, 1851, in *Vår frelsers* cemetery, the last resting place of the capital city's most prominent citizens. Mor

Sæther (Anne Wiger) had come a long way from Grue in Solør, a journey that documents the desperate need for health care felt by her fellow citizens regardless of their social class.[26]

Anne Brandfjeld (1815–1905)

Like Mor Sæther, the young woman later known as Anne Brandfjeld came to the capital city armed with knowledge of medicinal herbs and the desire to learn more. Born to Anders Didriksen and Marte Olsdatter, servants on the Mustad farm in Vardal near Gjøvik, she was baptized Anne-Marie Andersdatter. Her story is the story of many almue sons and daughters whose parents lacked the resources to keep them at home after Lutheran confirmation granted them adult status around age fourteen. These young people typically went into *tjeneste* (service), working for room and board on more prosperous farms, but as the century wore on, they increasingly sought employment in Norway's growing towns and cities.[27]

Anne-Marie left Vardal for Christiania at age twenty-five. Lack of schooling limited her options, and like many other young women, she found work as a housemaid. Employed by Herman Øyseth, a Kristiania goldsmith seven years her senior, Anne—again like many others in similar circumstances—"got into trouble," bearing the child of her married employer in 1843.

Anne's relationship with the goldsmith continued, for church records show that she gave birth in 1845 to a second son fathered by Herman Øyseth. Childless in his marriage, Øyseth seems to have

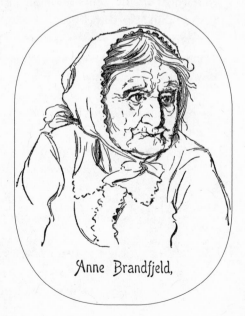

Anne Brandfjeld,

The aged Oslo healer Anne Brandfjeld continued to receive patients though confined to her bed until 1905.
(*Urd*, Jan. 14, 1905)

supported Anne financially and may even have given her the cotter's place where she lived for thirty-seven years after leaving his employ. Known as Ekeberglien, the place was a tiny section of the Brandfjeld farm, itself only a small portion of the sprawling Ekeberg estate that covered the ridge rising high above the capital-city neighborhood known even then as *Gamlebyen* (old town).[28]

Over the years writers have published much mistaken information about Anne Brandfjeld. In 1999, Anne's great-great-granddaughter Berit Øiseth Bakken delivered a lecture presenting new evidence about the healer's past and displayed the confirmation certificate of her great-grandfather, Christian Olsen Øiseth, Anne's first child with the goldsmith. Noting that the certificate identifies Christian's father as "Ole Hansen," Bakken turned the document over to reveal the following note written in Christian's hand: "Ole Hansen does not exist. I was born of Anne Marie Andersdatter and am the illegitimate child of the goldsmith Herman C. Øyseth. My mother was lured into writing a false name by my real father by the promise of marriage. NB. The person I am named for was believed to have drowned and that is why she used that name."

Mystery surrounds Herman Øyseth. Born in 1808 in Nes and trained in his craft in Kristiania and Moss, Øyseth received his professional *borgerbrev* (credential of guild membership) in 1833 and must have enjoyed enormous respect as a goldsmith. In 1846, he received the commission to make the crown for Sweden's crown prince, still the only item of Scandinavian regalia produced by a Norwegian craftsman, and that same year he became a leader in the city's goldsmith guild. Three years later, however, Øyseth inexplicably left Kristiania, giving up his borgerbrev as a goldsmith. His name reappears in the city records as a malt and liquor inspector in 1852 and again in 1881 when he died. By then he was a wealthy man and the owner of Nedre Slottsgate 19 on the corner of Karl Johansgate, the city's main thoroughfare.

When Øyseth moved, Anne found herself alone with two *uekte* (illegitimate) children, surely an enormous social stigma in her society, which emphatically excluded unwed mothers and their offspring. Yet records show that in 1849, the year Øyseth left Christiania (now Oslo), Anne at age thirty-four married a stonemason named Christen Evensen at the venerable Aker church (now *Gamle Aker kirke*), built around 1150. Evensen, eleven years her junior, came to live with Anne and her children at the Ekeberglien place, where the couple had at least three children of their own.

Thirty-five years later, at age sixty-nine, Anne became a widow and moved down the hill to a working-class neighborhood just outside the town limits (near Oslo Hospital). Anne's oldest son, Christian, had already moved to the same street (Gravergaten, known after 1901 as Konowsgate), an area of one- and two-story wooden houses below Ekeberg Ridge. Christian ran a grocery store next door to Anne's house at Gravergaten 23, which he also owned. Christian had by this time adopted the name Øiseth, and his improved finances suggest Øyseth's support.[29]

Anne had been successful in her own right, having become a folk healer of considerable renown. Walks on Ekeberg Ridge had supplemented her herbal knowledge, and she continued this favorite pastime until a broken hip confined her to bed. Still, she continued to see patients.

"Of every thirteen people who came to the capital city for their health," Bakken declared in her lecture, "eleven came to see Anne Brandfjeld." Though perhaps exaggerated, the claim accurately reflects Anne Brandfjeld's status as the most famous Norwegian folk healer of her time. The common assertion that she had "permission from the king himself to do her doctoring" was reiterated in Anne's 1905 obituary by a woman who claimed she had "seen with her own eyes" the king's large diploma "complete with seven wax seals."[30]

Most people who consulted Anne Brandfjeld brought children suffering from rickets. But Anne treated other ailments, as well, especially scrofula (a tubercular condition enlarging the lymph nodes and causing a pernicious rash) and other skin diseases, for which she relied on medications she made from juniper.

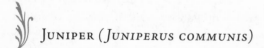

JUNIPER (*JUNIPERUS COMMUNIS*)

Juniper, whose berries lend their distinctive flavor to gin, has long been considered a sacred plant with magical, protective qualities. Norwegians traditionally burned juniper branches to drive away evil spirits thought to cause disease and fumigated sick rooms with juniper into the nineteenth century. The walls of St. Jørgen's Hospital in Bergen (now Norway's leprosy museum) retain a juniper odor to this day. Centuries earlier, Norwegians had also burned branches of juniper during childbirth, perhaps persuaded by its crackling sparks that it had power to protect mother and child from witches and *huldrefolk* (hidden people) who might cause them harm.

Nineteenth-century Norwegians used *einerlaag* (water infused with juniper branches and berries) as an all-purpose wash to purify their wooden dairy and beer-brewing containers, while folk healers used it to treat a variety of hair and skin ailments. A popular doctor book, Mangor's *Lande-apothek*, recommended daily drinking of six to eight glasses of lye made from juniper ashes and old beer; Mangor also advised soaking crushed juniper berries in wine for an hour and applying them to the temples for a headache. These applications may have had some effect, for recent research shows that its volatile oils and tannins have mildly antiseptic and anti-inflammatory qualities, although herbalists today advise against taking juniper internally.[31]

Able to soothe the pain of rheumatism, juniper became the basis of a cottage industry in several parts of Norway by the end of the nineteenth century, as workers earned extra income by distilling and selling juniper oil (*briskeolje*). In addition to treating muscle pain, this oil was commonly used for bladder infections by having the patient sit on a pail of boiling hot water to which juniper had been added.[32]

Anne prided herself on avoiding the strong chemicals favored by the doctors of her time, believing that these medicines did more harm than good. Toward the end of her life, however, she began consulting doctors, deeming them more "capable and insightful" than they once had been. She continued to oppose the use of strong medicines when an old-fashioned household remedy would do. "Providence has wisely arranged for the illnesses that occur in Norway to be healed by the very herbs that grow here."[33]

Anne's burial, arranged by her faithful son Christian, took place near their home at the cemetery known as Oslo Kirkegaard. Her grave has by now long since been replaced—Norwegian burial plots are reserved for only twenty years, unless payment is made—and her house on Konow Street was torn down in the 1970s. A large white sign lettered in green was ceremoniously placed on a tree at Ekeberglien in 1998, identifying the site as the cotter's place where the folk healer had lived for thirty-seven years.[34]

Almost a century before this posthumous recognition, Anne Brandfjeld

gained fame of a different sort when Jon Flatabø, a prolific writer of popular literature, published a fictionalized version of her life. He did not know
Anne personally when he wrote the novel, *Anne Brandfjeld, eller Hvad den
vise Kvinde alene vidste* (Anne Brandfjeld, or what only the folk healer knew),
but he met her on October 27, 1899, shortly after it appeared. "Over eighty
years old, but seeming no more than sixty or seventy," he wrote, Anne
Brandfjeld was "far finer" and "infinitely more wise than her stubborn, God-
denying critics imagine." The folk healer's story fit perfectly the agenda of
Flatabø's novel, which contrasted faith and intuition with the scientific ma-
terialism he felt was destroying other ways of knowing.[35]

Flatabø portrayed Brandfjeld as a seer who could predict the future and
who used her keen insight to defeat a villainous banker from Hamburg. The
intuitive knowledge possessed by women like Brandfjeld, Flatabø argued in
the novel's preface, was as precious as the scientific knowledge possessed by
doctors who refused to learn from her experience. Instead of appreciating
her gifts, they demonized her and cast her in the role of "a common witch
or exorcist." Poor and rich alike needed her gifts, he believed, though the
latter shunned her in public, loathe to acknowledge their reliance on her
help. "If it was a better class family . . . Anne was brought up the kitchen
stairs and discretely slipped into the living quarters," he wrote. "But once
inside there was no end of the delicacies she was plied with or kind words
uttered by the gentlefolk while she prepared her medicaments."[36]

In another scene from the novel, probably influenced by Mor Sæther's
experience, Anne Brandfjeld waves a bottle of her medication under the noses
of intimidating medical authorities as they gruffly demand to know its contents. "You're the doctors," she taunts, "smell it for yourselves and then tell
me what it is!"[37]

"Far too often the learned underestimate common people simply because they do not know them," wrote Flatabø in his preface. "How many of
the learned who denounced her activity knew anything about Anne Brandfjeld and her special talent for diagnosing illness and its cause?" Contending
that even those born to privilege could learn from her, Flatabø's book also
championed Norwegians who lacked the formal education increasingly demanded by society but which was denied to women and the almue. Competence, argued Flatabø, can come through experience and aptitude as well
and is not limited to a single class or gender.

Flatabø's novel, however reassuring, was no literary triumph, and it had little impact in its own time or today. As a portrait of a nineteenth-century Norwegian folk healer, however, it is incomparable. In real life, Anne Brandfjeld succeeded in establishing a useful position for herself, despite poverty and social stigmatization, because she was able to help fill the void in medical care that extended far beyond the workers and craftsmen of Graver Street.

Valborg Valand (1812–93)

While Anne Brandfjeld and Mor Sæther treated their patients in Norway's capital city, Valborg Torkelsdatter, like most nineteenth-century Norwegian folk healers, cared for her charges in rural Norway. Taught by her mother and grandmother, Valborg began treating patients in her childhood home at Holmen in Søgne, where the nearby ferry probably drew many people needing care.[38]

At age twenty-three, Valborg married Aanen Vatne, who had bought the Valand farm near the south-coast town of Mandal. It was to this farm that Valborg moved, as custom decreed, bringing along as part of her dowry an impressive array of legebøker (doctor books).

A strong, sturdy woman, Valborg took active part in the daily operation of the farm, helping her husband to fell the trees and build the house they would live in. (Painted yellow and attractively trimmed with wood, it still stands beside Highway E-39 at Valand). Valborg also attended to more traditional women's chores of caring for the cows, sheep, and goats and making butter and cheese. At the same time she kept busy treating her neighbors' maladies, for her reputation as a folk healer had preceded her to Valand.

As stories of her cures circulated, more patients came. Among them was Edvard Hansen (born 1843 in Sør-Audnedal), who as a young man suffered from a life-threatening chest ailment that Mandal physician Dr. S. Roscher had failed to cure. According to Hansen's daughter, when the doctor later met Hansen on the street, he blurted out in astonishment, "Can Valborg Valand raise people from the dead? If you had continued in my care, you'd be a dead duck by now!" Hansen lived to be eighty-two.[39]

Another of Valborg's patients, Sigvart Skeie (born 1882), had injured his ankle as a boy of ten. When it became infected, Dr. Roscher opened the wound to drain it, but the infection spread up to the boy's knee. When Roscher decided to amputate the leg to save the boy's life, the child's father took him to Valborg. "We can manage this," she said as she examined the limb. Inserting a length of straw into the base of the sore, she dripped her homemade medicine through it to make sure it reached the bone. Valborg had to repeat this treatment many times, said Skeie, before the inflammation finally gave way to healing, but in 1965, he could happily report having walked "on two healthy legs for the next seventy years."

Sigvart Skeie and Edvard Hansen's daughter told their stories to Alv Sverre Hvidbergskår, a Norwegian schoolteacher who traveled around Agder country during the 1960s collecting bits of information still remembered about local folk healers. Without Hvidbergskår's efforts, these few stories would likely have been lost forever.

Older residents told Hvidbergskår of watching Valborg drive off on lengthy "doctor journeys" in her *kariole*, a two-wheeled, horse-drawn conveyance. Northeast along the coast to Grimstad and Arendal she traveled, and up the long and steep-sided Setesdal valley to Valle.

Supplementing her herbal knowledge, Valborg learned a great deal from an apothecary chest she bought at an auction of goods rescued from a Dutch or English sailing ship that sank off Norway's southern coast. Valborg got help translating the instructions that accompanied these medications and learned how to use them. When her original supply ran out, she made similar compounds, obtaining ingredients not available at the town's apothecary shop from skippers of boats that docked in Mandal. In this way Valborg learned to use *blysukker* (sugar of lead or lead acetate), a medication she later ordered in quantity. Diluting it with water, Valborg prepared *blyvand* (lead water) to make poultices for treating bruises, skin inflammations, sore eyes, and ruptures, a common condition for people who regularly lifted heavy loads.[40] People also came to Valborg to be treated for boils, tumors, swellings, scrofula, and broken bones. In addition to the apothecary chemicals, Valborg continued to rely on medicinal herbs, reportedly favoring *ryllik* (yarrow), *tepperot* (tormentil), and *høymol* (dock), each deeply rooted in Norwegian folklore and medicine.

 ## Valborg Valand's Herbs

Yarrow's Latin name, *Achillea millefolium*, attributes the plant's "thousand leaves" of dark green, feathery foliage to the Greek warrior Achilles, who became invincible when his entire body, except for his right heel, was rubbed with this herb. The overlooked heel caused his famous downfall. The Vikings (ca. 800–1000 AD) salved their warriors' wounds with a balm made of tallow mixed with the dried leaves of yarrow, also known as milfoil, and for centuries afterwards the ability of this herb to staunch blood flow and ease pain kept it in demand as a wound dressing, not least by soldiers in the American Civil War. Pharmacologists today credit yarrow's anti-inflammatory and antiseptic properties to its volatile oils and add that its tannins and resins act as astringents and its high silica content promotes the repair of wounded skin tissue.[41]

Tormentil (*Potentilla erecta*), though less prominent in international folk medicine, ranks among the most often used medicinal herbs in Norway. Its solid red rhizome initially attracted attention because of the "doctrine of signatures," leading early folk healers to believe it would treat disorders of the blood. While that notion proved false, the herb's red dye, known as tormentil red, came to benefit medicine in quite a different way. Increasing the visibility of bacteria, whose movements could be detected under advanced microscopes by the 1870s, tormentil red aided in their identification.[42]

Centuries earlier, tormentil, whose four-petal yellow flowers are easily recognized among many other yellow plants, was used by healers to cure diarrhea because tormentil's red dye readily invaded and killed bacteria. Reflecting this use, the herb's Norwegian name, *tepperot*, means "stopper root," *teppe* being a cognate of the English word "tap," or a plug that stops liquid flowing from a barrel.[43]

Dock (*Rumex longifolius*; *Rumex domesticus*; *Rumex crispus*) has the opposite effect of tepperot. Resembling rhubarb in both appearance and result, dock plants act as mild laxatives and were used by the ancient Greeks for digestive disorders. In more recent times, Norwegian and other folk healers used dock to treat skin inflammations, burns, sores, and wounds, steeping the plant's roots in sweet or sour cream to concentrate its astringent tannins and produce soothing salves.[44]

Valborg probably treated the inflamed skin of her many scrofula patients using dock, making an ointment by boiling the roots in vinegar (a solvent she favored) to soften the plant fibers before mixing them with lard. American Indians made a similar dressing from the cooked roots of dock, which they applied as a dressing to cuts and wounds.[45]

Valborg specialized in deep cuts and wounds, a fortunate thing for Ole Johnson Ørbek when his axe slipped in the woods not far from Mandal. It took him almost five hours to get to the doctor, and his treatments with warm porridge poultices in the weeks that followed only made the wound worse. When his doctor said he could do no more, Ole went to Valborg, who significantly improved his condition within eight days and declared him completely cured after eleven weeks.[46]

Alcohol probably played a major role in Ørbek's recovery. "*Sprit paa steder som verker*" (alcohol on pus-producing places) was Valborg's mantra, and she ordered alcohol by the keg, said her neighbor Oskar Torkelsen Valand. Ninety-seven years of age when Hvidbergskår visited him in 1964, but still clear in mind and memory, Torkelsen told Hvidbergskår that Valborg removed patients' tumors and other unwanted growths using "surgical knives stored in alcohol." Others, too, remarked on Valborg's use of alcohol. A patient being tended by one of the many assistants that Valborg trained noticed that the water she used to wash his wound smelled like alcohol. Experience had no doubt taught Valborg the benefits of alcohol, and she apparently knew that sugar could fight infection, too, for the same patient was advised by the assistant to shave loaf sugar into his wound if any "white" appeared.

It was Valborg's *trekkplaster* (drawing plaster, from *å trekke*, meaning "to pull") that made her famous. To her neighbors, the apparent ability of this dark brown, smelly salve to pull infection right out of wounds was nothing short of miraculous. In addition to the expected alcohol and sugar, Valborg's plaster contained *harpiks* (pine resin, another antibacterial agent), sheep tallow (to soften the skin), ashes (to treat itching), *rigabalsam* (a popular aromatic mixture of volatile oils, alcohol, and exotic herbs), and a concentrated decoction of common healing herbs. But the secret of Valborg's trekkplaster was tobacco.[47]

Norwegians have cultivated *tobakk* (*Nicotiana tabacum*) since the 1700s. Smoking and chewing it for pleasure, they also used it extensively as a medicine. To soothe a child's earache, for example, Norwegians blew tobacco smoke into the ear or dribbled into it some *pipesaus* (liquid residue left in a pipe after smoking). They also placed tobacco leaves directly on sores and boils to "draw out" their infection.[48]

By 1915, even the popularized *People's Home Medical Book* warned against applying tobacco to broken skin: "Symptoms of poisoning sometimes result when it is thus used, and it is not utilized so much now as formerly."[49] Better alternatives existed by then, but in Valborg's day, her tobacco plaster could stop the all-too-familiar progression from infection to gangrene to amputation.

The efficacy of Valborg's drawing plaster also made it a *trekkplaster* (draw or attraction) in the modern sense of the word, as the farmyard at Valand filled each morning with the horses and carriages of patients who traveled great distances to see her. To accommodate them, Valborg arranged a waiting room and treatment area on the first floor of the spacious house. She used the many alcoves and small rooms on the second floor for patients who needed to stay for several days or even weeks.

This activity flew in the face of the *kvaksalverlov*, of course, and, like Mor Sæther, Valborg Valand was sued three times (in 1855, 1862, and 1865) for quackery.[50] Valborg easily paid the fine assessed in the 1855 case, but when the 1862 hearing resulted in a six-month jail sentence at hard labor, many felt the time had come to reassess the law. "If a person is not permitted to help a neighbor with simple remedies," argued a subcommittee charged with formulating the official opinion of Mandal and Lister counties, then the law is too strict. Given the country's topography and the almue's poverty, permitting respectable persons of proven ability to provide needed health care was not only reasonable, they found; it might even help prevent those of more evil or selfish intent from "taking advantage of people's gullibility and naiveté." The law rightly protected citizens from charlatans, but it did more harm than good if it punished such a "noble and humane" individual as Valborg Valand, the committee concluded. The law should state instead that a healer whose treatments benefited the sick should be permitted to continue. When the committee shared this statement with the full county council, however, the council rejected it, deciding they wanted no part of formulating the new law even though they agreed that a new law was desirable.

By 1863 Norway's desperate medical situation had begun to receive national attention, and when the quack law came up for discussion in *Stortinget* (parliament), O. G. Ueland, representative from Rogaland County, opened the debate. Speaking with eloquence and conviction, he drew a parallel between the quack law and the country's midwifery law of 1810 that had required every woman to choose a professionally trained midwife, despite the country's dire shortage of midwives. Only after several women were sued for helping deliver a neighbor or family member when the woman had no access to a professional midwife did the university's medical faculty and the government agree to change the law.

Fortunately, said Ueland, the quack law was enforced in only about one of 1,000 cases. If it had been consistently applied, it would have sent most of the clergy and their wives to jail, since they had been the principle "doctors" available in rural areas. Though more district doctors had been hired, Ueland observed, the almue lacked confidence in them and had no funds to pay their fees. "Who can afford a doctor that must be fetched from sixty to seventy-five miles away? And what person who owns a home medicine chest (*husapotek*) along with any measure of Christian charity can help but give assistance when it is needed? Ought this to be a punishable offense?" Ueland concluded, "If ever there was an unreasonable law, it was the quack law."[51]

Most representatives agreed with Ueland. Forbidding use of self-taught healers in rural areas amounted to forbidding medical help of any kind, and after lengthy debates in both houses, parliament agreed to support the change. After the medical establishment launched massive resistance, however, the government dropped the idea of changing the quack law.

In 1865, Valborg Valand found herself back in court because of a tragic accident. A young girl's head had become caught in a rotary saw and injured so severely that although Dr. Roscher had immediately come from Mandal, there was little he could do. When the girl survived the accident, her father received permission to bring the girl to Valborg. During the first eight days of Valborg's care, the patient seemed to improve, but then she suffered a relapse and died. Valborg offered to have a proper casket built the next day, but the father chose to take the body home that same evening. Eleven days later, the local magistrate demanded an autopsy and the next day exhumed the body against the family's wishes. On November 14, at the behest of Dr. Roscher, Valborg's hearing began.

Had Valborg done anything to cause the death? Why had the corpse been taken away under the cover of darkness? The court searched and found no guilt on Valborg's part, yet in accordance with the quack law, it sentenced her to a fine and two years in jail at hard labor.

Political agitator Søren Jaabæk, a native of Holum parish (to which the Valand farm belonged), who published the newspaper *Folketidende* (The people's times) in nearby Mandal, wrote bold editorials in defense of Valborg Valand and mocking the medical establishment for "working so hard to find fault with one of the most helpful human beings that ever lived." Along with numerous patient testimonials to Valborg's work, Jaabæk published the parish minister's declaration that she was a "woman worthy of respect." Noting the numerous petitions in her favor signed by local authorities and officials, he urged that Valborg's punishment be dismissed.[52]

Eventually Valborg's jail time was converted to a fine, but that, too, Jaabæk considered unfair, since the doctors had found no action worthy of punishment. "Yet how many wishfully worked to find it?" he asked in a May 1, 1867, *Folketidende* editorial. "Two sheriffs, two witnesses, half a score of judges, three lawyers, two doctors and at least two gravediggers, a half dozen medical school professors, four parliamentary representatives, in sum the efforts and expertise of at least thirty more or less learned individuals all attempting to find wrong-doing on the part of one of the most helpful individuals in existence. All that energy plus thirty-four specie daler in cash expended because bad laws protect the few who have special advantage from them."

Jaabæk had represented Lister and Mandal in parliament since 1845 and listened sympathetically to the 1863 discussion of the quack law, though he had taken no action. But when it came up again in 1871, he jumped into the debate. Medicine is a matter of experience, he argued. "Patients can be equally well served by someone who knows no Latin. Certain individuals with no formal education have a natural genius for healing the sick. But if they use their knowledge, they are punished, even if they do no harm!"

What if Norwegians were willing to have a middle class of healers, Jaabæk wondered, so that health care could be cheaper and more available in thinly populated rural areas? Seeing the battle between the district doctors and folk healers as part of the larger class war then being waged, Jaabæk weighed in on the side of "*de simple*" *mot* "*de fine*" (the "plain" against the "fancy"), as he put it.[53]

Though Norway's larger class war would rage on for many years to come, the skirmishes surrounding the quack law achieved lasting results in 1871 in the form of new legislation. "The new law has granted almost full freedom," cheered Jaabæk in the April 29, 1871, *Folketidende*. Certain self-trained healers with documented qualifications could now carry on their work under limited circumstances, provided they asked no payment and the district doctor had already declared the case hopeless. Slight as this victory may seem, it removed the constant threat that formerly had dogged folk healers' every move.

Valborg apparently lost no time in taking advantage of the new law. "The independent doctor Valborg Valand has been very active in Arendal

and Drammen and in great demand in Bergen, where she makes several annual trips," reported the June 6, 1871, *Folketidende*. A later issue included a
letter from Telemark about a successful operation Valborg had performed
to remove a growth just below a woman's jawbone, a procedure none of the
doctors had dared attempt.[54]

If Valborg's visit brought a pilgrimage of patients, it also unleashed the
gossip mill. "The woman who with the assistance of parliamentary representative Søren Jaabæk has become a national celebrity credited with the
recent reform of the quack law that has liberated medical care," reported
the July 2, 1871, *Drammens Tidende*, "has in her capacity of miracle worker
arrived in our town." And the July 17 issue announced that Valborg had left
town after a successful stay, her landlord having charged her extra "in consideration how much she made here."[55]

Valborg *was* well-to-do. Several individuals told Hvidbergskår they estimated her net worth at 100,000 kroner, a great fortune at the time. Valborg
managed her money well, making judicious loans and good investments in
farmland and forests. Both she and her husband dressed in finer clothes
than their neighbors, she in silk blouses and sporting a heavy gold chain
necklace, said to be a gift from the Swedish king Oscar himself—others
said it was from his queen—for curing him of some ailment.

The Valand couple generously established two annuities to benefit the
poor of their parish and to reward elderly servants who had demonstrated
loyalty and dependability by the time Vatne died at the age of sixty-four,
some sixteen years before Valborg. He had been a successful farmer, well
respected in the community and regarded as a deputy by the local sheriff.

Though Valborg did not practice medicine to make money, taking no
payments from the poor and even giving them free medicine, she asked
wealthy patients to pay what they could afford. "She never lost on that," says
Else Valand, who married the son of Valborg's nephew and most immediate descendant. Writing in 1985, she noted that "even today, a hundred years
later, stories of Valborg's ability live on in oral tradition." She used "the gifts
the creator had so richly bestowed upon her," Hvidbergskår observes. "She
could have avoided the attacks and simply sailed smoothly through life, but
felt an obligation to use her skills."[56]

After Valborg's husband died, writes Else, Valborg lived alone with her
housekeeper, Maja Auensen, who helped make the medicines and salves
needed in Valborg's practice. Several years later Valborg had a driving acci-

dent on the way to the magistrate's office in Mandal. Annoyed about some legal matter, she was driving too fast for the sharp corner of the block now occupied by Mandal Sparebank. Her kariole tipped over, sending Valborg to the ground, and she broke her hip in the fall. Refusing to see a doctor, Valborg tended the injury herself but never completely recovered. In 1893, at age eighty, she contracted pneumonia, but still refused to see the doctor.

Valborg's niece, Abel Jørgensen Føreid, took care of her, writes Else, and it was she who on the morning of April 20 sent a note in a beautiful hand on unlined stationary bordered in black informing Valborg's twin brother, Torkel Holmen, that "Valborg Torkelsdatter Valand died today at 5:30 in the morning." Valborg's grave, marked with a prominent headstone, stands in the Holum churchyard not far from that of her champion, Søren Jaabæk, and is similarly maintained at public expense.

Valborg's work continued after her death, carried on by the many assistants she had trained. Maja Auensen, who had lived with Valborg for forty years, practiced as a folk healer long afterwards. Valborg's niece Abel had already become a folk healer in her own right by the time of her aunt's death, and so had Abel's housekeeper of thirty-three years, Johanne Johansen (born 1864 in Fåberg). Johanne became especially well known for curing "blood poisoning," as people called seriously infected wounds that would not heal. When Johanne subsequently emigrated to America, she continued to make Valand's famous trekkplaster for sale as "Mrs. Olsen's Salve." Available at drugstores in Brooklyn (according to Else Valand), it also appeared in a Norwegian-language advertisement in the July 1908 issue of the Norwegian American *Kvindens Magasin* (Woman's magazine): "Mrs. Olsen's Valuable Salve (trademark), price 25 cents, is excellent for burns, boils, sores that will not heal, beard fungus, chapped nipples, frostbite, eczema, and all other skin ailments. Ask your pharmacist for Mrs. Olsen's Valuable Salve. Accept no substitutes. If he will not get it, write directly to me and enclose 25 cents in 1 or 2 Cent stamps, and I will send you a box postpaid."

Ivar Ringestad (1812–92)

As Valborg Valand's salve crossed the ocean to America, several little-known Norwegian American folk healers continued her calling in the rural Midwest. Among them was Ivar Guldbransen Ringestad, an emigrant from Valdres in 1849 who first settled in Koshkonong, Dane County, Wisconsin. Information about him has been preserved because fellow Valdres emigrant Anna Mohn later shared her memories of early immigrant life with the editor of *Samband* and included details of Ivar's interest in doctoring that otherwise would have gone unrecorded.[57]

Shortly before leaving Norway, Ivar Ringestad married Anne Brandt (1812–84), the sister of famous pioneer pastor Nils Brandt (born 1824). In Koshkonong, the Ringestads lived at the parsonage of Pastor J. W. C. Dietrichson (1815–83), the organizer of several Norwegian American Lutheran congregations.[58]

Interest in medicine ran in Ivar's family, said Mohn, but Ivar did not put his knowledge to practical use until a dynamite charge seriously injured a well digger's hand. "Ivar saw to healing the hand himself, since there was no doctor, and it went well. This was the beginning of an activity that proved helpful to many settlers. Ivar had brought along some good *doktor bøker* (doctor books) from home, and on the basis of their instructions, he made salves and pills." Through a combination of interest, aptitude, and self-instruction, she continued, "Ivar managed to save many a limb that would otherwise have been amputated."

Ivar Ringestad's interest in medicine may have been stimulated by his father, Sgt. Gulbrand Iversen, who would have received rudimentary medical instruction in the army. Ivar gained additional exposure to military life during a brief stay in the home of an army captain (on whom novelist Jonas Lie later based the father character in the popular classic *Familien paa Gilje. Interiør fra 1840-årene* (The family at Gilje. An interior from the 1840s).

Ivar's neighbors sought his help, too, in Winneshiek County, Iowa, after the Ringestads moved there in 1851 to claim land of their own. The Ringestads finally settled northeast of Decorah in Madison Township, which consisted of nothing more than "a couple of log houses and a mill," said Mohn. Ivar's wife, who "lacked the strong constitution of the peasant wives," belonged to the kondisjonerte class, her father having been a schoolteacher and church *klokker* (deacon) in Vestre Slidre, and she herself was the widow of a local Valdres official. Though Anne's "nature and frailty did not ideally suit her to frontier life," said Mohn, she nevertheless pitched in "as a matter of course," especially taking care of women and children and assisting her neighbors in childbirth.[59]

In Norway, rural women of the almue class traditionally assisted each other in childbirth, while women of the kondisjonerte class increasingly used professionally trained midwives. Anne Ringestad consequently lacked the experience possessed by most almue women, but she must have learned fast. When husbands came to fetch Anne, "even if they came for her amid violently raging storms," wrote Mohn, "she didn't let that stop her from going with them to provide assistance."

Settlers continued to come to Ivar, too, "in case of accidents and when treatment of a medical nature was needed. . . . He was usually quite lucky [in devising an appropriate treatment], and always put his own work aside when someone needed advice or medical assistance," according to Mohn. "He did not do this for pay, as there was little 'cash' among the settlers."[60]

Olava Wick (1807–1904)

Another little-known Norwegian American healer named Olava Wick also emerges from the historical shadows. The story of her service to the early settlers of Tumuli Township near Fergus Falls, Minnesota, was reported in a 1937 interview with her granddaughter Oline Dahl Skrove.[61] Before emigrating, Olava had lived in Trondheim with her husband, Mikkel Yttervik, a small landholder, who supplemented his farm income with carpentry. The couple had three children, and like most nineteenth-century Norwegian women, Olava helped her neighbors through childbirth. But Olava's interest in medicine went further, for she is said to have consulted the local doctor to obtain formulas for compounding salves and lotions. Though no records remain to document this activity, she may very well have begun

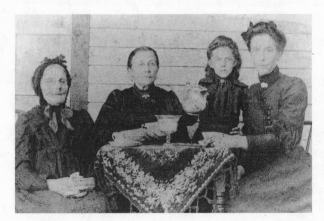

Olava Wick, better known as "Doctor Gamla," or the old lady doctor, tended her patients in Dalton, Minnesota. She was photographed with her daughter (born in Trondheim), her granddaughter (born in Hesper, Iowa), and her great-granddaughter (born in Dalton).

devising and dispensing remedies long before she departed from Norway for America in 1866 at age fifty-nine.

Tragedy surrounded Olava's departure, according to family tradition, for Mikkel hanged himself "in grief over his family leaving Norway." Emigrating with Olava were her daughter, Anna, and Anna's husband, Borre Dahl. Borre's seven-year-old sister Tilda Dahl (born 1860) emigrated, too, and in a 1940 memoir she described sailing to Quebec on the decrepit immigrant ship *Harmoni*, then proceeding by a horse-drawn canal boat along the St. Lawrence River, and finally by railroad in a cattle car. On the train, when Anna found herself starting labor with her first child, the family debarked in rural Hesper (near Decorah), where Olava delivered Anna's child, Oline.[62]

The family's stay in Hesper extended to two years, and it was not until May 1868 that the party resumed their interrupted journey to Dahl Town in Otter Tail County, Minnesota. They traveled the several hundred miles by ox-drawn prairie cart to the home of Borre Dahl's brother, Sigmund, who had settled there a few years earlier. He housed them until they could build a log cabin on their own homestead land (and also provided the town's name, Americanized to Dalton in 1880 when it became a stop on the Great Northern Railroad).

Here it was that Olava became "Doktor Gamla" (the old lady doctor), known for her interest in medicinal herbs and skill at healing wounds, sores, and burns. Stories of her healing abounded. There was the little boy who nearly severed his hand while running with a sharp ax. His parents bundled him off to the trading post at Pomme de Terre, where the doctor brought out his instruments to amputate, insisting that the hand would never heal and the child would die from blood poisoning. Refusing to believe this, the desperate couple drove eight miles farther to Olava Wick. She dressed the wound with a special salve she concocted and bandaged the hand with a piece of cardboard. It healed without further complication.

Olava also saved Erik Bergerud's hands, which were badly burned after he ran into a flaming stable to save his brother's hogs. When the doctor recommended amputation, Bergerud asked instead to see Doktor Gamla. Olava used her salve to treat Bergerud's severely burned face, but even more significant was her success in healing his hands, which enabled Bergerud to continue supporting himself.

Like Mor Sæther and Valborg Valand, Olava Wick took patients into her home. After the three-day blizzard of 1873, one of the worst in Minnesota history, Olava treated Matthias Halvorson for several weeks at her home. Halvorsen had used the unusually mild January day to do errands in Fergus Falls, and the unexpected storm caught him far from home. Without shelter, Halvorson froze his legs so badly that doctors planned to send him to St. Paul to have them amputated. Olava, however, determined to try to save the legs although she recognized that his toes would have to be amputated. Lacking a suitable instrument, she had her son-in-law fashion a fine-toothed saw blade about eight inches long from a hoop skirt's steel ring and mount it between the ends of a pail handle. With this crude but sturdy implement (now at the Otter Tail County Historical Society), Olava performed the operation with success—and no anesthesia. "It was up to the patient to grit his teeth and hold still during her none too gentle manipulations," wrote Olava's great-grandson Nils J. (Benny) Johnson in the 1936 Fergus Falls *Daily Journal*. To distract patients from their pain, Olava would "get their dander up by making some sarcastic remark." (Olava evidently knew something about adrenaline, too.) "Her many cures were far from painless," Tilda Dahl Rustad conceded, "but it was surprising how effective they were in many cases."[63] Because of her ability to help people with "problems of sickness beyond their own knowledge to cope" and since her help was "given freely and usually without any pay or remuneration," wrote Rustad (whose family had also settled in Dalton), Olava's reputation grew.

Settlers frequently appeared in Dalton seeking Olava's help, and her reputation even added a branch to the family tree. On the western Minnesota prairie near Doran (about thirty-five miles west of Dalton) lived sixteen-year-old Ida Skrove, whose ulcerated leg refused to heal. When her parents, Norwegian homesteaders who immigrated in 1867, heard about Doktor Gamla in Dalton, they delegated Ida's older brother, Sigurd, to hitch up their horse and buggy and take his sister for treatment. Sigurd's willingness to make the long journey to Dalton whenever his sister needed additional treatment initially puzzled his parents. Then they learned of the young widow in the Dahl household. (Olava's granddaughter Oline, born in Hesper, had grown up and married but lost her husband and young daughter to diphtheria.) By the time Oline married Sigurd on October 1, 1893, Olava's medicines had healed Ida's leg so successfully that she could dance at the wedding.

Having had no formal training, Olava based her treatments on careful observation combined with trial and error, wrote her great-great-granddaughter Viola Johnson Behrends. But superstitious neighbors thought she used magic. "They called Olava a witch doctor," said an incredulous Mrs. Behrends, and "did not realize the depth of interest, experience, and intuitive knowledge that guided her in finding effective cures and knowing the right thing to do." As a child, Tilda Dahl Rustad heard neighbors claim that Olava "could stop the bleeding of a bad cut just by being told about it. She would 'mumble' a few words after being told, and many persons who had experienced 'her power' to do this testified to the truth of it." This ability to stop excessive bleeding was commonly attributed to especially talented folk healers, although bleeding usually stopped by itself—in about the time it takes to recite a magic formula.

Many healers in preindustrial Norway, in fact, employed such formulas. Some used them because they believed their incantations had real power. Others used them to increase their patients' faith in their treatments. Charlatans, of course, dramatized their "magical healing abilities" to fatten their wallets.

Without testimony from those who knew these healers personally, it is difficult to know what to make of these claims of witchcraft. The words of Olava's descendants therefore have special value, showing as they do that even folk healers who used purely rational remedies rarely escaped being branded as witches.

Fortunately, Olava's descendents preserved information about her rational means, including the precise composition of her most valuable medical secret, the "magical" salve that saved so many lives and limbs and consisted entirely of everyday ingredients. Aware of its value, Olava bequeathed the recipe in her will to her great-granddaughter, Anna Martha Johnson, whose daughter, Viola Johnson Behrends, included it in her family history.

Olava Salve

· 1 pound fresh butter
1 pound sheep tallow
rosin 10 cents worth
beeswax 10 cents worth
1 loaf sugar crushed
pinch of powdered alum.

Melt butter in double boiler, keeping stirring. Add remaining ingredients. When cool, add one ounce Riga balsam.

Containing no "tongue of bat" or "eye of newt," as Olava's neighbors may have suspected, the ingredients resembled those of other nineteenth-century salves: butter and tallow to keep the skin soft and supple; rosin and sugar to kill germs; astringent alum to remove both excess moisture and "*villkjøtt*" or "*dødkjøtt*" (dead skin tissue thought to cause blood poisoning); beeswax to stabilize and add body to the mixture; and Riga balsam to add alcohol and aroma.

"This recipe makes a thick smelly salve," wrote Behrends, who had "proved time and time again that it pulls adolescent pimples or felons [infected abrasions on hands and fingers] to a head and drainage in no time at all." Known in Norwegian as *verkefinger*, such infections disrupted the work of home, farm, fishery, and forest, and they demanded an effective cure. "If you can stand the smell and the discomfort of the drawing, you are healed," Behrends continued, noting that her father would say that Olava salve "could pull a tenpenny nail out of the wall."

Concluded another of Olava's descendants, Mrs. Julius Johnson, in a 1939 interview some thirty-five years after her death, "Although she had no diploma or legal standing, she was held in high esteem for what she accomplished." A simple gray obelisk marks Olava's grave in Dalton's intimate St. Olaf Cemetery.

The Folk Healer as Witch

Mother had pinched her finger and raised a blister. . . . With two little girls in diapers, she had her hands immersed in hot and cold water many times each day, not to mention washing for three boys and a husband—and the dishes. The blister turned into a good-sized sore that none of Mother's remedies would heal, and neither Doc Picett's wisdom nor his salves helped, either.

Doc burned the sore with silver nitrate, causing a deal of pain but no cure and, as a last resort, offered amputation as the only cure. He would have done it, too, but then I remembered Mrs. Shoemaker Riley. We neighborhood children were afraid of her and made ourselves scarce whenever we saw her. She spent a lot of time hunting for herbs, and when she came out of the weeds with a bundle in her apron, she really did look like a witch—just as we thought she was.

Someone suggested that mother should try her. Art and I went along as interpreters since Mother couldn't speak English. She told us that she was sure that she could heal Mother's finger, but didn't have the necessary herbs on hand, for she had to pick them when they were wet with dew early in the morning. We went to her house the next evening and she gave us a sackful of grey weeds and told us to go out into the woods and collect the soft pitch from pine trees, too. The herbs were to be steeped in hot water, and Mother was to wash her finger in this tea. The pitch was used as a salve. In a short time the sore finger was entirely healed, and I, for one, was never again afraid of Mrs. Shoemaker Riley.

Eivin Bakken, born 1900 in Wilson, Wisconsin,
quoted in Del Matheson, Reunion East of the Sun ❧

Anne Ludvikke Løberg (1871–1955)

Anne Løberg neither saw nor marketed herself as a healer, yet desperate people found their way to her Milwaukee, Wisconsin, home in their search for reliable medicines. Even after germ theory became widely known in the late-nineteenth century, new medicines were slow to reach the public at large.[64]

Anne settled in America in 1902, and the medicine that her Norwegian American visitors considered miraculous came from an older doctor book. Originally written in French and translated into Danish in 1863, it was used for many years by Anne's family in both Norway and the New Land. Anne had worked at Skien's prestigious *Svane Apotek*, or Swan Apothecary (now at the Telemark District Museum), in Norway. Perhaps it was there she obtained the book cumbersomely named *Huuslægen. Anviisning til selv at tilberede og anvende de vigtigste Lægemidler der tjene til at helbrede og beskytte mod de hyppigst forekommende Sygdomme* (The house doctor: directions for preparing and using the most important medications that serve to heal and prevent the most commonly occurring ailments). Only slightly less unwieldy than its title, the popular 292-page tome, written by François Vincent Raspail, had been issued in three editions prior to the 1863 version Anne owned.

As a young man François Raspail (1794–1878), a French statesman, physician, and chemist, had founded an important branch of science known as "histochemistry," or the chemistry of tissues and cells. Later, however, he became the purveyor of a purported cure-all based on camphor, for which he made amazing claims. In a sense, Raspail's career reflects the crisis experienced by medical professionals in the mid-1800s, when many people turned to unorthodox cures. Apparently, profits in the lucrative proprietary-medicine market tempted even regular physicians who had begun to doubt their profession's future.[65]

The cure-all that Raspail called *Sedativvand* (sedative water) would eventually make Anne known as a folk healer, but it was her father, Lars Thorsen Løberg (1839–1904), who first taught her to use it. Anne's parents emigrated to America in 1892 at the urging of their older son, Thor, who had already left Norway. Anne and her fiancé, Peder Kristoffersen Hvaal (born 1866 in Vestfold), accompanied her parents to Milwaukee, but when Peder could not find suitable employment, the younger couple returned to Norway, where they married and settled down in Notodden. Peder worked as a mechanic at the Tinfos paper factory (now home to a trendy art gallery and café). Anne and Peder had three children, and two more were born after they returned in 1902 to Milwaukee, where the family name Hvaal was Americanized to Waal.

Though Anne did little to promote herself as a healer, word of her Sedativvand quickly spread. People came to the Waals' household near Greenfield Avenue on the south side of Milwaukee, asking her to apply the fabled medicine to their infected sores and wounds. "The first time you see for yourself the quick and certain remedies effected by Sedativvand," Raspail told his readers, "this medication will seem miraculous." Extolling Sedativvand as a cure for everything from the bites of snakes, scorpions, and poisonous insects to blood clots, poor circulation, inflamed breasts, stiff muscles, and fever, he further claimed it could bring a drowned person back to life and cure insanity!

Curing infection remained only slightly less sensational in Anne's day, when limbs and lives were still being lost to "blood poisoning." To prevent this infection, Anne made her own Sedativvand using the ingredients Raspail recommended: spirits of camphor, spirits of ammonia (not household ammonia, but spirits of hartshorn, purchased at a pharmacy), kitchen salt, and ordinary water. Anne's recipe differed somewhat in proportions from the one in Raspail's book, her father having undoubtedly modified it over the years. In 1994, Anne's granddaughter, Carla Waal (born 1933 in Milwaukee) provided this version of Anne's recipe:

Sedativvand

1½ oz. spirits of camphor
3 oz. aqua ammonia
3 level Tbsp. table salt
3 cups water

Dissolve salt in some of the water. Add ingredients a little at a time and shake, shake, shake. Be sure to put olive oil on skin first; then soak clean *white* cloths with Sedativvand and wrap well. Resoak cloths as often as necessary to keep moist.

"'You can't shake it too much,' Grandma used to say, as she walked around the house, shaking and shaking the bottle," Carla wrote. "Grandma felt that her Sedativvand was very potent and should be applied with great caution." She continued, "One day a stranger came to the house and showed Grandma a horrible sore, about the size of a silver dollar, on her arm. Many doctors had tried to cure it, but it kept getting worse. She begged for 'that water.' After she left, Grandma admitted being concerned about the responsibility, but said she had promised her father she would never refuse to supply Sedativvand when it was needed."

Though Anne's father urged her to help those who needed it, he also made her "solemnly promise that she would not pass the recipe on to anyone else, because using Sedativvand was too serious a responsibility." Anne extracted the same promise from her daughter-in-law, Carla's mother (Esther Christiansen Waal, born 1906), when she entrusted the recipe to her. "One reason for the tight control," Carla explained, was so that "strict instructions could be given to *always* apply olive oil to the skin first and to use a clean *white* cloth soaked in the Sedativvand." The olive oil protected the skin from being burned by the mixture, and the white cloth probably helped engender cleanliness at a time when germ theory was still in its infancy.

Several weeks after Anne had treated the stranger's arm, according to Carla, the woman returned and gratefully showed her how well it had healed. "This woman was from Milwaukee," remembered Carla, "but people phoned or came from other towns in Wisconsin to get Anne's Sedativvand." Anne used it to cure a serious infection in a boy's hand caused by fishhooks, and "for many years the family saved the letter sent by a grateful mother thanking Anne for saving her child's life." Another letter writer credited Anne with curing him when a doctor wanted to amputate his arm.

Anne's family used Sedativvand, too. Twice Carla asked her mother to make it for her, once to treat an infected spider bite and the other time for "a really bad pimple" on her face. But on that occasion "the compress with ammonia and spirits of camphor proved to be too strong and I looked worse with my skin peeling!" Carla's inflamed skin and Anne's cautionary warnings attest to the perennial problem with folk medicines of determining a proper dosage.

In the absence of alternatives, Sedativvand worked remarkably well for a wide array of maladies. Both Carla and her mother recalled Anne putting a "compress with Sedativvand on her forehead when she had a headache," and Carla's father and uncle "allowed" Anne to apply this treatment when they had a headache. "My father and his brother Roy used to joke about Grandma Waal making Sedativvand," says Carla, but they occasionally asked for it "as a last resort." (Maybe they had read Raspail's claim that those who used Sedativvand for headaches were often "surprised to find that their hair is growing thicker where the compress has been!")

Even after the advent of penicillin in the mid-1940s, Carla's family occasionally used Sedativvand, once for a persistent infection in her mother's finger. Carla recalled that "as a child Mother once stuck her middle finger in a cigar cutter and sliced off the tip! For years the finger bothered her. Finally a doctor said he could easily relieve her of that pain. His surgery was not a success, however; infection set in. After about three weeks, Grandma asked if Mother would like to try Sedativvand, to which she agreed with enthusiasm. About three times she sat soaking her finger in Sedativvand—it drew out a little yellow lump, and the finger healed."

Raspail's extreme claims for Sedativvand notwithstanding, he actually had made an important discovery. Twenty years before Pasteur discovered the existence of bacteria, Raspail found a way to kill them, as Valborg Valand and Olava Wick would also do with their salves. Though nineteenth-century folk healers treated a wide array of ailments, including digestive disturbances (probably the most common nineteenth-century ailment), their skill in treating infected wounds seems to have made the greatest impression on contemporaries. Preventing infection from ending in amputation seemed such a miracle that these stories live on.

With the acceptance of germ theory in the late nineteenth century, professional medicine diverged dramatically from folk medicine, and scientific discoveries brought reliable remedies for formerly fatal infectious diseases.[66] Yet as the story of Anne Ludvikke Løberg and her Sedativvand demonstrates, the benefits of the medical revolution only slowly reached the larger public, and well into the twentieth century, self-trained healers valuably continued to bridge the gap in available health care.

· 3

The Pastor as Doctor

A matter of trust

"People came to the parsonage wanting medicine from my mother's supply or they asked for communion wine to give to the sick and dying, regarding it equally as medicine and sacrament. Some of those who came for medical advice had the idea that studying for the ministry was the same as medical training. 'You've gone to the same school as the doctor,' one man told my father."

Prost Henrik Seip, son of Jens Arup Seip, pastor at Åseral, 1885–97

MINISTERS AND MINISTERS' WIVES did much of the doctoring and dispensing of medicine in rural nineteenth-century Norway and Norwegian America. As the most educated members of the community, they naturally asssumed this role. The clergy's superior education also gave rise to legends of black-book ministers who could conjure up the devil and force him to do their bidding.[1]

The association of medicine with religion has ancient and international roots. In Norway this linking predates the country's eleventh-century conversion to Christianity. Foreign monks began establishing monasteries, whose charitable infirmaries in Oslo, Bergen, Trondheim, Stavanger, Tønsberg, and Hamar long provided essentially all of the institutional health care available. Destruction of the monasteries in the wake of the Lutheran Reformation of 1537 left a serious void in the country's medical care. Perhaps it was to meet this need that King Christian V (1646–99), in the so-called "Norwegian Laws" promulgated after 1687, directed the clergy to visit and treat the ill in their parishes. This law also gave ministers the responsibility of instructing midwives.[2]

Readily accepting this new medical role, prominent Sunnmøre pastor Hans Strøm (1726–97) treated parishioners in Volda, and on the basis of his experience he wrote one of Norway's first books of popular medicine. Appearing in 1778, his *Kort Underviisning om De paa Landet meest grasser-ende Sygdomme, og derimod tienende Hjelpe-Midler* (Short instruction on the most common illnesses of the countryside and their cures) gives a valuable picture of the medical conditions of his time.

Like Strøm, pastors Niels Schytte (1692–1739) and Niels Jensen (1693–1764) had no formal medical training, yet both became notewor-thy healers and eventually passed down their medical interest, along with their parishes, to their sons. Erik Gerhard Schytte (1729–1808), who trav-eled extensively to tend the sick in vast areas of North Norway, worked with his wife, Anna Jentoft (1743–1818), to convert their Bodø parsonage to a hospital before founding and directing the town's permanent hospital. Niels Jensen's son, Peder Harboe Hertzberg (1728–1802), made medicines using local herbs and water from a healing spring he found near the parson-age at Finaas in Hardanger. As one of Norway's renowned *"potet prester"* (potato pastors), Hertzberg worked to overcome his parishioners' long-entrenched refusal to eat potatoes or any other vegetable, significantly im-proving their general health.[3]

Hertzberg's son Niels (1759–1841) continued his father's work, "sooth-ing and even curing the ills of the country folk," as his autobiography says, "in our isolated area that is served by no district doctor." One of Norway's first vaccinators, Niels Hertzberg began inoculating parishioners against smallpox as early as 1803, just seven years after Edward Jenner published his groundbreaking work in England.[4]

Though less famous than the Hertzbergs of Hardanger, a host of other clergymen around Norway similarly stepped in to fill the void in health care. As formal medical education gradually became more available and, then, re-quired of ministers, some young pastors studied theology and medicine at the university. Many joined physicians in hailing the 1794 quack law, which banned individuals without formal training from practicing healing, medi-cine's first official step toward professionalism.

But the quack law was far more often broken than observed. Avoiding doctors because of distance, expense, and inadequate results, the almue more-over held the conviction that disease was something ordained by God. They saw illness as "divine retribution for their sins," complained Dr. Alexander Møller (1762–1847) in an 1803 Norwegian chancellory report, and incurable "without their own and the minister's prayers and supplication."[5]

These beliefs clearly gave ministers the advantage over doctors among the almue, who also found ministers to be more approachable. When the syphilis-like disease known as *radesyken* raged in Setesdal, for example, afflicted parishioners rebuffed the aid of the district doctor and openly confessed their affliction to Pastor C. T. Aamodt (1770–1836). Aamodt subsequently traveled to nearby Kristiansand, visited a doctor for training and medicines, and then returned home to treat his parishioners.[6]

The greater confidence enjoyed by the clergy also enabled them to act as vaccinators during the early nineteenth-century smallpox epidemic. Authorities granted ministers official dispensation from the *kvaksalverlov*, Hertzberg said, because "doctors would not as soon have gotten popular opinion on their side as ministers—even though this was a disease everyone was deathly afraid of."

So it was that nineteenth-century Norwegians in need of medical care consulted folk healers, for their supposed witchcraft, and ministers, for their close contact with God, whom they saw as the ultimate arbiter of health. Not surprisingly, emigrants carried this magical-religious view of medicine from Norway to America.

The pastor as doctor on the American prairie

Along with their concept of illness, many Norwegian immigrants brought the expectation that their minister would be involved in their health care. "Everybody around here turns to us when something is the matter," wrote Caja Munch, wife of pioneer pastor Johan Storm Munch, from their Wiota, Wisconsin, parsonage on August 12, 1857. To Caja, as to other new pastors' wives, this came as a surprise.[7]

Pastor's wife Oline Muus had, by contrast, prepared for this role and arrived in the New Land equipped to fill it. Married to pastor Bernt Julius Muus (born 1832), who emigrated in 1859 and is best known for founding St. Olaf College in Northfield, Minnesota, Oline had outfitted herself with a portable medicine chest and medical instruments in Norway. She had also learned from her brother-in-law, a professional doctor, how to do bloodletting and assist in medical emergencies. Her letters mention that she was treating a young man at the parsonage. Out in the community, too, Oline became an active health care provider who even received payment for her services.[8]

As in Norway, the pastors themselves often provided medical care. "We never had a doctor and no medicines," wrote a member of Iowa's St. Ansgar settlement, founded in 1853 by Pastor Claus L. Clausen (1820–92), "but Rev. Clausen helped those who were sick as far as he was able." When smallpox threatened Dakota Territory in the 1880s, Pastor R. O. Brandt "had a talk with the doctor at Estelline and brought back a supply of vaccine points," said his wife. "Many people, both old and young, came to the parsonage for free vaccination."[9] As in Norway, authorities in the New Land relied on the strong bond of trust between clerics and their communities.

While Oline Muus, Claus Clausen, and R. O. Brandt expected parishioners to come to them for care, Elisabeth Koren initially found this new role overwhelming. Born in the town of Larvik by the Oslo Fjord, Elisabeth, age twenty-one, married Vilhelm Koren in 1853, shortly before he accepted a call to minister to congregations in northeast Iowa. When the couple arrived in Iowa on Christmas Eve that year, Elisabeth was unseasoned as a pastor's wife and unacquainted with the customs of the rural peasantry.

One of the first parishioners to call upon Elisabeth in her new surroundings astonished her by expecting medical assistance. The visitor, Mrs. Dysja, belonged to the newly organized Little Iowa congregation (now Washington Prairie, near Decorah) that Vilhelm had been called to serve. She came to get Elisabeth's help in treating her father-in-law's chronic eye and facial pain. Flustered, Elisabeth asked if "there were not some other people, older, more experienced who might be consulted?" "It would hardly be of any use to go to others," retorted the parishioner, "if you did not know what to do." To her diary Elisabeth confided on January 25, 1854, that Mrs. Dysja "could hardly have turned to anyone more inexperienced in such matters."[10]

Moreover, the Korens had their own troubles, having arrived in northeastern Iowa to find no parsonage ready for them. They spent much of their first year sharing quarters with other immigrant families, often feeling out of place and sorely missing their privacy. They also missed their belongings, having left their heaviest trunks filled with their beloved books in Wisconsin.[11]

Among these treasured volumes, Mangor's *Lande-apothek*, written to assist with medical matters in the absence of a doctor, no doubt occupied a

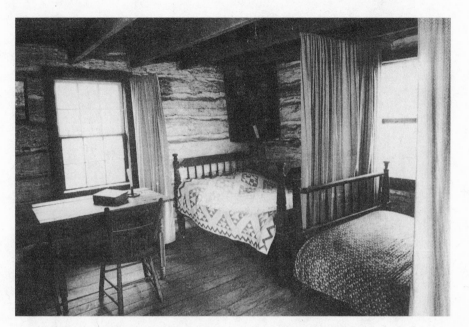

Elisabeth and Vilhelm Koren shared this cabin with the Egge family in 1853–54, when parishioners began coming to Elisabeth for medical advice. The cabin is now part of Vesterheim Museum.

prominent place and is surely the "medical book" Elisabeth refers to in her diary. Lacking access to this volume must have made it hard for the Korens to provide the medical assistance expected of them.[12] Not until the young couple moved to the farm of Erik and Guri Skaarlia on May 2, 1854, could they finally unpack. Gone were the days of sharing the small cabin of the Erik Egge family, as they had from December 24, 1853, until March 10, 1854, and past now, too, were the seven weeks they had lived with Embret and Eli Sørland. On the Skaarlia farm, living in a small, unoccupied house recently built by the Skaarlias, the Korens would at last have some privacy. Elisabeth could arrange her belongings that had arrived in trunks from Dodgeville.

With Mangor's doctor book at hand, the Korens could more readily assist the parishioners who continued to seek their medical advice. "People come and ask for help," wrote Elisabeth on June 16, 1854, noting that these requests sent her "searching through my medical book." Although Elisabeth termed Vilhelm and herself "only indifferent [medical] counselors," her diary belies that characterization, for it records treatments that were appropriate to her time and usually effective. "Yesterday Iver Kvale was here for advice and medicine for his child," reported the June 16, 1854, entry. "That medicine [probably multipurpose tartar emetic, frequently recommended in Mangor's book] came in handy indeed, and I wish we had much more of it."[13]

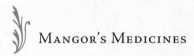

MANGOR'S MEDICINES

Mangor's recommended medicines offer a vivid insight into nineteenth-century conditions. The often selected tartar emetic caused patients to vomit before emptying their bowels. Made of antimony and potassium tartrate (cream of tartar), it also stimulated urination and induced profuse sweating, thereby conveniently delivering all four of the time's most trusted treatments.

Spanish fly plaster, Mangor's favored blistering agent, was a soft, dark-green substance consisting of ten parts yellow beeswax or tallow, three parts turpentine, six parts freshly pulverized Spanish flies, and three parts olive oil. Glittering with green iridescent beetle bodies, the plaster's irritating chemicals would "draw the infection of the illness out of the body and through the skin," said Mangor, "and thereby save the patient's life."

Lead water was "a wonderful remedy for almost all external injuries such as red eyes, for deafness and ringing in the ears, swollen glands, and as a gargle for throat conditions," said Mangor, "and at the same time is the easiest medicament to make and which no household should be without." He advised that it be made by dissolving in a whole bottle of water just one teaspoon of lead subacetate and two teaspoons of French cognac.

Mangor's Lande-apothek ✎

Recording the full range of the couple's experiences, Elisabeth's diary also traces her gradual growth as a self-trained healer. On June 18, 1854, for example, she "got busy at once and made a plaster to send to Sørland's," after learning that Eli Sørland's husband had cut his hand. A week later she made a plaster of the highly irritating Spanish fly to treat John Dysja's seventy-year-old father. Spanish fly relieved pain by establishing a counterirritation that distracted the patient's attention from the initial ailment. In her diary on Monday, June 26, 1854, she wrote: "The one-eyed man from Dysja's was here this forenoon and asked whether 'the mother' could advise him what to do for the neuralgia in his head. Well, 'the mother' looked in her book and then put a Spanish fly plaster on him, and gave him a rag with salve on it for the sore, and explained how he should take care of himself. The old man seemed to have great faith in my skill in the art of medicine and left with many expressions of thanks." (Dysja referred to Elisabeth as "the mother" in deference to her status as the pastor's wife or, perhaps, since Elisabeth seems to find it comical, he was using the title customarily applied to talented folk healers like Mor Sæther.)

Following Mangor's recommendations, Elisabeth would have left the Spanish fly plaster in place from six to twelve hours to ease Dysja's pain before she cut the resulting blister. Her salve-coated cloth was probably to soothe the resulting sore and, if based on Mangor's book, would have been made of tallow or basil, to keep the sore open and draining, or wax, to close the wound.

Two later diary entries show Elisabeth, with increasing dispatch, dispensing both the familiar tartar emetic and a popular patent medicine known as Hoffmann's drops: "Wednesday, July 5, 1854: I had a visit from Ole [Bergan, a local farmer] who asked my help for his sick child and took an emetic powder back with him," and "Friday, July 7, 1854: After breakfast a messenger came from Ole Bergan to get help for their child and later one from Suckow's asking for some Hoffmann's drops. I am glad I could help them." The *Hoffmannsdraaber* requested by Lars Johan Suckow, the local shoemaker, consisted of one part ether and three parts alcohol. "Everyone ought to keep Hofmanns drops on hand," advised the 1883 domestic medical manual *Huslægen* (The house doctor), published in La Crosse, that recommended the aromatic and stimulating drops to treat "fainting, nervousness, convulsions, nausea and indigestion." The 1879 *Lægebog for hvermand* (Doctor book for everyone), published in Chicago, observed that they "come in especially handy for colds." It further advised that a dose of fifteen to thirty drops be taken in water or dribbled on sugar and added that "if the patient can't swallow, the drops may be smelled or rubbed into the temple."[14]

Busy at home with her healing work, Elisabeth Koren kept an eye out for Vilhelm to return from his seemingly ceaseless ministering to the settlers in his enormous parish. On the days he was expected to return, she would go out to the road to meet him, knitting as she walked. That was her plan on Monday, July 10, until her doctoring took precedence. "Wednesday, July 12, 1854: Late Monday afternoon I was on the lookout, and was just thinking of taking my knitting and going for a walk, when a woman came to ask advice for her husband, who had an inflammation of the eye; so for one day the medicine books took the place of the walk. They were consulted a good deal while Vilhelm was away. While I stood mixing a blister plaster for her, Caroline [Linnevold, a neighbor's teenager and the Korens' hired helper] ran up and said the pastor was coming."[15]

The entry suggests that Elisabeth did considerably more medical consulting than her diary details and, further, that eye ailments were common complaints. By now Elisabeth must have known Mangor's instructions by heart: "If the eyes are running constantly and you cannot get advice from a doctor, try tartar emetic and apply a Spanish fly plaster on the back of the neck. You ought to bathe the eyes frequently with soothing eye wash of lead acetate as well." Unaware of the potential for lead poisoning, Mangor and his contemporaries routinely recommended "lead water" to soothe sore eyes and all other manner of wounds, bruises, and irritations to the skin. The striking number of eye ailments Elisabeth treated conforms to the 1879 *Report of Disease in Minnesota and the Northwest* that lists "opthamalia" among the most commonly occurring disorders. Unhygienic conditions in the settlers' cramped, smoky cabins certainly contributed to this statistic.[16]

That the parishioners so often sought Mrs. Koren's help for their eye ailments suggests they regarded her as a specialist. Wives and mothers took care of routine health needs, but for more serious afflictions and sophisticated treatments, families consulted healers with known expertise and proven ability to interpret the doctor books. Elisabeth had shown facility with such sophisticated remedies as tartar emetic, Spanish fly plaster, and lead acetate, and her diary entry for August 3, 1854, a day she treated another eye ailment, shows that the couple's reputation as healers was on the rise: "Going home I met the man [Dysja] I had given medicine for his eye; he was also coming to thank me and to get help for his daughter, who also was having trouble with her eyes. To judge by what he said, people believe we are skilled in medical matters; he also said he had heard that the pastor had been trained as a medical doctor."[17]

Having known ministers with medical training in Norway, the parishioners probably assumed that Koren had this background, too. Their assumption also confirms that the Korens were living up to expectations. Care of the parishioners' physical, as well as spiritual, needs remained as essential to the pioneers on the prairie as it was to the almue of rural Norway.

The black-book minister

As seen by parishioners, nineteenth-century pastors possessed exceptional skill with words, intimate knowledge of sacred objects and spaces, and unquestioned authority. These attributes seemed to endow some ministers with supernatural powers, as expressed in the ubiquitous legends of the "black-book minister" (*svarteboksprest*). Said to "know more than the Lord's Prayer," the legendary black-book minister was believed to have gained his skills at Wittenberg, where in 1517 Martin Luther had posted his theses about reforming the Catholic Church.

The legends evidently arose in the wake of the Lutheran Reformation, which emphasized the authority of the Bible and of books in general. Lutheran ministers, adhering to a section of Christian V's 1687 Norwegian law that clergymen should "have and use in addition to the Bible other good and useful books," kept substantial libraries. These libraries mightily impressed their parishioners. Among those volumes, many people believed, the pastor surely had the magical, mystical "black book," a compendium of magical formulas, some dating to ancient Egyptian magical papyri (ca. 1500 BC). Actual black-book formulas addressed problems of daily life such as making a soldier bulletproof, protecting livestock from predators, or stopping excessive bleeding from a wound.

Legends of the black-book minister, however, focus on his power over the devil. If a wheel fell off a black-book minister's carriage, for example, he could simply conjure up the devil and force him to carry the cart to the appointed destination. Compelling thieves to return stolen goods was also within the black-book minister's purview, as was exorcising the devil from troubled households and curing diseases.[18]

While mere mortals could obtain the black book only at the cost of their souls, black-book ministers used it with impunity. This folk belief probably reflected the reality that pastors usually avoided the lawsuits that plagued other self-trained healers. "I marvel that I never was arrested and sent to jail for *kvaksalveri*," observed Hardanger minister Niels Hertzberg (1759–1841), "for all the years I impersonated a doctor."[19]

The notion of the black book itself seems to have been revived by the sixteenth- and seventeenth-century witch trials, which overwhelmingly targeted self-trained healers whose cures had gone wrong. While so-called "witches" were presumed to perform black magic in service to the devil and,

Beret Hagebak outside her sod house in western Minnesota. Rugged homesteads in the New Land reinforced the Old Country tradition of relying on minister and neighbors for medical care. (*Photo by Hugh J. Chalmers*)

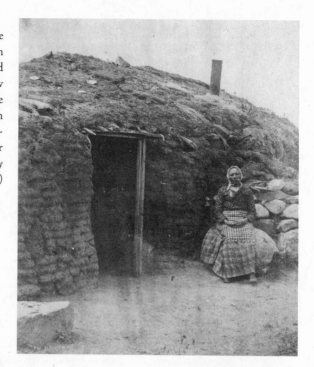

accordingly, were made to suffer by being burned at the stake, ministers escaped this fate, being presumed to perform "white magic" empowered by the word of God.[20]

Social clout probably accounts for the minister's privileged treatment, but legend had its own explanation, told in this version from south Norway about Søren Schive, who served as the pastor of Bjelland from 1670 to 1705: "At Wittenberg the Black Arts were studied with the rule that one of the students would subsequently belong to the devil. Lots were drawn to decide who that would be, and it fell to Sir Søren. One day as he was out walking in the sunshine the Evil One came to take him. 'Take the one standing behind me,' said Sir Søren, and the devil was tricked into taking Søren's shadow instead."[21]

Germany's Wittenberg University probably figures prominently in legends of the black-book minister because of the 1627 church ordinance that required prospective ministers to have a university degree before they could be ordained. Such an education, available only to the privileged class, had to be pursued abroad because Norway had no university before 1811. This created a chasm between the clergy and the almue they served. With vastly superior schooling and a continental lifestyle, the minister was sufficiently clever, the legend suggests, to rob even the devil of his due.

Pastor Schive, a renaissance man, engaged actively in the timber trade in addition to his clerical duties, and another legend claims he used magic to clear a logjam. Schive trapped the devil in his snuff box and threw it into the river, where the devil's pent-up fury exploded and released the jammed logs. In yet another account, Schive hosted a dinner party for some of his upper-class cohorts, who habitually mocked his leather lumbering britches. After his guests dined heartily and robustly complimented the fare, Pastor Schive quietly informed them that they had eaten the controversial trousers.

One Valdres pastor believed to possess the black book was Hermann Ruge, who served the Slidre parish from 1737 to 1763. He had received some medical training and cared for the sick in his home, which according to his supervisor, Prosten Dorph, "resembled more a hospital than a parsonage." Though "many were cured there by his doctoring," Dorph observed, "they believed less in his medicine and doctoring skills than they 'knew' that he had studied at Wittenberg and used the black book." Ruge could "make the devil dance, if he wanted," parishioners insisted, firmly believing that "it was this supernatural help that enabled him to heal."[22]

While the claim of "having the black book" had tainted self-trained care-givers such as Anne Brandfjeld and Olava Wick with the aura of witchcraft, it seems to have left the black-book minister unscathed. In fact, parishioners usually attributed the status of being a black-book minister to the most out-standing clergy. Ruge, as described by Dorph, certainly qualified, being "exceptionally learned" and "one of the most exceptional ministers who ever served Slidre and perhaps the most knowledgeable of his time." Similar superlatives were applied to Petter Dass (1647–1707), the renowned pastor at Alstahaug parish and probably the most famous black-book minister of them all.

 ## "WHEN PETTER DASS PREACHED IN COPENHAGEN"

In Kabelvåg, North Norway, people told this story of Petter Dass, who possessed the black book and used it decisively.

> Once, the devil himself arrived with a summons from
> the king in Copenhagen ordering Dass to preach at the
> palace church the very next day, which happened to be

Christmas. Seeing his cloven hoof, Dass realized who stood before him. "Yes, I'll go," he replied, "but you will provide the transportation." Now with black book in hand, Dass transformed the Evil One into a horse, and, climbing on its back, took off like the wind.

Dass preached in Copenhagen, all right. He delivered a sermon such as no mortal has heard before or since, even though the big shots down there had placed some blank sheets of paper on the pulpit instead of the finished sermon they had promised. They had wanted to make a fool of a "poor country pastor from Ultima Thule." Dass rode the same horse home and preached in Alstahaug church on Second Christmas Day (December 26), and these trips gave rise to the expression *"Petter Dass skys"* (Petter-Dass ride) to describe a journey that proceeds at breakneck speed and at the risk of one's life.[23]

Stories of black-book ministers that flourished in seventeenth- and eighteenth-century Norway lingered on in the nineteenth century. "My father's parishioners were totally convinced that he had *svarteboka*," said Kirsti Magelssen, the daughter of Nils Stockfleth Magelssen, whose nine-year ministry in Gildeskål ended in 1906.[24]

Given the vital role Norwegian American pastors played in dispensing medical care on the prairie, it might be expected that parishioners would continue believing that certain ministers possessed the black book. Several folk-healer immigrants, notably Hans Haaga in Coon Prairie, Wisconsin, and Peder Enger in Spring Grove, Minnesota, were said to use the magical tome. Yet no accounts associate the black book with Norwegian American ministers.[25]

The belief in magic began to fall away in the Old Country at century's end in the face of education, industrialization, and science, and magical thinking receded even earlier among immigrants to the New Land. Yet while stories of the black book survived in the New Land, those of the black-book minister did not. Norwegian American parishioners apparently no longer found the black-book minister legends relevant.

If this lore arose from the difference in life experience that separated the almue from the kondisjonerte pastor and if the belief expressed the ambivalence people felt toward him, its absence on the prairie suggests a less ambivalent relationship between the congregation and their pastor. An 1878 letter from a Norwegian immigrant living in Wisconsin supports this theory. Detailing the new and, in his eyes, "more desirable" relationship between pastors and their congregations in the New Land, the letter writer forthrightly observed: "One does not fear the pastor other than as a messenger pointing to the Lamb of God who bears the sins of the world. He is not an aristocrat. One dares to speak to him and ask him about everything. There can be no doubt that the pastors are in a better position to counsel people here than in the Norwegian state church."[26] The greater openness between minister and parishioner would make meaningless the intimidating figure of the pastor seen in legends of the black-book minister. The shared challenges of prairie life must have done much to remove the distance between the pioneer pastor and his immigrant congregation.

Still, many similarities remained between Old Country and New Land pastors, not least being the willingness to address the parishioners' ills, even when doctors were readily available. Rev. N. E. Bøe (1846–1925) continued this part of his calling, and his parishioners usually consulted him first before going to the doctor. "He delighted in reading doctor books and was well supplied with them," wrote his daughter, adding that he regularly treated his patients with "Fluss plaster [a treatment for blood poisoning], quinine and liniment," all purchased in the local drugstore. "Whether it was faith or the medicine itself is hard to say," she concluded, "but it was really remarkable how many cases he helped."[27]

More likely the faith than the medicine, trust was the basis of the Norwegian and Norwegian American clergy's medical activity. Doctors in mid-nineteenth-century America certainly had better repute than their counterparts in Norway. "Perhaps no profession, art, or even trade," John Mitchell, president of the Wisconsin Medical Society, could remark at the 1856 annual meeting, "is looked upon with as much distrust as that of medicine."[28]

Even after professional medical care began to improve, the Norwegian immigrants' faith often stayed with the minister. The 1882 annual report of the Wisconsin State Board of Health actually singled out Norwegians as being "next to impossible to treat" because they listened "too extensively to the preachers' rather than the doctors' directions."[29]

Parishioners' reliance on pastors in matters of health could even outweigh the divisive doctrinal disputes that otherwise destroyed the unity of the Norwegian immigrant church. "Even those who were actively opposed to the Synod and regarded [Rev. J. M.] Dahl as a blind guide in spiritual affairs," wrote Laurence Larson in his *Log Book of a Young Immigrant,* "sought his parsonage in quest of healing or sent for him to visit their sick relatives." Although Dahl had training in the rudiments of domestic medicine, it was rather his cheerfulness and the way his broad countenance radiated hope and assurance, Larson suggested, that won him adherents. "He understood his people, he could look into their troubles, he could explore their imaginations."[30] Clearly, some pioneer pastors, though no longer assisted by the magical black book, ably used their understanding of human nature and their willingness to serve wherever and however they were needed to provide "more than the Lord's Prayer" in the New Land.

·4

The Black Book

Magical, mystical medicine

> "Who as a child did not hear about the black book and then quake in terror at the 'true' reports of this book's magical, mystical powers?"
>
> *Skilling Magazin, 1859*

*F*OR NINETEENTH-CENTURY NORWEGIANS, the simple name "black book" raised goose bumps and conjured up thoughts of the devil. Stories about the black book accompanied Norwegian emigrants to America, where, according to Carl Roan (born 1878), they might even talk about the book at social events such as a quilting bee. In his memoir of life in Glencoe, Minnesota, during the 1880s, Roan wrote that after women spent the day piecing together a decorative coverlet, they would make dinner, and, as "the men visited with each other while eating supper and looking over the women's handiwork, they would talk, among other things, about the *svartebok*, a volume purporting to reveal various tricks accredited to the devil."[1]

The terror that once surrounded the black book had faded by Roan's time, and the magical tome had come to seem more legendary than real. "Very few *if any* have ever seen it," wrote Roan, whose cavalier tone sharply contrasts with that of Carl Nyerup, a Dane who wrote in 1816 about the *Cyprianus*, as the black book was also known. The name Cyprianus referred to the church patriarch Thascius Caecilius, Bishop of Antioch in the third century, who inexplicably became the subject of medieval stories alleging that he attended a school of black arts and wrote the original black book. According to an early nineteenth-century history, the book was the "horrifying, nefarious tome known by everyone in the countryside as Cyprianus, whereby one can conjure up and put down the devil and get him to do just as one commands, and whose pages teach how to recover lost goods, cure all kinds of disease, remove curses, find buried treasure, turn back the attacks of snakes and dogs, and more."[2]

While some associated the black book with Cyprianus, others believed it to be "the sixth and seventh Book of Moses that had been left out of the Bible by the learned, so that simple folk shall not get to know the things written there." (Norwegians know the first five books of the Bible as the Books of Moses.) While the Bible never had a sixth or seventh Book of Moses, the allusion to the black book as something people have lost suggests a link to the Catholic healing prayers that constituted an integral part of church ritual before they were rejected by Lutheran doctrine. "Luther didn't translate the 6th Book of Moses because it dealt with magic," held a tradition from Nordmøre. "The Catholic Bible had a Sixth and Seventh Book of Moses, and those who went to the Wittenberg School [Martin Luther's university] have certainly read them; these books comprise the black book," held a corresponding tradition from Valdres.[3]

Once a constant kindler of conversation and controversy, the black book accompanied emigrants to America only to retreat into oblivion after the 1920s. But while few Norwegian Americans today have heard of it, awareness lives on in Norway. "I have wondered where people get hold of the black book," said a man from Fjærland in Sogn (born 1914) during an interview in 1996. "I've thought about that often." But many Norwegians doubt such a book ever existed in reality. "I've heard about the black book," said another informant (born 1920 in Fjærland), "but I have never seen one and don't think there was such a book."[4]

No single black book did exist—hundreds of them did. Most were handwritten compilations of advice and magical cures, items people copied down as they came across them by word of mouth or in written form. About 150 individual black books, mostly compiled between the late 1700s and early 1800s, are known today. Museums, archives, and libraries own some; private collectors have others; and new ones still occasionally come to light, such as the two black books that recently surfaced in a dusty attic near Elverum, some seventy-five miles northeast of Oslo.[5]

Mary Rustad (born 1952 in Minneapolis) found them one rainy day in 1994 at Nord Rustad, the farm left by her great-grandfather in 1879 when he emigrated to America. Mary came to Nord Rustad as a new bride in 1977 at age twenty-five, having married her third cousin, Nils. "One year after I was married," she wrote, "my husband and I found a black book in the storage room of the old barn. Nils noticed it had something to do with black magic and quickly put it away. 'We won't look at that now,' he said. I was pregnant with our first child and the black book would bring bad luck." Years later, Mary finally looked again for the book among things that had been moved to the attic.[6]

The attic was humid from rain. Mary found a child's stool and sat down under one of the eves, her head just below the ceiling. The first box she looked through contained discarded shaving equipment and a few old books. She picked up one that had thick, yellowed pages sewn together by hand. "*En Liden Kunstbog*" (A little book of skills), someone had written on the first page, though Mary could not decipher the gothic handwriting just then. On the second page, however, she made out the name "Cyprianus," and on a later page, the even more demonic "Belsebub." The second tome, hardbound in an aged cover, seemed to be blank until Mary noticed that the edges of the middle section of pages were soiled from use. Opening to them, she found the same type of handwriting as in the first book. The volume consisted of seventy-eight incantations; the first volume had thirty-four.

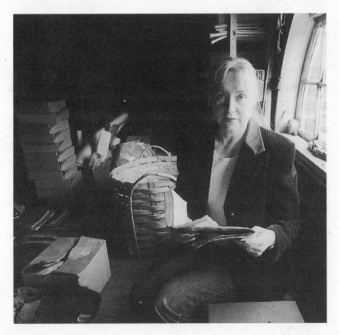

Mary Rustad holding two black books of magical incantations discovered in a farm attic near Elverum, Norway

FORMULAS FROM THE RUSTAD BLACK BOOKS

To heal an eye infection:
"Jesus and St. Peter were walking down a road and met a blind man.
The man said, 'Heal my eyes as you healed your good mother's eyes.
In the name of the Holy Trinity.'" Then say the Lord's Prayer.

For a toothache:
Write these words on a piece of paper. Then cut it into three pieces.
Have the patient place the first piece on the bad tooth in the evening
and in the morning quietly spit the paper on the fire. Do the same
morning and night with the other pieces. The words are these:
"Agerin, Nagerin, Vagerin, Jagerin, Ipagerin, Sipia." You should write
these words with a new pen.

For a woman having a difficult labor, so that the baby will be born quickly:
Take two pieces of a white lily root. Give it to the woman to eat.
Soon the baby will come and then the afterbirth. The woman will be
unharmed.

Or:
Take two eggs, let them cook to the consistency of hard-boiled eggs.
Have the woman, on an empty stomach, take a couple of good-sized
spoonfuls of the water that the eggs were cooked in. The birth will
then soon commence. This has been used with very good results and
is harmless to the woman.

To cure a fever that begins with chills:
Write this on a piece of bread and give it to the patient for eight
days, one piece each day, and on the ninth day, burn the last piece,
which is C x: Colameris x, Colameri x, Colamer x, Colame x, Colam x,
Cola x, Col x, Co x, C x. After doing this, the fever will be gone.

For airborne pestilence:
"Our Lord Jesus and St. Peter and St. Andrew walked with the
other disciples along a river. Up from the water like a fish came a
terrible being that tried to devour them. Jesus grabbed it by the tail,

asking 'Where are you going?' The evil spirit answered, 'I am going to the farm of N.N. (insert the appropriate person's name) to harm the horses, swine, goats, and sheep. Their bones to break, flesh to eat, and blood to drink.' 'No! You will not!' said Jesus. 'You shall return to those who have released you, down into the river again, and to its greatest depth. In the name of the Three.'" Then recite the Lord's Prayer three times.

So that lice shall not thrive on you:
Take a human bone from a graveyard and sew it into your clothes, but do not take the bone on Tycho Brahe days [unlucky or dangerous days named by the Danish astronomer Tycho Brahe (1546–1601)].

When your churning won't make butter:
Throw a piece of silver into the churn, even if it's only a silver two-shilling.

"Now two wasps started buzzing around my head," Mary recalls. "Oh, wow, I thought, this is a sign that I'm looking at or doing something that I shouldn't. My heart was in my throat and I felt sick to my stomach." Then she realized she was only imagining things; the wasps were just irritated because of the humidity. "I killed the wasps and went down stairs to tell my husband what I had found."

Uneasy about their discovery, the Rustads took the books to Per Sande at the public archives in Hamar. They also consulted a local black-book expert, Ottar Evensen, who readily understood their apprehension and said: "I know one owner of such a book who dares not sleep in the room where it is kept."[7] Mary admitted that after finding the books, she started thinking of people being "punished for possessing the black book, even burned at the stake." In fact, one of her husband's ancestors, Ingeborg Økset, had been convicted of witchcraft in 1625 and executed in just that way.

Norwegian witch trials

Ingeborg Økset was one of 1,750 Norwegians accused of witchcraft between 1550 and 1700. About one-fifth of the accused were executed, according to the Norwegian witch-trial scholar Hans Eyvind Næss. In most cases their crimes consisted of nothing more than using magical healing incantations of the sort contained in black books.[8]

Witch-trial transcripts provided many of the black-book formulas now known, such as the one used by accused witch Lisbet Nypan. At her hearing on May 30, 1670, Nypan freely admitted using this incantation to treat her neighbors for *grep* (arthritis or rheumatism), a common ailment of her time: "As Christ walked to church with book in hand, the Virgin Mary appeared and inquired about his health. 'I am seriously afflicted with rheumatism, my blessed mother.' To this she replied, 'Incantations against rheumatism I will read for you: from joints and bone, to shore and stone, in the name of God the Father, Son and Holy Spirit.'"[9]

The formula portrays Christ afflicted with the same condition the healer seeks to remedy, and many Norwegian black-book formulas consist of comparable stories featuring sacred personages curing disease by magical means. Like them, Nypan's words appeal to the Virgin Mary to repeat on the patient the miracle that Mary used to cure Christ.

Nypan's formula employs "transference," magic that removes the disease from the patient's body ("from joints and bone") and transplants it to another location ("to shore and stone"). Like Nypan's incantation, black-book formulas often conclude by quoting the Catholic mass, sometimes including fragments of the Latin: *In nomine patris et filie et spiritus sancti.* Although Danish king Christian III converted Norway to Lutheranism by royal fiat in 1537 and Catholicism was officially banned until 1842, remnants of Catholicism persisted for a long time among the almue.

Black-book formulas were often accompanied by rituals. Lisbet Nypan testified that she "read her formula over salt," which she smoothed onto the painful areas of the patient's body. The warmth and massaging action of her hands probably provided some measure of genuine relief. Between each reading of the formula, Nypan recited the Lord's Prayer. She repeated the entire ritual a total of three times. While the ritual was meant to intensify the effect of the material remedy (in this case, salt), it also worked to intensify the patient's faith in the remedy. "The belief in a thing's healing power often works better than the best apothecary medicine," one nineteenth-century folk healer observed.[10]

On the day Nypan confessed and made public her formula, the authorities said little, but when her trial continued on August 10, they asked if she was "knowingly serving Satan with these disgusting, illicit prayers." Nypan denied serving Satan in any way. How could these formulas possibly be viewed as such, she asked, "since they were, after all, the word of God."[11] The authorities saw things differently. Condemning Lisbet Nypan to be burned at the stake, they carried out their judgment on September 5, 1670.

From a modern perspective it is difficult to imagine what had brought Lisbet Nypan to trial. Historian Hans Næss blames intensely stressful circumstances prevailing in Norway during the sixteenth and seventeenth centuries, when exploding population resulted in too many families living on farms too small to support them. Scarce and dwindling resources pitted neighbor against neighbor. Shortages and starvation raised anxiety, and illness fueled these fears. Unhygienic conditions spread disease of all kinds, and few ailments had an objectively identified cause or cure.[12]

Believing that malevolent spirits or supernatural beings cast infirmities upon them, the almue turned to neighborhood healers, convinced that some had magical means to cure them. But if the cure proved unsuccessful, desperation drove them to accuse the failed healer of witchcraft.

Consider the case of Osmand Gildal, who accused neighbor Inger Roed of witchcraft in 1617. Having suffered several mysterious ailments earlier that year, he had paid Roed, reputed to have powers of supernatural healing, one bushel of grain plus twenty shillings for a cure. When his health did not improve and Roed could not return his payment, Gildal reported her to the authorities. Significantly, Gildal's accusation of witchcraft made no mention of a pact with the devil. Nor did Roed acknowledge any such pact, though she willingly admitted that she could lese (recite magical incantations) for a variety of illnesses.

Supernatural healing of the sort practiced by Inger Roed and Lisbet Nypan, known as signeri, played a role in the vast majority of Norway's 263 documented witch trials. In trial after trial, accused "witches" came forward and freely testified about their healing methods, telling about the salves they made and the bønner (prayers) they read over them to enhance their potency. These individuals must have thought they had nothing to fear, for the Church taught that prayer promoted healing.

Like many sixteenth- and seventeenth-century healers, Roed and Nypan apparently failed to realize the danger of their actions. How could they have foreseen that witchcraft accusations unleashed latent aggressions among neighbors struggling to survive? How could the healers have known that Lutheran clergy who dominated these hearings would regard their work as

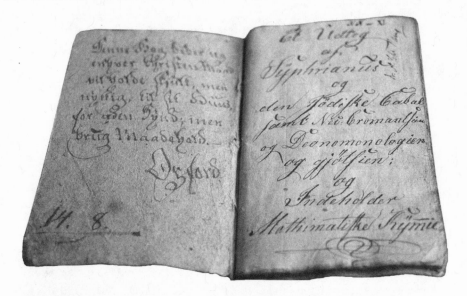

In these pages from a handwritten Syprianus (Cyprianus) or black book, the left-hand page urges the user to employ its power with care.

satanism? How could they know that their ready admissions of using prayers and remedies traditionally viewed as *trolldom* (magic or witchcraft) would backfire in the atmosphere of church reforms? "Thou shalt not allow a witch to live," commanded Exodus 22:18. This biblical injunction assumed fatal dimensions in the context of a Lutheranism that interpreted the Scriptures literally and viewed Catholic elements of healers' prayers as heresy.

The black book and the clergy

The healing formulas used by the unfortunate Roed and Nypan made no mention of conjuring up the devil or of selling one's soul. Formulas of a more demonic nature do appear in Norway's classic collection, *Hexeformularer og magiske Opskrifter* (Witch formulas and magical incantations), published in 1901–02 by Bishop Anton Christian Bang, but these examples come from German and Latin sources.

Ironically, it was probably Lutheran clergy themselves who imported this type of formula to Norway, along with the diabolic view of healing formulas in general. The Church Ordinance of 1627, which made a university degree prerequisite to a Lutheran minister's ordination, resulted in prospective

Norwegian clergymen being sent to study in Denmark's Copenhagen or in Rostock, or at Luther's own university in Wittenberg, Germany. (Catholic priests, by contrast, were trained by apprenticing to an older priest in their own parish.) While abroad, prospective Lutheran pastors could hardly have avoided the talk of devil conjuring that was popular among the European elite. Books like the *Malleus Maleficarum* (The hammer of witches) specified lawful procedures to torture and kill suspected witches, and interest in witchcraft permeated the literary world, as well. The familiar German legend of a sorcerer who sold his soul to Mestopheles in return for supernatural power was widely circulated in 1587. Translated into English in 1592 as *The Damnable Life and Deserved Death of Doctor John Faustus*, it provided the core of the wildly popular play, *Dr. Faustus*, written shortly afterward by the renowned Christopher Marlowe.

While the "diabolism" (appealing to the devil for power) that infused these works was foreign to the Norwegian healers' formulas, Lutheran clergy came to see all healing formulas as diabolism, and it was probably on this basis that they condemned the healers to horrible deaths. Though the folk healers' formulas appealed for power not from the devil but from the Christian trinity, Lutheran doctrine rejected such direct supplication to God and repudiated the notion that man-made rituals could influence God. Instead, Lutheranism emphasized the far more abstract concept that individuals received grace by their faith alone.

The Norwegian almue had little concept of such intellectual refinements. Without access to academic education, they relied on traditional beliefs and ancestral ways. "With regard to medicine," observed one contemporary, "they have the same prejudice as in other matters, namely that their forefathers knew best."[13] Moreover, given the dearth of doctors and medicines, most people had no alternative other than to cling to healing prayers and past practices. If the church had formerly promoted such rituals, how could they become evil?

Lutheran clergy, however, argued that attempting to alter God's divine providence was evil, that healers' formulas desecrated the sacred Word of the scripture and defied the second commandment's injunction against taking the name of the Lord in vain. Blinded to the almue's sincere Christian piety and intent on establishing the legitimacy of the new worship, clergy insisted that the accused folk healers used Catholic ritual merely as "powerful words intended to multiply the healing strength of their formulas."[14]

Two hundred years after the last witch was burned, Norway's Bishop Bang still agreed with the clergy who conducted the witch trials. "In the formulas," he asserted in 1885, "we see the darkest regions of the spiritual life of our people." Bang's words carried the weight of authority in Norway, for besides being a Lutheran bishop, he had collected and studied the black-book formulas as no one else had done. While Bang suggested that authorities had "over-reacted" when they executed innocent people, he found their actions "entirely justified" because of "the evil nature of the black-book formulas they had employed."[15]

In his strong condemnation of healing formulas, Bang shared the view held by many nineteenth-century clergy. Proud products of a privileged social background, these ministers had so little in common with their parishioners that they regarded them "less as faithful Christians than as exotic workers of magic," to quote the Norwegian theologian and folklorist Arne Bugge Amundsen.[16]

On September 6, 1825, for example, the otherwise compassionate Telemark pastor M. B. Landstad, compiler of a still-used Lutheran hymnal, entered in his diary some "amusing evidence of the local peasants' enormous superstition." He wrote: "A woman came here recently with an extremely ill child, believing a magic experiment conducted in the church could heal him. Three men brought the child into the church at midnight. Without uttering a single word to disturb the sacred silence, they wound the altar cloth around the child three times, then placed the child in the pulpit and left the church."[17] This ritual that Landstad regarded as an entertaining "experiment" was to the woman a desperate attempt to save her child's life based on her sincere faith in the healing power of holy places and objects. A similar combination of desperation and faith drew the Norwegian almue to sacred springs and to lovekirker (devotional or "promise" churches) throughout the 1800s, three hundred years after the Reformation had banned such pilgrimages. Clearly, Catholic customs lived on in Lutheran Norway.

Continuing Catholic customs

"There was healing water in Olavsgryta [St. Olav well] at Letnesholmen," said Andreas Ystad (born 1879), "and down through the ages many from Inderøy fetched water there for those who were sick, a practice that has continued until recent times." Sacred springs can still be found in all parts of Norway. ,

Many, like the one at Inderøy, were dedicated to Norway's patron saint, Olav, though the veneration of springs predated Christianity. The Vikings had attributed the springs' healing powers to Odin, Thor, Frey, and other gods.[18]

Olav Haraldsson (King Olav II, later St. Olav) died in 1030 at the battle of Stiklestad, and Norway's fledgling Catholic church subsequently portrayed the Viking warrior as a Christian martyr who died for his faith. Historians have argued about Olav Haraldsson's motives ever since, but the vital role his church-created image played in Norway's Christian conversion is beyond dispute. For five hundred years, the shrine of St. Olav in Nidaros (now Trondheim) attracted pilgrims from around the Christian world, putting Norway on the medieval map. Centuries after the Reformation of 1537 officially banned the veneration of saints, popular legends about St. Olav lived on, and many of these involved sacred springs. (Norwegians and foreigners alike have again begun following the recently restored pilgrim routes to Trondheim and visiting the St. Olav springs along the way.)[19]

"That water had healing power," said Ystad of the spring at Inderøy, "because St. Olav rode his horse down into it and washed away the blood from his wounds." Even better known is the spring near the Vatnås church in the Grenskogen woods between Sigdal and Eggedal. "Local farmers kept bottles of water from the St. Olav spring and used it like any other medicine, rubbing it on for pain and sprains, drinking it for sickness in the body," wrote local historian Andreas Mørch in 1932. He noted that the water was "especially effective in treating skin rashes and sores, as well as lice and itching." Given the low standard of hygiene that characterized many parts of Norway well into the 1900s, the water's simple ability to clean would have proved beneficial.[20]

The nearby Vatnås Church had its own power. Many believed that prayers said there would be answered if accompanied by the promise of a gift to the church. Å love means "to promise," as well as "to praise," and lovekirker received support from gifts given in hope of healing and in thanksgiving for having been healed. During the Middle Ages, pilgrims stopped at these churches on the long, perilous journey to Nidaros. Though pilgrimages to Olav's shrine officially ended with the Reformation of 1537, the almue continued to bring prayers, gifts, and promises to the lovekirker for hundreds of years to come.

Today the best known of the lovekirker is near the remote mountain village of Røldal between Telemark and Hardanger, which had been the site of a secret midnight mass held annually on Midsummer's Eve until 1835. Hundreds came to Røldal expecting to see a miracle and hoping to be healed by the "tears" that on that one night alone came from the church's medieval crucifix. Many of these pilgrims left behind their crutches along with small votive gifts: carvings of arms, legs, and other body parts where their illnesses had dwelled. (Bergen's Historisk Museum has preserved a sampling of these offerings.)

"There are still old inhabitants in Røldal who remember the strange scenes that took place within the little sacred edifice each St. Hans aften (Midsummer Eve), and the collection of crutches and other wooden aids to locomotion laid up in the church rivals the one at Lourdes," wrote British traveler A. F. Mockler-Ferryman in his 1896 Hardanger account some sixty years after clerical authorities had put an end to these masses. "The annual gathering on the outskirts of Røldal must have been a marvelous sight, but until the sun went down no one was permitted to enter the village, and before the sun rose again, the pilgrims had to be gone, leaving only a few short hours for the healing of the sufferers."[21] The cover of darkness and Røldal's remote location apparently helped the pilgrims escape official detection. Though the church now lies beside a highway, in former times visiting was not easy. Pilgrims from Telemark had to traverse the difficult and dangerous Dyrskar Pass before making the precipitous descent to Røldal, while visitors from Hardanger faced an equally perilous route. Yet they came, crawling and limping by the score, driven by faith in the healing power of the crucifix and convinced that the difficulty of reaching such a goal was healing in itself.

Clergymen, meanwhile, had only limited contact with the old church at Røldal. The parish minister lived miles away in Suldal and visited the church only three times each summer. Decades could pass between visits by his supervisor, or prost. Thus it was a rare occasion, the night before July 7, 1835, when Prost Ole Nicolai Loberg (1804–68) and the Suldal pastor wound their way up the rough mountain road. They had chosen this night instead of June 23, the usual date for celebrating St. Hans, because July 7 marked the old midsummer date observed before 1700, when Norwegians had adopted the Gregorian calendar.

Pilgrimages to Røldal predated the calendar change and retained the old date, another factor that helped them avoid detection, though word did occasionally leak out. (When Oslo bishop Niels Glostrup visited Vinje,

Telemark, as early as 1622, he was told by the minister of "great idolatry in Røldal concerning a crucifix that the almue seek when they are ill.") Now the Suldal minister and his prost intended to put a stop to it.[22]

Lodging for the night at the Gryting farm, Prost Loberg was just getting into bed when he heard church bells ring. From his window he could see light streaming from the church. He fetched the minister who was staying at Saltvoll, and the two set out to investigate. What they saw must have astonished them and probably resembled the eyewitness account quoted by Mockler-Ferryman:

> Within the church at midnight all was dark save the confined space of the chancel, where the pilgrims awaited their turn to touch the crucifix, which lighted by six candles stood on the altar. A drop of the holy moisture that, on one night only of the year, issued from the crucifix, was sufficient to cure the most malignant disease. The incurably lame cast aside their crutches and unaided left the church; the blind received their sight; while those affected with grievous sicknesses of every kind and description were immediately cured. Each person as he left the altar made an offering, for which purpose a large iron-bound chest was placed close by, and the sums collected were often considerable.

Was the drop of moisture only condensation of air warmed by the many pilgrims as it contacted the cold wooden cross of the church so high up in the mountains? Whatever the explanation, the mass celebrating the weeping crucifix defied the Reformation for three hundred years.

The mass that attracted pilgrims to the lovekirke at Vatnås was probably less spectacular, but it may have featured equally venerable remnants of Norwegian Catholicism. Local legend associated the church and spring at Vatnås with St. Olav and the Christian conversion, as reported in this version from Andreas Faye's well-known 1844 collection: "When King Olav traveled around Norway to enforce the Christian faith, he also came to Sigdal. After baptizing the inhabitants, he and his retinue went hunting but they lost their way. Exhausted and thirsty, they eventually came to a narrow valley. As the king dismounted, he promised that if he now found water, he would have a church built on the very site."

No sooner had Olav spoken these words than a spring began to flow from the hard rock, the spring whose water local farmers were still using as medicine in the late 1800s. A short walk on the well-worn path behind the church today brings visitors to the rock outcropping that gave the church its name. *Vatnås* or "water hill" suggests that veneration of the spring predates even the original stave church that was replaced by the present yellow, wood-paneled, cross-shaped structure. Named for the substantial *staver* or log pillars at each corner, stave churches have been termed "a genial translation of the Romanesque basilica from stone to wood."[23] Engineered by descendants of the Vikings between 1100 and 1300, their construction shows the influence of masterly ship-building techniques.

Extending from the gables of many stave churches are dragons with poisonous tongues to protect the sacred space from attack by demons. Similar dragons project from Norway's medieval reliquaries (repositories for the sacred remains of Christian martyrs), such as the one that according to legend inspired the design of the original Vatnås church. Faye's version continues: "The king and his men, all about to perish from thirst, rejoiced and drank merrily and King Olav repeated his promise. Preparing to leave, he saw a grouse on a tree branch and took aim, but then he spotted a tiny church of pure gold suspended above the bird. The king ordered that the church be built in its image."[24]

Thus, legend accounts for the Catholic saint's reliquary that must have mystified the workers who found it in the woods behind the church two centuries after the Reformation had banned the veneration of saints and made Catholicism illegal in Norway. With its rectangular base and peaked lid from which dragon heads project, the foot-long reliquary looks like a miniature stave church. Its wooden frame is covered with shiny metal pressed into reliefs depicting Christ, the Virgin Mary, and the apostles. Another relief shows a pilgrim on his way to Nidaros Cathedral, where Olav's body lay encased in a similar, though much larger, shrine.[25]

"Vatnås church lay abandoned after the Black Death of 1350 until 1665, when the altar and a crucifix, as well as a miniature gilded-copper church, were found in the overgrown forest by the church," wrote Pastor Nils Bernhoft in his 1745 description of Sigdal parish. "This miniature church was placed on the church altar when the building was restored in 1665," he concluded, seemingly unaware of the reliquary's significance in Catholic ritual. The almue themselves, meanwhile, probably continued Catholic practices as part of their heritage and as a link to their ancestors.[26]

Supplementing official religious doctrine with ancestral ways was nothing new. Long after the Christian conversion, Norwegians had similarly retained pre-Christian practices such as paying homage to the *gardvord*, the spirit of the one who first cultivated the family farm. Well into the 1800s, many believed this guardian spirit dwelled in the farm's ancestral grave mound, and they continued to honor it with Christmas tributes of beer or porridge, despite ecclesiastical laws that since the Middle Ages had expressly forbidden the veneration of spirits.[27]

The almue's constant attentiveness to the *huldrefolk* or hidden people, and the way they tailored their actions to meet these hidden beings' expectations, is similarly rooted in pre-Christian practice. Apparently the almue found no conflict between their folk beliefs and the pious Christian faith that they observed with equal devotion. Rather than resisting official church doctrine, the almue simply supplemented it with traditional beliefs and practices that addressed the practical needs of their daily lives. In the wake of the sixteenth-century Reformation, the almue similarly supplemented the official faith with customs—including pilgrimages to St. Olav springs and lovekirker and Catholic healing prayers—that featured the direct appeals to the deity that Catholicism had encouraged but Lutheranism denied.

Using the black book

The Lutheran clergy's condemnation of Catholic practices and demonization of Catholic healing prayers in the witch trials forever changed the way people regarded folk healers and their incantations. Subsequently associated with the devil, these formulas came to be known collectively as the black book. Popular legend accepted this diabolical association, as evident from these instructions for obtaining the black book:

> If you want the black book you must go to the church three Thursday evenings in a row. Each of the evenings you must walk three times counter-clockwise around the church, and after doing so the third evening, read the Lord's Prayer backwards. Then the Evil One himself will appear with the black book in hand. But before you take it, you must cut yourself in the finger and write your name in blood in another book the Evil One holds out. When this is done,

you get the book. But once you have it, you can never get rid of it, and from that time on, you will belong to the devil.[28]

Recorded in Østerdalen in the early 1900s, these directions leave no doubt about the terror the black book aroused. Obtaining it perverted both nature (walking against the sun) and the Church (reading the Lord's Prayer backwards), and to use it was to give up one's soul to eternal damnation ("from that time on, you will belong to the devil").

Similar instructions from one of the Rustad black books used even more diabolical terms:

> When you want to release the angels from hell, then say when you arise in the morning: "I renounce you, God and Father that has made me. I renounce you, Holy Spirit that has blessed me. I will never worship or serve you after this day, but completely swear my allegiance to Lucifer, ruler of the dark abyss. To his rule I swear, and he shall serve me and do what I ask of him. In exchange I give my own blood as insurance and pledge. This binds me to him, body and soul, for all eternity, as long as he does what I ask, order or command of him. And to this pact I sign with my own hand and with my own blood that this be certain and true in every possible way."[29]

Could it be put more plainly? To use the black book, one had to renounce the Christian faith, an unspeakable act to most nineteenth-century Norwegians.

Given the dire consequences of association with the black book, Norwegians were remarkably quick to accuse their neighbors of owning it. "My grandmother used rational medicines, but people insisted she had the black book," said Andreas Eliasson Aanen (born 1858), the grandson of a well-known folk healer from Vefsn in North Norway. "They said that about anybody who knew just a little bit more than others; such people were always accused of having the black book."[30]

Aanen's grandmother, Karen Bentsde (ca. 1790–1863), lived on the Smed-seng farm. Neighbors relied on her cures—and gossiped about her magic. They alleged she went to the "church tower every Christmas Eve to scrape metal from the bells for her medicines." They also suspected her of sneaking to the cemetery for another staple of magical cures, graveyard soil: "Smedseng-Karen took dirt from the church yard at Dolstad.... Since it was only powerful on Midsummer Eve, she had to take enough that night for the whole year through." Midsummer's Eve (*jonsok* or *St. Hans*), like Christmas Eve, enhanced the power of ritual, as did any item associated with the dead.

People sometimes resorted to magical cures for mysterious ailments and when rational remedies failed. "For colds, people used elderberry tea, hot milk and pepper, hot beer or French cognac, and aromatics like ether and rigabalsam," said Ludvig N. Holstad (born 1885 in Hareid, Møre og Romsdal), "but when it came to the kinds of pains that no one understood, more mystical methods came into play." Pulled muscles and tendons and other strains and sprains, made all too common by the rough, rocky Norwegian landscape, seriously disrupted the physical labor required of most people in preindustrial times and demanded immediate attention. Having no other remedy, Holstad's neighbors "*leste*" (read or recited incantations) for them.[31]

As a boy in Trøndelag, Andreas Ystad (born 1879 in Inderøy) also encountered these "*vreilord*" or healing incantations: "Many a time when I had sprained a hand or a foot, one of my aunts or another woman in the neighborhood would read *vreilord* over the injured joint. She didn't read out loud, just mumbled something so softly I couldn't hear a word of it. She read the formula three times, each time spitting a little on the wrist or ankle and stroking her hand counter clockwise over it. Then it felt better." Spittle frequently accompanied magical formulas, as did silence and secrecy, all believed to enhance the incantations' power.[32]

Though secrecy prevented the young Ystad from hearing the words, he later managed to learn one of these formulas:

Jesu rei over ei hei
Fållån snåva og foten vrei,
Jesus steig av og la foten an
som den tilforn var
i namnet Gud, Fader, Sønn og Helligånd.

(As Jesus rode across a stony plain,
his horse stumbled, its leg did sprain.
Jesus dismounted to cure the pain
And he made the injury good again.
In the name of God, Father, Son and Holy Spirit.)

Like the incantation used by the "witch" Lisbet Nypan, this formula appeals to the power of Christianity to heal the sufferer as Christ healed his own horse.

Who had the black book?

Healing incantations seem to have been quite common, but the tremendous secrecy that until recently surrounded the black book has concealed the identities of those who compiled them. A considerable amount, however, is known about one black-book owner, Ole Toftelien. Born around 1810 in Dovre, Gudbrandsdal, Ole Toftelien impressed his neighbors not least because of his enormous library. The ability to read was not unusual among nineteenth-century almue, who "read for the minister" in preparation for Lutheran confirmation. But laboriously spelling one's way through the Bible, hymnal, and catechism was altogether different from reading the treatises on natural and cultural history, geography, religion, and art history that Toftelien's library contained. Few among the almue had the opportunity to learn to write, and they certainly did not use foreign words, as Toftelien liked to do.

Baptized Ole Hansson Åkerjordet, Toftelien was the son of a schoolteacher. His father, Hans Hanson Åkerjordet (born ca. 1775), augmented his meager income through decorative painting and sign lettering. It was Hans who compiled the four-by-six-inch, fifty-nine-page black book inscribed "15 August 1807" that Toftelien inherited. Toftelien took his name from the tiny cotter's place that barely supported his growing family. Ole married Eli Samuelsdatter Ekrehagen (whose father was also a teacher) in 1837, and the couple had several children. To eke out a living, Ole also did ornamental painting, gracing some of the most prosperous farms in Dovre.[33]

Just how skillfully Ole's father could wield a quill pen is evident in the precise script of the black book's first forty-one pages, which almost appear to be set in gothic type. Another hand, probably that of Toftelien himself, has added several formulas in more ordinary script, including one for protecting a farm from malevolent beings that appears to emanate from the master sorcerer himself: "I, Cyprianus, servant of Jesus Christ, command that all the evil that has infested this farm, its buildings and its grounds, shall hereby and forever more be expelled. Like the cold at springtime and salt in a running stream, as snow beneath the sun and all that is bound by *jordfast* [immovable] stones, this evil shall henceforth disappear from sight, exiled to the place whence it came. And this shall be in the name of the Father, Son and Holy Ghost. Amen."[34] Using simple images (snow melting, water dissolving salt, earthbound stones) to express extraordinary power, this incantation reveals the terrifying threats its users feared from all manner of forces. The familiar closing words, *I navnet fader, sønn, hellig ånd amen* (abbreviated by Toftelien as *I:N:F:S:H:A:A*) confer a final measure of comfort and control.

As a black-book owner and by virtue of his unusual talents, enlightenment, and personality, Toftelien naturally became the subject of neighborhood gossip. Some emphasized the single-minded focus on his work. An old, tall, dark, and terribly thin man when he decorated the house at Øvre Lindsø, says John Meyer, Toftelien seemed to forget everything else while painting. Children watched from a respectful distance, wondering if he would ever be through mixing his paints in oil and trying out the various shades. Though they freely played around the old carpenter, Tjøstol, as he worked and even dared to touch his tools, the youngsters quickly learned to stay away from the secretive magician of a painter who evidently considered each of his paint pots sacred.[35]

Others told about Toftelien's irreverence, such as the time he was trying to finish up a job at the Toftemoen farm on the eve of Ascension Day and realized that no matter how fast he worked, he could not possibly complete the task before all work had to stop for the holiday. "*Fand brenne meg*" (May the devil burn me), Toftelien exploded, "I could have gotten done if that rascal hadn't been in such a rush to get up there!"[36]

His rough reputation not withstanding, it was to Ole Toftelien that the neighbors turned when illness struck. After all, he had the black book. When Ola Sætrom's cow got sick, Sætrom set out for the Toftelien place. The healer paced the floor several times before he turned to Sætrom and said: "Go straight home, and if the cow hasn't recovered, come back here as fast as you can." When Sætrom got home, he found the cow had recovered at the very moment he was with Toftelien.[37]

Identical accounts of other folk healers were told across Norway, but in Dovre such stories still evoke the memory of Ole Toftelien. In 2005 the family who lives on the Toftelien farm, though no relation to Ole, knew the old stories about him, including the familiar incident of Toftelien using the black book to stop thieves in his turnip patch. "There they stood," the story concludes, "each holding a big turnip and unable to budge. 'You'd better put the coffee pot on,' Toftelien called to his wife. 'The two out there in the turnip patch will probably be wanting some.'"[38]

Stopping thieves dead in their tracks is a common motif of Norwegian black-book legends. Its continued association with Ole Toftelien suggests the vivid impression he made on his neighbors. So it must have been with mixed feelings that they learned in the late 1860s of Toftelien's decision to take his wife and youngest daughter, Marit (born 1844), to America. In preparation, Ole sold most of his fabled library, including his father's black book.[39]

FORMULAS FROM OLE TOFTELIEN'S BLACK BOOK

For sprains:

"Jesus was out riding with Saint Peter when his horse slipped. Jesus dismounted and said, 'The leg is sprained.' Sprain in sprain, joint in joint, and blood in blood. Today N. N. [patient's name] will be cured. In three names."

To drive rickets from a child:

Take some soil from a grave and replace it with a pin. Place the soil in brandy and have the child drink it. It helps.

To protect livestock from harm:

"Jesus and the Virgin Mary were walking along the shore and saw a fine stand of valerian. Jesus dug up some roots to give to St Peter. The troll in the mountain called to them: 'The root will not help.' St. Peter replied that the root could cure many ills, such as listlessness, dysentery, the tooth of wolf or bear, and the hand of the witch."

To get butter from cream:

"God the father gives me my bounty. I put my churn to the ground, I bless it with God's word. God give me butter of the earth's bounty, God give me the dew of the earth. God the creator in my hands. *In nomine Patris.*"

To bind a thief:

Take your own blood and write the following on a slip of paper, put it in a human bone and place it where you fear the thief will come:

"And when Apylon who is the thief's headmaster binds his blood vessels and tendons, his feet and throat, let him be bound in teeth and tongue until he puts down the goods he has stolen. In three names, F. S. H. G. [Father, son, holy ghost]. Amen."

To stop bleeding:

"I bid you stop as surely as one is forbidden heaven's door who goes to court knowing right but swears false. In three [names]. Stand still blood, not one drop more."

Or:

"Stand still the bleeding of N. N. just as the current stood still when Jesus with his twelve disciples walked through."

When the Tofteliens reached the New Land, they settled in Hanska, Minnesota, where "Old Man Tuftali," as people called Ole, once again became the subject of neighborhood lore. In one story, told by Hanska native Doug Becken, "Old Man Tuftali" was staying overnight at a stranger's home. When he started up to bed he left his suitcase unattended downstairs in the entryway, prompting his host to ask if he didn't want to take the bag to his room for safe keeping. Tuftali answered that it would be all right just as it was. "Early the next morning a young boy in the family took a notion to look in the suitcase, thinking there might be something in there for him, but after he opened it, he found himself unable to move away from the suitcase. And that's how Old Man Tuftali found him when he got out of bed: red-handed, wide-eyed, and soon with a backside that was red, too."[40]

The story bears a close resemblance to the turnip story told back in Dovre, and Ole Toftelien's habits also remained remarkably consistent. In Hanska, he assembled an impressive library and again became known for having the black book. Although how he acquired another black book is unknown, one in the collection of the Norwegian-American Historical Association in Northfield, Minnesota, is inscribed by Ole Toftelien.[41] In Hanska, the Tofteliens became founding members of Nora Free Church, the Unitarian congregation served by Kristoffer Janson from 1882 until he returned to Norway in 1893. When Nina Draxten completed her biography of Janson in 1976, she deposited her research materials at the Nora church. Rev. Sarah Oelberg later transferred these materials to the association's

This black book, published in Chicago in 1892, is allegedly based on an original from the 1400s. It promises to confer upon the buyer a "key" that will reveal the book's many secrets. (Photo by Stokker)

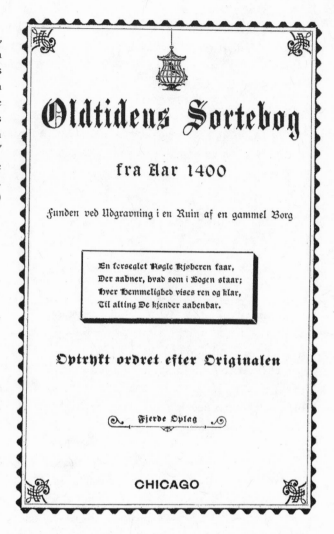

Oldtidens Sortebog

fra Aar 1400

Funden ved Udgravning i en Ruin af en gammel Borg

En forseglet Nøgle Kjøberen faar,
Der aabner, hvad som i Bogen staar;
Hver Hemmelighed vises ren og klar,
Til alting De kjender aabenbar.

Optrykt ordret efter Originalen

Fjerde Oplag

CHICAGO

archives, including Toftelien's books that once constituted the core of the town's lending library.[42]

Thanks to the efforts of these two women, we know which books Ole Toftelien owned. In addition to the black book (titled *Cyprianus* and published in Copenhagen in 1870), there is an 1865 history of witchcraft and magic in Norway written for the general public (*Hexevæsen og troldskab i Norge; medelt til læsning for menigmand*). Beyond these two esoteric volumes, Toftelien's collection ranges widely to include language books, religious tracts, sermon collections, travelogues, and histories, along with manuals on science and geography, volumes of fairy tales, literary works such as Swift's *Gulliver's Travels*, and a primer on the finer points of aquavit and other liqueurs.[43]

Did Toftelien conceive of his remedies as witchcraft? Public opinion proves unreliable, given its tendency to see all folk healers in that light. On the other hand, Toftelien did not distance himself from that image. Nor did his daughter, Marit, whose medications generations of townspeople relied on even as they feared her as a witch.[44]

Children ran in fear past Marit's house, and at least one of them, Clara Becken (born 1895), saw Marit's black book, though she wished she had not. At age thirteen, Clara was sent by her mother to fetch some medicine from "Mati Tuftali," as Becken's grandson, Doug, heard the Norwegian name. In 1986, he recorded the story his grandmother told him about Mati's black book.

"MATI'S BLACK BOOK," BY DOUG BECKEN

Clara had walked up the flat-stone path from the dirt street, and had knocked lightly at Mati Tuftali's door, secretly hoping she wouldn't be home. But the door had pulled open on the third rap, and there stood a small, quick Norwegian woman with twinkling grey eyes and a smile like a troll's. "*Hvordan har du det idag?*" (How are you today?), Mati had asked. Clara couldn't remember speaking, though she must have answered because now she was in here, and the old woman was upstairs "working." She heard terrible words drifting down the steep, narrow stairs. They were being read in a slow, even tone, not quite loud enough for her to grasp at their meaning.

Mati was reading from that *Svart Boken*, Clara knew, because she had seen her take it down from its place in the cupboard above the kitchen pump. It was old and looked well-used, not tattered or frayed, but as if it would open naturally to the pages with favorite recipes, like her own mother's cookbook opened to "Butter Cookies" or "Krumkake."

The recipes in Mati Tuftali's black book weren't for cookies, though. It was about the size of the Old Testament Bibles the peddlers all tried to sell, and the recipes were for curing babies of colic, among other things about which God only knew, if even He was allowed to know.

Some folks said the medicines she made did the curing. You would rub them on the ailing parts and the sickness would get better. Other people claimed that the power must lie in the words she spoke over her concoctions. They said it was dangerous to listen to them. Everyone who knew Mati at all seemed to agree without saying that there was a curse on the Svart Boken; anyone who read it, besides Mati herself, would go mad and do away with himself. Clara closed her eyes and tried hard not to listen. "Clara? Clara, here is the medicine for Marvin. Tell your mother to rub the green one on his stomach at night, and the clear amber one in the morning." Clara's eyes snapped open and the "old witch" was handing her two small bottles. She took them from Mati very carefully, not wanting to break them and have to risk hearing the words from the black book all over again. ᴂ

Is it coincidence that Marit's grave in Hanska, with a stone dated August 5, 1934, lies in the farthest row of the cemetery away from town, the position traditionally reserved for social outcasts and miscreants? What has become of Marit's black book, which would reputedly drive anyone who read it to "go mad and do away with himself," according to Clara's daughter, Lorraine? After Marit's death, reported Clara's daughter, Marit's belongings were sold in an auction in October 1934. Pastor George Whalen, a native of Haugesund, purchased some of her Norwegian books, including, it was said, the black book. Those who believed that "something tragic might happen to whoever got Marit's black book" interpreted the pastor's subsequent drowning in light of the curse.[45]

Black books in America today

No one knows what has become of Marit's black book. The Toftelien *Cyprianus* now in the Norwegian-American Historical Association archives is neither Marit's book nor the one so finely lettered by Ole Toftelien's father. Instead, it is a pamphlet of three-dozen pages published as a curiosity in 1870 by the Danish philologist L. Pio and based on a 1607 manuscript found in the Royal Danish Library.[46]

Surely the hand-lettered black book meant something personal to Ole Toftelien, so why had he left it behind in Norway when he emigrated? Perhaps he shared the once common belief that owning a black book at the time of death automatically excluded one from salvation. For, as the people of Eidskog believed, "the worst thing is that the one who has gotten hold of this book from the Evil One must forever belong to him." To avoid this fate, many Norwegian emigrants apparently disposed of their black books before embarking on the perilous journey across the ocean.[47]

Erik Kvennerud did. Much in demand throughout Eggedal as a *kjøgemester* (master of ceremonies at weddings and funerals), he was no less renowned for having the black book. Yet "before Erik Kvennerud left Norway," said Tormod Skatvedt, "he burned his black book together with a *Fadervorblad*" (page on which the Lord's Prayer was written). No ordinary fire could consume the black book, according to well-established lore. Terrified owners reportedly saw their black books reappear after they thought they had destroyed them. "It's no use thinking of throwing it in the fire, for it jumps back out of the flames. Nor does it help to throw it in north-running water. It comes right back," they said in Eidskog. Knowing the power that folk belief attributed to items associated with sacred objects, Kvennerud apparently had reason to believe that adding the fadervorblad to the fire would make the flame strong enough.[48]

As for Toftelien, who sold his black book in Dovre, he must have acquired a new one after he arrived in Hanska, for the *Cyprianus* in the Norwegian-American Historical Association archives was not published until 1870. Toftelien's inscription—written in a fine, even hand on both the first and final pages of the book, "*Denne Bog tilhører Ole Hansen Toftelien*" (This book belongs to Ole Hansen Toftelien)—includes the date 1874.

As the stories of Toftelien and Kvennerud suggest, few black books from Norway came to America. Perhaps it was to meet the demand of those who had left their black books in Norway that the well-known Scandinavian American book dealer, John Anderson, published a few of them, though none that displayed his name or imprint. Born in Voss in 1836, Anderson emigrated with his parents in 1845, and in 1866 he started the Norwegian language newspaper *Skandinaven* in Chicago, soon the most widely circulated publication of its kind. Anderson eventually became the largest purveyor of Scandinavian publications in America. He imported books directly from Norway and Denmark, reprinted titles in his own establishment, and also published original works by Norwegian American authors. Birger Osland, who as a young man worked for Anderson, mentioned in his 1945 memoir that "*Svarteboken*, dealing with witchcraft" ranked among the firm's best sellers in 1899.[49]

John Anderson probably published the *Oldtidens Sortebog* (Ancient black book) bearing the imprint "Chicago 1892," the only known copy of which now resides at Luther College, Decorah, Iowa. This American edition duplicates an undated black book published in Copenhagen, allegedly "written in the year 1400 and found while excavating the ruins of an ancient castle." Publishers of black books often made claims of venerable origin to spur sales by increasing the potential buyers' faith in the product.[50]

Effective use of the black book traditionally required a "key," to be obtained by performing a ritualized ceremony. A black book for Sigdal instructed the reader to "remove slivers of wood from the church door and place them in a nearby stream while reciting an oath of allegiance to the powers of darkness."[51] More commercial, *Oldtidens Sortebog* has a verse on its cover touting its key as justifying the price of purchase:

> To the buyer a sacred key is sold
> to open up secrets concealed of old.
> Containing arts, pure and bold,
> that through this book all are told.

The "key" in question—a folded sheet of paper "concealed" inside the back cover—"reveals" that the book's formulas must be read in reverse, and it is signed, "Cyprianus."

Cyprianus

The identity of the mysterious figure Cyprianus varied wildly. People in Holsten, Denmark, imagined Cyprianus to be a fellow Dane so evil during his lifetime that when he died the devil threw him out of Hell. This act so enraged Cyprianus that he dedicated himself to writing the nine Books of Black Arts that underlie all subsequent Scandinavian black books.[52] The Cyprianus of Ole Toftelien's 1870 black book, by contrast, is a "tender and decent" student who, when compelled by the devil to attend the Black School and use his knowledge to do evil, made amends by explaining in his black book how to undo all the evil formulas it contained.

In stark contrast, the Cyprianus of *Oldtidens Sortebog* is a ravishingly beautiful, irresistibly seductive, prodigiously knowledgeable, pious Mexican nun. The nun's gory story, dated 1351, details her mistreatment by a debauched cleric whose advances she steadfastly refused—to her peril. Brutally cast into a dark dungeon from which she feared she would never escape, Cyprianus shredded her clothing to form pages and wrote upon them in her own blood the secrets known only to her, "the wonder-woman whose wisdom and renown are honored by the learned monks of all Eastern lands."[53]

These secrets are the magical healing formulas contained in *Oldtidens Sortebog*, which further distinguish themselves, as the "key" foretold, by words appearing in reverse order and to be read from the bottom up, right to left:

succeed. will work your strong is belief if things all in Remember . . .
bid. I as do blindly and silence in me keep you when need every in
you help will I

The ailments these formulas address range from relatively minor (ringworm, scabies, warts, rashes, corns, dog bites, colds, sore throats, headache, earache, toothache, stomachache, hernia, cramps) to life threatening and fatal (fever, tapeworm, gangrene, epilepsy, cholera, and cancer). The list accurately reflects the afflictions commonly suffered by nineteenth-century Norwegians on both sides of the Atlantic.

Many of the remedies *Oldtidens Sortebog* contains rely on "sympathetic magic," a pillar of international folk medicine holding that objects once in contact continue to be related even after they are separated. What happens to one of the objects therefore influences the other, as in the *Sortebog's* "Cure for chest inflammation" (read backward).

consumed. is egg the when well get will person sick the and current
the with water running into thrown is pot The anthill. an in egg the
Bury pot. the in phlegm more no is there until again it cook and it
peel boiled, hard is it When person. sick the by up coughed phlegm
the in egg an Boil

When the egg, boiled in the patient's phlegm, has been consumed, the patient recovers. However unappetizing, the formula sensibly allows nature and time to take care of the ailment, while assigning patient and caregiver participatory roles in the cure.[54]

Equally fundamental to folk medicine, "transference cures" transplant the illness to an object in the nearby landscape (like Lisbeth Nypan's remedy for rheumatism). An example from *Oldtidens Sortebog* is the "Cure for stomach inflammation, dropsy and such":

well. gets patient the but dies, animal The—eat. to meat the dog a give then away; cooked is urine the until time each urine, person's sick the in times three pork of piece a Boil

Urine as well as feces, phlegm, and other bodily excretions and secretions have figured in folk medicine since ancient times. Their use relates to a principle expressed in Norwegian as *"ondt skal ved ondt fordrives"* (it takes evil to drive out evil). The more repulsive the medicine, the more efficiently it will repel the evil causing the disease. "No pain, no gain," we would say today, still more likely to ascribe efficacy to bitter pills than sweet.[55]

Transference lived on, too. "I never thought of my mother [Hjordis Elfreda Buck Olsen, a registered nurse, born 1901 in Trondheim] as being superstitious," wrote Phillip Buck Olsen, the retired dean of an American university. But in an attempt to cure his childhood warts, "she once used a remedy from something called the Old Book. . . . When all else failed, she applied the old cure to me. It consisted of using a piece of salt pork which she rubbed over my warts on a night of a full moon, and which she buried in the garden beside Lake Superior in Duluth, Minnesota, where I was born. I recall no ritual accompanying the remedy, only the provision that I must not watch where Mother buried the salt pork." This transference ritual, traditionally enhanced by the full moon and secrecy, proved effective. "The warts withered and fell off," wrote Olsen in 1996, "never to reappear." (Because the viral cause of warts long remained unknown, their seemingly inexplicable appearance and disappearance made them the frequent focus of folk remedies all over the world.)[56]

Changing perceptions of the black book

Over the years, the terror and distaste once aroused by the black book has abated. The Norwegian folklorist Håvard Skirbekk (born 1903) experienced this change firsthand, noting that when he began collecting folklore in Solør during the 1920s, people refused to mention the black book. By the

1960s, however, two black books arrived, unsolicited, in his mail, two separate donors having apparently come to regard their grandparents' formula collections as no more than interesting curiosities of historical value.[57]

Norwegian Americans had their own qualms about the black book, but for the Thompson family of Moorhead, Minnesota, the attitude seems to have gone from acceptance to rejection. Thorvald Thompson (born 1895 in Valdres) enjoyed telling colorful stories about the black book, but when it came time to inherit the one owned by his father, he flatly refused. His son, Harry Thompson (born 1928), believed his grandfather had used his black book "honorably for medical purposes," but Harry did not want it either, seeing it as "an evil power and of the devil."[58]

Growing up in Moorhead during the 1930s, Harry heard plenty of stories about the black book owned by his grandfather, Ole Thomason (born 1867 in Hedalen, Valdres). Ole emigrated to America with his wife, Kjersti, and their two-year-old son, Thorvald, who became Harry's father.

Nor was Grandpa Ole the only member of Harry Thompson's family who possessed a black book. "This power was also held on my grandmother Kjersti's side, by her father's mother Kristi Ellingsdatter," wrote Harry, and by his own great-great-grandmother, Kari Larsdatter Lybekk (1825–92). "A large woman with a big lump under one arm, on which she carried her SvarteBoken," Kari managed her farm with unusual skill, producing more milk and butter than her neighbors. Such superior results fueled fantasy and envy. "Stories passed on to us," said Harry, "say she would pour cream into the churn and put the cover on and read her magic words, and the cream would turn to butter."

As Kari's impoverished neighbors saw it, only witchcraft could account for the abundance of Kari's butter. The always quirky business of churning became even trickier when small farms and frequent crop failures forced peasants to practice "starvation feeding," giving cows minimum fodder to survive the winter. The milk given by the undernourished cows when they haltingly emerged from the barn in the spring contained very little fat, and when the arduous job of churning failed to produce butter, peasants blamed witches for having "spirited" their neighbors' butter into their own churns.[59]

Harry's father had a different explanation. When the witches were "mad at a neighbor, they sent their *trollkatt* to drink the milk before the cow was milked." Witches made a trollkatt from discarded rags, fingernails, and hair, adding a few drops of their own blood to give it life. Then they sent it rolling from farm to farm to gather the neighbors' milk, a scenario that explained why the witch prospered while neighbors stayed poor.

"I was about five or six years old when my dad would tell me all these scary stories," wrote Harry Thompson. "I can still see my mother getting angry with him and having to take me upstairs to bed because I was afraid to go alone." Yet, when the time came for Ole Thompson to pass the black book down to his son, "Thorvald refused to take it." When "Grandpa Ole died in 1952, Aunt Olive and Aunt Clara burned the book when they cleaned his little house on Fifth Avenue and Nineteenth St. North in Moorhead" (now the site of a church).[60]

Fortunately, reports of Ole Thompson's prowess in using the black book live on. "Grandpa could be covered with bees," writes Harry, "and he would not be stung," and he could also stop the flow of blood, a feat formerly considered magical: "Russell Hovdestad said that when he cut his arm, Grandpa said something and the bleeding stopped. My dad said when he was sticking turkeys, and accidentally struck his chest, Grandpa made the bleeding stop without touching him."

Without question, the black book with its magical formulas occupied a more significant place in the minds of Norwegian and Norwegian Americans than has been publicly acknowledged. Despite a terrifying reputation, it provides unparalleled insights into Norway's traditional remedies and rituals, while its associated lore helps illuminate a way of life distant from our own.

·5

Doctor Books
Mirroring the march of medicine

"You did not go to a doctor unless you really had a very serious problem, so like many other farm mothers, my mom invested in a couple of very nice, leather bound 'Doctor Books' to take care of her family."

Paul "Bud" Hanson (born 1923)

WHEN ILLNESS STRUCK, nineteenth-century Norwegians on both sides of the Atlantic relied on doctor books (*legebøker*). "We read in the medical manuals and used everything suggested there we could get hold of," wrote Caja Munch from the Wiota, Wisconsin, parsonage on August 12, 1857. Caja had confessed earlier that year how "frightening" it was to be "so absolutely devoid of a physician's aid." She added, "*Mangor's Country Pharmacy* stands us in good stead," showing the consolation a good doctor book could bring.[1]

Immigrants gradually replaced the well-worn volumes brought from Norway with English or Norwegian editions published in America. Some of these books arrived as premiums for subscriptions to Norwegian American newspapers such as the Chicago-based *Norden*, whose editors distributed *Lægebog for hvermand* (Doctor book for everyone) in 1879. The La Crosse, Wisconsin, newspaper *Fædrelandet og Emigranten* similarly issued *Huslægen* (The house doctor) as part of its 1883 *Husvennen* (Home companion), and the *Decorah Posten* produced *Før Doktoren kommer* (Until the doctor arrives) as its "*Præmeiebog for 1890–91.*"

American volumes like John C. Gunn's *New Domestic Physician* (1862) and "People's Home Medical Book" (1915) eventually replaced ethnic doctor

Much used by Norwegians on both sides of the Atlantic, Mangor's 1835 *Lande-apothek* (Country apothecary) helped rural dwellers with no access to doctors and recommended plants the people could grow themselves. *(Photo by Stokker)*

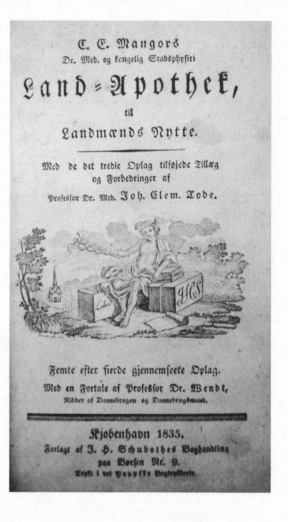

books. Their stained and tattered pages vividly testifying to years of constant consultation, copies of these publications now reside in the libraries of Norwegian Lutheran colleges and in Vesterheim Museum in Decorah, Iowa.

"I remember poring over the 'doctor book,' the big thick black 'bible' for anything and everything related to health," wrote Muriel Vollum (born 1928 in Albert Lea, Minnesota). She may have meant the "People's Home Medical Book" that constituted the first third of the hefty, black-bound *People's Home Library* (published in Cleveland, Ohio, in 1915). Once a familiar fixture in many family circles, this three-hundred-page doctor book combined the "latest professional medical advice" with a "broad sampling of home remedies from all parts of the world." It thereby symbolized, as much as it assisted, the immigrants' adjustment to the New Land.[2]

Whether in English, Norwegian, or another immigrant language, the home-health manuals that proliferated in nineteenth-century America derived from the same ancient source. The shared origin of these books—and of the cures they contained—accounts for the remarkable continuity in international folk medicine, something that must have made it easier for the immigrants to exchange remedies across cultural lines.

Far into the past century, Norwegian Americans continued to rely on doctor books. They used the remedies already printed there and inserted additional tips of their own, whether handed down in the family, clipped from the newspaper, or obtained from neighbors and friends. Some families even used the doctor book as a repository for recording the dates of family births and deaths, confirmations and marriages, information otherwise entrusted to the family Bible.[3]

As medicine became increasingly professionalized, doctor books reflected the change, evolving from hands-on manuals for do-it-yourself care to theoretical works designed to explain the treatments administered by the physician.

Historic doctor books

When friends with different ethnic heritages talk about their grandmothers' home remedies, they quickly discover how much these remedies have in common. Some identical cures may have arisen independently of each other, but most can be traced back almost two thousand years to the same source, *De materia medica* (The materials of medicine) compiled by Pedanius Dioscorides (ca. 40–80 AD). Born in Asia Minor, Dioscorides trained as a doctor in Alexandria and Tarsus. Perhaps as Nero's military physician, he traveled extensively throughout the Greek and Roman world, seeking out information about curative substances wherever he went. Between 50 and 70 AD, Dioscorides published five volumes that listed the medicinal properties of more than six hundred plants, eighty animals, and fifty minerals, in all describing some 950 curative substances and 4,470 medicines that could be made from them.[4]

Subsequent generations based their pharmacies on Dioscorides' work. Translating his original Greek text into Latin, Arabic, and Armenian, they disseminated the information widely, and by the Middle Ages it was known from the Viking North Atlantic to the Islamic territories on the Indian and Pacific Oceans. Interest in Dioscorides reintensified during the Renaissance (1450–1600), when the newly invented printing press produced imprints of the original Greek text along with countless translations into Italian, French, German, Czech, Spanish, Dutch, and English. Often containing artful woodcuts of the herbs and animals they described, these volumes and their imitators secured Dioscorides' place as the central pharmacological authority in Europe and the Middle East for 1,600 years.[5]

The compiler of the first Scandinavian doctor book copied Dioscorides, too. Danish cleric Henrik Harpestreng (1164–1244) was known as an astrologer, but his *Liber Herbarum* (Book of herbs) reflects the strict academic style of the renowned medical school at Salerno, Italy. Since 800 AD, this school had continued the healing practices of the ancient Greeks, and during the Middle Ages, when medicine languished in Europe, healing received new impulses from Arabia, where medicine still flourished. Though Harpestreng essentially copied his predecessors, his work broke new ground in Scandinavia. The book also described an herb no earlier book had included, *kvann* (angelica), thereby introducing Norway's most significant contribution to international folk medicine.[6]

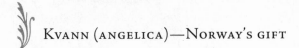

Kvann (angelica)—Norway's gift

By the Viking era (ca. 800–1000 AD), *kvann* (*Angelica archangelica* or angelica) was already an important item of trade. Snorri's medieval *Saga of Olav Tryggvasson* describes the king buying it at the market place in Nidaros.[7] The 1164 Law of Gulating emphasized kvann's continued importance, urging landowners to set aside special *kvanngårder* (patches to grow these leafy stalks, which in western Norway reached six or seven feet tall). Strict punishments were imposed for stealing kvann from another farm. Place-names such as Kvannagrø and Kvanndal further attest to the importance Norwegians once accorded this herb.

Monks grew kvann in Norway's medieval cloister gardens, and many wore it as a protective amulet or carried it in their pockets to ward off sickness and danger. It may have been a visit by kvann-

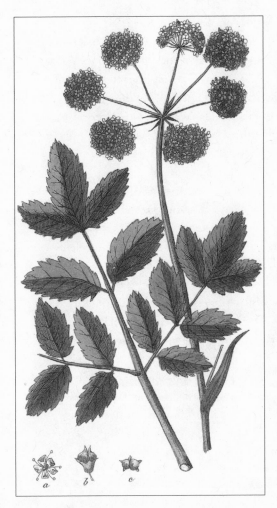

Kvann (later known as *Angelica archangelica*) was introduced to Europe in the thirteenth century by Dane Henrik Harpestreng in his *Liber Herbarum* (Book of herbs).

carrying monks to Harpestreng in Roskilde that prompted him to include the herb in his *Liber Herbarum*. "Kvann is an excellent plant," he wrote. "It shields wearers from evil incantations, and eating it in the morning protects one from poisonous food or drink, driving out their toxins by means of its virtue." In addition to warding off food poisoning, kvann could be eaten to cure *gikt* (rheumatism) and *tæring* (consumption), said Harpestreng, advising that dog bites and other wounds be cured by placing slices of kvann root directly on them.[8]

After being introduced by Harpestreng's Latin text, kvann's healing properties quickly became known beyond Scandinavia. When the Black Death struck Europe in the late 1340s, kvann gained a reputation for curing the afflicted and stopping its spread. Desperate for this protection, people clamored for the small cakes that apothecaries rushed to make from distilled aromatic oils of kvann.[9]

According to legend, it was at this time kvann got its Latin name,

Angelica archangelica. Seeing piles of plague corpses grow high, an archangel appeared to pious monks and revealed that God had sent kvann to cure the terrible scourge. The line "pocket full of posies" in the children's rhyme "Ring around the Rosy" may refer to the kvann that people carried in hopes they would not "all fall down" dead from the plague. Throughout the Middle Ages and long afterwards, Norway continued to supply Europe with kvann, sending it by ship-load from Bergen and other west-coast towns as various pestilences continued to rage.

Kvann's antibacterial properties may have had a slight limiting effect on the plague's contagiousness, but kvann's greatest effect came in treating another scourge—scurvy (*skjørbuk*), once as dread a disease as it was widespread. "The skin turns blue, hard and swollen, and in some can resemble leprosy, though without the contagion," wrote an observer in 1744.[10] Poverty and lack of sanitation often exaggerated the symptoms, which more typically include weakness and malaise, soft gums, bleeding hair follicles, anemia, and diarrhea. Considering scurvy worthy of note, the great Bergen humanist Peder Claussøn Friis (1545–1614) included it in his *True Description of Norway and Surrounding Islands* (1632), observing that the almue customarily treated it by eating the stalks and roots of kvann. "Drinking an occasional glass of brandy infused with *kvannerot* will prevent scurvy," advised I. F. Munthe one hundred years later in a handwritten book of eighteenth-century remedies from Hardanger.[11] Not until the 1920s would researchers identify Vitamin C and explain its role in alleviating scurvy, finally providing the scientific basis for centuries of home remedies based on kvann.

In addition to its high Vitamin C content, kvann has aromatic oils and tannins that stimulate digestive juices. Along with its sweet taste and fragrance, these properties have long made kvann an important component of the French liqueurs Chartreuse and Benedictine, along with their Norwegian counterpart, *St. Halvard likør.*[12] ⚞

Writing his book by hand on parchment, Harpestreng had to depend on monks to copy it, also by hand, for its distribution. After the printing press was invented in the mid-1400s, doctor books joined the Bible as the earliest and most frequently published volumes and those most often translated into the vernacular.

The earliest preserved Scandinavian example of a printed doctor book, *En nyttelig lægebog for fattige og rige, unge og gamle* (A useful doctor book for poor and rich, young and old), appeared in 1533. "There aren't many doctors in these lands to help the common man in time of illness," wrote its Danish author, Christiern Pedersen (1480–1554), to justify the publication that he based on the best Latin and German doctor books available, all originally inspired by Dioscorides.[13] Pedersen, originally a canon of Lund Cathedral, became a committed protestant and collaborated on the first Danish translation of the Bible. In 1532, he established his own press in Malmø (then a Danish city) and published numerous volumes including two doctor books, *En nyttelig lægebog* and one on herbal extracts (*Om UrteVand*) in 1534, together containing 250 medical herbs, 140 of them domestic.

Henrik Smid (ca. 1495–1563) continued the tradition of Scandinavian doctor books, copying long sections from Pedersen and other sources for his own *Skøn lystig ny Urtegaard* (Beautiful, merry new herb garden), which appeared in 1546. Like Pedersen, Smid was a committed protestant and collaborated on the Danish Bible translation, but unlike previous writers of Scandinavian doctor books, Smid had a formal education in medicine.[14] Though Smid briefly practiced medicine in Malmø, he had trouble succeeding as a doctor because of the public's preference for self-trained healers. "Unlearned monks, ministers, and corrupt merchants," Smid sniped, were overrunning the country, "deceiving the simple almue in order to sell their medicines for more money." Ironically, Smid's books became the mainstay for the self-trained healers he so despised.[15]

Originally published as six separate volumes between the years of 1535 and 1557, Smid's work appeared as a single edition in 1557 and 1577, and subsequently in frequent reprints as late as 1870 and even 1923. In the books, Smid declared that disease was a punishment sent by God but that God provided its cure in plants, whose use Smid promised to teach. Smid focused on domestic herbs that the sick could gather for themselves and which "God has created for our benefit and whose power and virtue we would honor if we but knew them."[16]

The popularity and longevity of Smid's book no doubt helped sustain the belief that sickness was part of God's divine plan, an article of faith among the Norwegian Americans into the late 1800s. "Providence had destined only a short stay at the Parental home," James Berdahl repeatedly wrote in describing the deaths of five of his nine children on the South Dakota prairie.[17] Despite an extensive education at Wittenberg and Rostock, Smid held the mystical concepts common to his time, believing that some people have magical powers such as the evil eye (the ability to do harm by means of a glance), that herbs had to be gathered at special times to achieve their power, and that natural catastrophes, eclipses of the sun, and the position of the planets foretold epidemics. These calamities, he asserted, could only be prevented by the confession of sin, penance, and prayer, acts that he also deemed necessary for effective use of his doctor books.

Since Smid included plants from foreign sources in his book, we cannot assume that all plants listed therein were actually used in Scandinavia, but he valuably described 250 domestic plants and his own observations about them. For 350 years after Smid's death from the plague in 1563, his books continued to be handed down through the generations, remaining in use longer than any other Danish or Norwegian volume.

The prolonged use of Smid's books came in for harsh criticism from the Norwegian pastor Hans Strøm (1726–97) in his own book published in 1778 in Bergen. "The lack of good doctor books makes our healers resort to Smid, by which they only are betrayed and often don't rightly understand," he wrote in his own volume titled *Kort Underviisning om De paa Landet, I Bergens Stift, meest grasserende Sygdomme, og derimod tienende Hjelpe-Midler* (A short instruction about common sicknesses in the area around Bergen and their most common remedies). More a report than a doctor book, it describes the living conditions and medical remedies of his time. Strøm, who served as a parish minister in Volda from 1764 to 1779 and in Eiker from 1779 until 1797, was considered among the best scholarly minds of his time and had already established his reputation with a multivolume topographical description of Sunnmøre (1762–66). He authored several other books in science, theology, and social science and in 1790 earned a doctoral degree in theology with a volume on early Christianity.[18]

"It is difficult for a doctor in this country to gain knowledge and experience of illnesses and remedies," writes Strøm in the preface, and his book shows the challenge presented even to someone of his keen intellect, dedication, and determination. Strøm cites the almue's lack of trust in doctors and belief in inescapable fate as two reasons the almue avoided professional medical help. "But if new remedies are to be found," he observes, "one needs to have the sick constantly at hand and always be able to visit them, while here in Norway, the dwellings are so spread out, doctors seldom have the opportunity for such observations." He therefore reports with regret having "no new or less costly medicines to recommend."[19]

Strøm admits that some self-trained healers deserve praise, but generally disparages the plethora of "blood-takers" and their "outdated doctor books, written when medicine was in a sorry state." These healers lacked insight into the body's structure and nature and have no knowledge of the effects of medicines, yet they dare to give advice for all kinds of ailments enabled by the blind faith of the almue who regard them as "oracles." Strøm blames the healers for allowing the public to keep this faith and for strengthening their belief that illness is caused by evil spirits.

Strøm visits coastal fishermen's cabins, where cleaning fish and producing cod-liver oil proceed amid the smoke of hearth fires and tobacco. Wet clothes hang to dry, milk and other foodstuffs await preparation, leftover food remains in cooking pots between meals, and the never-washed floor is usually wet or damp. The almue survive, says Strøm, only because of their strong constitution and lesser sensitivity. The old-style cabins helped, he notes, since their roof smoke holes had to be opened whenever a fire burned on the hearth, forcing inhabitants to get some fresh air. These cabins also provided more light than the newer windowed cabins with chimneys, since the almue insist on keeping windows tightly closed.

When illness strikes, the almue's lifestyle sabotages the positive effects of even the best medicine, says Strøm, who criticizes doctors for not providing information about diet and a regimen for the sick. Considering such a regimen important and as poorly understood as the medicines themselves, he suggests one regimen himself: opening the doors and windows and sprinkling vinegar on the floor and stove to freshen the air. Replace rich food, brandy, and strong beer that peasants prefer with barley and oat water (made by boiling oats or barley in water until half the water is cooked away), barley and oat soup, or sour bread boiled in water until it dissolves. By thinning the "feverish blood," these liquids enabled the harmful material in the stomach and intestines to be more easily expelled through sweat, urine, and feces. Strøm also recommended a daily enema (which, he said, the almue and their "blood takers" usually rejected in favor of bloodletting, though the procedure is no more difficult). "No household should be without an enema syringe," he adds, noting that it can be used either as a purge for constipation (using a liter of hot water, a half-tablespoon salt, and four spoons of melted butter) or to soften the contents of the intestines (using a quart of sweet milk, six tablespoons of fresh butter or the same amount of oil, plus an egg yoke).[20]

Strøm names Spanish fly plaster, tartar emetic, and lead acetate as the "doctors' newest and best medicines." He also describes the home remedies used by the almue, further revealing the challenging conditions they faced. For the "putrid fever," a common, contagious, and debilitating condition believed to be due to overwork and abrupt change in temperature and which produced a thickening of the blood, fast pulse, high fever, terrible thirst, and headache, the almue "cook cow manure in milk and drink it," says Strøm, who found this a useful remedy in the absence of anything better because it caused profuse sweating. Others used a mixture of gunpowder and brandy to treat the condition, he notes with partial approval, since the gunpowder contains saltpeter, which has a cooling effect, and the sulfur produces sweating. "But the brandy ruins it," he declares, by making the blood more feverish. All in all, Strøm preferred his own remedy for fever: bloodletting—the sooner the better—followed by a cooling powder of saltpeter and sugar, along with large draughts of blood-thinning barley or oat water.

 HANS STRØM'S HOME REMEDIES

Pig manure gathered in the summer and crushed into powder works well for treating diarrhea and bloody dysentery, a disease the peasants' poor diet makes resistant to less potent medicine. Patients should avoid indigestible food and drink only barley water, which can usefully be mixed with some tartar emetic since a tincture of rhubarb (the usual cure prescribed for dysentery) is not usually powerful enough for the peasants. A little cinnamon or nutmeg can be added to the manure, which should be ingested as a tea three to four times a day.

For chest inflammation (pneumonia), drink a tea of elderberry flowers, ingest camphor powder three to four times daily, place poultices of chamomile and elderberry flowers or warm oatmeal on the chest, or—if nothing else helps—apply a plaster of Spanish fly. And with all of these, drink barley water or an øl-ost (two parts milk, one part beer, heated separately, then mixed).

For diseases of the throat, use bloodletting (to hinder the formation of a boil) along with a daily enema to remove toxins. Poultices of chamomile and elderberry flowers mixed with dog manure cooked in water or milk, and gargling with lead acetate (which no household should be without) and a little salt peter cooked in water.

For whooping cough in children, give rhubarb in sufficient amounts to move the bowels two or three times each day. Mix into the rhubarb twice a week an emetic and when the vomiting begins, give the child barley soup to drink.

For rheumatism, whose pains move from place to place and feel like a fire burning an entire side of the body, frequently repeated bleeding and purging along with drinking elderberry tea is most effective, along with a Spanish fly plaster on the affected areas.

For jaundice, Epsom salts or rhubarb, but as Mangor advises in his *Lande-apothek*, only goose manure in wine cures this disease in peasants whose hard nature does not respond to weaker remedies.

Advice from Strøm's 1778 Kort Underviisning
(*Short instruction on common illnesses*) ❦

Strøm considered Mangor's "Country Apothecary" (*Lande-apothek*) state-of-the-art medicine. Appearing in 1767, the book guided him through his first years of practice. Christian Elovius Mangor (1739–1801) based his book on a Swedish original, but revised it to suit Danish and Norwegian conditions. Mangor had studied medicine in Copenhagen, where he subsequently practiced as a doctor, but he originally wrote his *Lande-apothek* to enable readers to handle "sickness, accidents, and childbirth on their own." Mangor admits, "Visiting a capable doctor would certainly be the best and most certain remedy, but what is the rural dweller to do in cases that demand immediate assistance and those that occur in the middle of the night or in the dark of winter?"

"Especially in Norway," Mangor observed, medical need was acute, since "few can afford medicines from the apothecary, let alone the cost of a doctor's travel, time, and trouble." Clearly filling an enduring need, Mangor's book went through eight printings between 1767 and 1863. It also accompanied Norwegian emigrants to America. Caja Munch and Elisabeth Koren probably used the 1835 edition, the only one still found in the United States. "The many published and sold-out editions of this book seem clear evidence of its usefulness for rural people," writes J. C. W. Wendt (1778–1838) in that edition, which he apologizes for not having updated. Since the book received no update after 1803, much of its advice was archaic when used in the later 1800s.[21]

Mangor made a point of recommending domestic herbs that people could grow in their own gardens. He especially favored elderberry (*hylle*), which, he advised, "every landman should have growing on his farm because it is an irreplaceable remedy." Mangor used elderberry for respiratory ailments primarily as a sweating agent, and modern research confirms elderberry's effectiveness in soothing bronchial inflammation and points to its biburnic acid as the ingredient that promoted sweating. For conditions ranging from ruptures and swollen feet to colds and sore throat, Mangor recommended making poultices using a mixture of elderberry and chamomile flowers (also shown by modern research to have an anti-inflammatory effect) and cooking them in beer or water and vinegar, "a superb solvent with so many uses that I wouldn't think well of a housewife who wasn't constantly using it."[22]

 MANGOR'S METHODS

The treatments recommended in Mangor's *Lande-apothek* aimed to remove bodily toxins. They included: 1) bleeding by opening a vein, 2) bleeding with leeches, 3) bleeding by cupping, 4) blistering with Spanish fly plaster, 5) vomiting induced by tartar emetic or root of ipecac, 6) defecating induced by bark of elm or elderberry; tinctures of aloe, rhubarb, or mustard leaf; jalappe; and Epsom salts, 7) sweating induced by elderberry tea, sage tea, camphor powder, and 8) bathing (which was sufficiently uncommon to be regarded as medicinal).

Doctor books in the New Land

Mangor wrote his *Lande-apothek* to be used when no doctor was at hand, but doctor books written in the last three decades of the 1800s increasingly discouraged home treatment. "When one is sick and feeling ill, it is always safest to get help from a good doctor," advised the Wisconsin-published *Huslægen* (The house doctor) in 1883. "Those unable to consult a physician immediately have to help themselves with home remedies and doctor books," acknowledged the anonymous author, who nevertheless urged that readers "not use the little guide to treat their own illnesses. That can be just as dangerous as being treated by a *kvaksalver* [quack]. When readers or their family members are sick, it is best to consult a good doctor despite the travel and expense involved."[23]

Though medicine in the 1880s was rapidly becoming a profession with formal training and licensing requirements, the advice to consult a doctor is one of the few clues found in this book that a revolution was under way.

"Decorah-Postens" Præmiebog for 1890—1891.

For Doktoren kommer.

Letvint Lægehjælp og Sundhedspleie

—ved—

Fredrik Mohn, Cand. Med.

Decorah, Jowa,
Trykt i "Decorah-Postens" Damptrykkeri,
1892.

Until the Doctor Arrives, a doctor book published for subscribers by the *Decorah-Posten* in 1892, promised "simple medical aid and health care" and reflected the revolution in medicine that arrived with the germ theory of disease.

Neither *Huslægen* nor the Chicago-published *Lægebog for hvermand* (1874) make any mention of bacteria, continuing instead to regard inflammation as an excitation of the blood best treated by bloodletting, poultices, or cooling drinks.

Noting with regret that such popular remedies as Spanish fly, rigabalsam, and camphor drops were "only available at Scandinavian apothecaries," the 1879 *Lægebog* gives thorough directions for making warm poultices by wrapping in canvas a stiff porridge of oatmeal or the flour made by grinding *høyfrø* (hay seed). If the poultice was for treating infections like boils and tooth abscesses, one should add shredded onion, "drawing" herbs, or a salve made with peppermint and wormwood (sixteen parts each) and flowers of German chamomile, elder, and lavender (three parts each). For inflammations and contusions, headaches and fevers, meanwhile, the book recommended cold compresses made with cold water, vinegar, or lead acetate.[24]

Turpentine and tar continue as important ingredients recommended by the *Lægebog* for use in poultices to bring infections to a head, to treat ringworm, scabies, and scrofula, or, taken internally, to treat colds. Warning that "wounds on the extremities" are "always dangerous" because of the "infection that invariably accompanies them," the *Lægebog* expressed the accepted assumption of the time that infection necessarily accompanied the healing process. The 1883 *Huslægen* similarly recommended that pus be removed from wounds by means of "drawing" medicines and wisely advised that sugar be applied to sores that would not heal. Most significantly, when dealing with open wounds, it urged "above all, cleanliness!" Yet it barely hints at the revolution that had begun with the 1882 discovery by Robert Koch of the bacillus that causes tuberculosis.

By the time *Decorah Posten* published *Før doktoren kommer. Letvint Lægehjelp og Sundhedspleie* (Until the doctor arrives. Simple medical assistance and health care) in 1892, the revolution was well under way. Bacteria figure prominently in this book, whose author was no longer anonymous but a university-educated doctor, Fredrik Mohn. Confusion still reigned about the exact nature of bacteria, which Mohn described as "tiny plant growths present everywhere decay occurs," but Mohn admitted that "the extent to which bacteria are a result or a cause of decay remains unknown." The book nevertheless recognized the fundamental, new principle that "contagious illnesses derive from bacteria."[25] He continued, "We know that most bacteria cause sickness and death if they enter the body and are allowed to grow there," uttering in one quick sentence what had taken decades of international research to accomplish.

Three years later, *Det sunde og syge mennekse* (The healthy and sick person), published in Decorah in 1895, registered the full impact of this work. Medicine's "enormous progress" in "recent decades" had put a "definitive end to do-it-yourself medical care," declared the author, Matthias Johnson, M.D. "The human body is like an ingeniously constructed machine, whose composition is very complicated. If something goes wrong with this machine, the one who repairs it must understand the principles of its construction and operation in order to be certain what needs to be done and how to do it." "This is a job for the doctor," Johnson announced, dismissing the "many advertised quacks." Neither is "the patient's own description to be trusted, since he as a rule lacks the necessary qualifications to describe the case in sufficiently exact and certain terms." This is a far cry from carefully listening to patients describe their symptoms, so crucial to the success of folk healers like Mor Sæther, Valborg Valand, and Anne Brandfjeld. As if to discredit these healers' herbal remedies, Johnson writes that though all medications exist in nature, "they must be refined and prepared before they can be used. This is the job of chemistry and pharmacology."[26]

While folk healers had shared their patients' view of the disease, medical treatment was now to become the exclusive province of the professionals, and the patient's role was to consist solely of "understanding the doctor's intent and the necessity of following his prescriptions." Such an understanding required mutual trust, Johnson observed, even as he noted the absence of that trust and "the most varied and mistaken notions about doctors and medicines." Many people "have no confidence in doctors or medications, and simply give themselves over to fate. Others attribute magical powers to them and think that the more often they visit the doctor and the more medicine they can take, the more certain they are to be healthy."

It was to address these misunderstandings and to raise the professional profile of medicine that Johnson wrote his "brief, popularized presentation" of 450 pages (the new knowledge having doubled the size of previous volumes) that instructed readers on "the human body's structure and the function of its organs, as well as its illnesses and their treatment." Registering a shift away from the popular midcentury belief that disease was caused by miasmas or illness-inducing vapors, Johnson's book included "a supplement on air, sunlight and water as conditions for life and health."

Like the Norwegian-language doctor books, those written in English for broader American audiences had similarly evolved from self-care manuals to guides for understanding symptoms to be treated by professional doctors. Among the American do-it-yourself manuals, Dr. J. C. Gunn's 1862 *New Domestic Physician or Book of Home Health* attained special popularity. Promising to provide in "familiar and plain terms the causes, symptoms, treatment and cure of the diseases incident to men, women and children," it gave specific directions "for using medicinal plants and the simplest and best new remedies." But by the mid-1800s, as similar hands-on, self-care manuals flooded the American market, doctors increasingly doubted their merit. Some even blamed doctor books for diminishing popular reverence for medicine. "It would be impossible to exaggerate the trouble or harm produced by domestic health manuals," charged Dr. Walter Channing in a lecture at Harvard University in 1845.[27]

As physicians developed professional guidelines for their field, they reevaluated the kind of information they wished the public to receive. Most felt a duty to provide doctor books to enlighten the public but increasingly concluded that such works should not contain information that might tempt readers to treat their own conditions. As a result, doctor books published in the last quarter of the 1800s gave specific advice only for handling emergencies and minor ills. While providing a wealth of theoretical information about how the body works, they urged the public to leave its treatment to trained professionals.

The *People's Home Medical Book* (1915) that was a mainstay in the Toronto, South Dakota, childhood home of Milton Sorenson (born 1917) occupies a middle-ground between the do-it-yourself manuals and Matthias Johnson's more theoretical book. "Realizing that not all diseases can be treated at home, we have endeavored to make it clear when a physician is necessary and have advised sending for him in such cases." At the same time the book claimed to include "the most valuable collection of simple home remedies ever published," being "gathered from all parts of the world" and "universally in use among the people."[28]

The patient-centered focus of *The People's Home Medical Book* must have appealed to the many Norwegian Americans who continued to rely on selfcare. "We did not have many medications around the house," said Lynn Sove Maxson (born 1943 in Chicago). "My mother believed in a lot of orange juice or tea with honey to cure just about everything."[29]

By the 1900s, most Norwegians no longer needed the help of pastors' wives or folk healers to decipher their doctor books. "Whenever anyone in the family took ill, out came the doctor book and with a certain amount of research, Mom came up with the right diagnosis," writes Paul Hanson (born 1923 in Geneva, Minnesota). "Being a sickly child," Hanson was the "recipient of many of the remedies suggested," such as "a tablespoon of sugar dissolved in kerosene" to open breathing passages constricted by bronchitis or the poultice "made of hot fried onions and fastened to the chest" to treat pneumonia. "For almost all things from slivers to boils to carbuncles and shingles," Hanson's mother relied on a poultice consisting of bread soaked in sour cream. With his foot wrapped in this concoction, Hanson says he "walked the halls in high school." Awkward, to be sure, but "it worked," declared Hanson in his Albert Lea *Evening Tribune* column on September 12, 1996. "And to this day it is a favorite of our family clan."[30]

Hanson's words suggest that besides curing illnesses, home remedies sometimes evoke fond memories. "I enjoyed thinking back with my sisters to our childhood and the home remedies which we can remember," writes Crystal Lokken (born 1929) from Berkeley, California. "I had to chuckle remembering having fried onions applied in a poultice to my chest as a child," echoes Norma Bondeson Gaffron (born 1931 in Minneapolis). "I don't know if the smell or the warmth was helpful in curing a cold," Gaffron continues, "but I'm sure one or the other was. When my own children were little I used a piece of quilted flannel as a poultice over Vicks Vaporub on their chests. I told them it looked so cute, and this piece of flannel became known as our 'cute.'"[31]

Crystal Lokken and her sisters remembered home remedies they used growing up in McFarland, Wisconsin, with their grandparents from Sogn. "They were mostly home remedies, not herbal ones. . . . Baking soda for beestings and brushing teeth and mustard plasters for putting on our chests when we had colds. Grandma sliced up onions and fried them for us to eat when we had colds and chest congestion, and a few drops of brandy eased a sore throat."

While a few of the more specialized treatments, including Anne Ludvikke Løberg's Sedativvand and Mrs. Wick's Olava salve, were passed along to the next generation, most concluded their usefulness with the people who depended on them. Yet, to the extent that their stories live on, these remedies continue to have value, whether evoking family memories or putting

a face on the people from the past. They help us see them as human beings who suffered illness and injury and battled their afflictions as best they
could. Illuminating that battle, the doctor books and their outdated remedies mirror the march of medicine's revolution while documenting how
long it took to reach the larger public.

6

Birthing Children
Do-it-yourself delivery

"Beata was pregnant. The baby was expected in February [1880].
As the time drew nearer, Maria dug out the 'doctor book,' a treatise on the delivery and care of babies written by a Norwegian
midwife. It had been their comfort and help when Gust was born,
and by the time February came, both Maria and Andreas knew
the book by heart."

Borghild Melbye, in Borghild,
a memoir from Clay County, Minnesota

O N BOTH SIDES OF THE ATLANTIC, nineteenth-century Norwegian
women faced childbirth with a combination of fear and fatalism. "Childbirth is like standing a piece of flatbread on edge," held an old adage from
Aust-Agder, "you never know which way it will fall [toward life or death]."
Childbirth claimed some mothers, but most deliveries proceeded successfully. Assisted by good neighbors, informed by the wisdom of ancestral ways,
and comforted by traditional rituals, most women survived the precarious
process of childbirth—before hospitals or professionally trained midwives
became the norm—to tell an often incredible tale.[1]

"No midwife, graduate nurse, or physician was in attendance," wrote Dr.
Carl M. Roan (1878–1946) of his mother's experience giving birth in the
Big Woods of McLeod County, Minnesota. "Just a neighbor woman came
in—that was all." Writing in 1946, this typical physician of his time marveled at what once was the normal state of affairs. Throughout the 1800s
Norwegian women on both sides of the Atlantic delivered each other's babies at home, only rarely seeking professional care. "Mother never had a

jordmor" (professionally trained midwife), says Ludvik A. Hope (born 1879), describing her situation in Norway. "It was Grandma and the neighbor women who delivered the babies, and amazingly enough, everything went just fine."[2]

By the time Roan wrote his memoir, doctors had taken control, and women commonly went to the hospital to deliver their babies. Families had also grown considerably smaller than the thirteen children Roan's mother bore between 1853 and 1880, each less than two years apart. Happily, neither Roan's mother nor any of her children died during birth, despite the heartbreaking statistic of seven women per thousand dying in the late 1850s (compared to one per ten thousand in the United States today).[3]

"No surgical equipment was at hand to repair any bodily damage suffered during childbirth," Roan continued, and "such conditions had to be endured for the rest of her days." Helen Olson Halversen (who was in her twenties when she bore her first child in Leland, Minnesota, around 1885) candidly confirmed in a 1969 interview that she had been "torn clear to the rectum. I actually never healed up. Even today!"[4]

Roan greatly admired his mother's endurance and referred to it in his professional writing. "The reader will kindly overlook the digression that I make [from a general discussion of childbirth in *Home, Church and Sex*, published in New York in 1930] by referring to the pioneer women of the Middle West during the later half of the past century. . . . I am familiar with this history, as my own mother was one of them. . . . [If their] hardships could be adequately pictured, there would be a chapter written about their suffering, their struggles, and their childbearing that would be in a class by itself."[5]

Both of Roan's parents emigrated from Valdres in 1852. Ole Johnson from Hedalen and Berit Eggen from Tolgen met in America and were married in 1854 in Wingville, Minnesota, by a justice of the peace, because no church or pastor was yet available. Settling in the vast tract of hardwood timber that extended 125 miles northeast of Chaska, Minnesota, the Johnsons made their home in Bergen Township, fifteen miles due east of Hutchinson, a new town being established. "Clearing the deep woods, breaking the prairie, hewing logs for a cabin, fighting the Indians, mosquitoes and poverty, sending the husband and father to war," he marveled. "In most instances they had to bear their children under circumstances not much better than those under which animals bear their young—without help or aid of any kind."

Childbirth proceeded in much the same way in Trysil, Norway, during the

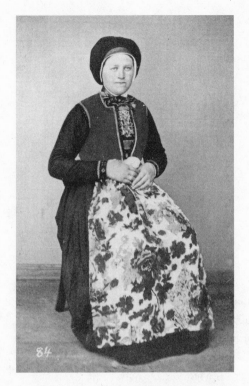

A young woman from Sammanger,
photographed in Bergen, about 1870
(*Photo by K. Knudsen*)

1850s, as Valborg Skåret (born 1910) wrote in a 1970 memoir of her grandmother's experience. "When they saw that the birth was close at hand, they
removed the bedding, which usually consisted of a ticking filled with hay,
or simply hay placed directly on the bed frame over a sheep or calf skin.
When this was removed and the boards washed, fresh spruce branches
were placed on the bed frame.... Then came a covering, usually some old
cloth that could be quite threadbare as long as it was clean. When the birth
was over, the bedding and greenery under the mother were removed and
replaced with fresh spruce branches and bedding that she would lie on as
long as necessary."[6]

HERB-ASSISTED CHILDBIRTH

In South and West Norway, pregnant women induced labor by
sitting on a steaming pail in which boiling water had been poured
over *høyfrø* ("hayseed," a common cure-all consisting of the seeds

of various herbs and grasses collected during haying). Women also encouraged contractions by rubbing themselves with pepper and other irritating agents mixed with milk or alcohol.

Of the various herbs used in childbirth, none played a more prominent role than the strongly scented *kamille* (chamomile, *Matriciani chamomile*). Norwegians used the daisy-like kamille for everything from soothing labor pains and stopping hemorrhage to treating postpartum depression. Chamomile roots resemble a uterus, and this similarity is reflected in its Latin name, *matriciani*, meaning "mother" or "womb." It was probably this resemblance that initially drew the attention of ancient midwives to chamomile, but its proven ability to reduce swelling and inflammation kept it in continuous use aiding childbirth the world over. Norwegian birthing assistants applied pouches of kamille flowers soaked in warm milk after the delivery to soothe the sore birth canal. The plant's high concentration of an anti-inflammatory agent known as azulene made it particularly effective.

In Norwegian tradition the stimulant known as *burot* (mugwort, *Artemisia vulgaris*) was both highly recommended—and strongly cautioned against. Midwives around the world have relied on mugwort for its ability to contract the uterus. Like chamomile, mugwort's Latin name suggests its use in childbirth, since Artemis, the Greek goddess of the hunt, was said to have helped her mother, Leto, deliver her twin brother, Apollo, shortly after her own birth. Norwegian lore advised using a sprig of the dark-green, sword-shaped burot leaves to strengthen the mother's contractions, but it also warned that prolonged exposure to burot could cause contractions so strong as to "expel the mother's intestines." Uncertain outcomes plagued the users of herbal cures but were particularly vexing in the case of burot, whose volatile oils and active ingredients varied radically according to the amount of rainfall, humidity, season, and storage time. A particular dose might not work at all or be fatally potent.

Mangor's Lande-apothek ⚜

Roan's memoir described the fourteen-by-twenty-foot, single-story cabin where a birth occurred, its logs mortared by mud and the rough floor and furniture made of hand-hewn, split logs. "The beds—oh yes, let us be frank—were made in like manner and blue muslin ticking provided the mattress bag containing hay, straw, corn leaves, and the like. Cooking utensils were few and scarce. The main trouble being that no money could be spared for the purchase of household goods. . . . Whatever equipment had been brought along from Norway was highly appreciated and utilized."[7]

Such desolate conditions naturally raised anxieties. "The anticipation of my wife to become a mother during the winter in this wilderness caused all but a pleasant feeling," wrote James O. Berdahl (born 1848), who had settled in a sod house not far from Sioux Falls, South Dakota, in the early 1870s. Fortunately, his wife's "dark hours of struggle" resulted in a "well matured and healthy" daughter, Christine, born in December 1873. By June 6, 1895, when Christine married Erick Langness, Mrs. Berdahl had given birth to eight more children, all but four of whom had died.[8]

Yet the Berdahls' "most severe and saddest grievance" still lay ahead. Christine, who was "in the family way," Berdahl said, fell ill with an extremely high fever. Doctors concluded her baby had died and was "decaying and poisoning her system." Thanks to the recent development of antiseptic surgery, the doctors could operate and remove the dead fetus. But Christine lingered for a few days with a fever of 105 degrees and died.

Death during pregnancy was far from uncommon. "Again we are called upon to announce the sad and hasty death of a young wife and mother," stated the October 10, 1884, obituary in the Blue Mounds, Wisconsin, *Weekly News* for Mrs. Lewis Gjesme (born 1861). At the age of twenty-three, she had died of eclampsia (convulsions caused by toxemia, a poisoning of the system) in her second pregnancy; she left behind a husband and one-year-old child.[9]

Newspaper obituaries and word of mouth added to women's uneasiness about approaching childbirth. Even thirteen-year-old Mary King (born 1869 in Fillmore County, Minnesota) grew alarmed upon hearing her mother was pregnant. "I knew what it meant by that time. Many of the women would talk in my presence and I began to worry for fear mother would die."[10]

Taking comfort

To calm fear and console sorrow, the Berdahls, like most other Norwegians, looked to their Christian faith. "In the midst of our grief we knew that our dear ones that were taken away by death were safely landed in the heavens above with their Lord and Savior . . . where with His Grace and blessing we shall meet them again."[11] A host of diaries, letters, and memoirs written by immigrants document a similarly steadfast faith that a heavenly afterlife would one day reunite the immigrants with each other and with those left behind in Norway.

Folk customs added their own comforts. Believing that women who died in childbirth were immediately transported to paradise, survivors placed baby clothes in the coffins of women who died undelivered so they could tend their infants when they were born in heaven.[12]

Mothers who survived the birth could look forward to the far more joyous custom of receiving *sengemat* (bed food), a tradition the immigrants continued in America. After Roan's mother bore her second child in October 1857, "the neighbor women came to see her and brought along *fløtegrøt* [sweet cream porridge], such as had been the custom on similar occasions in Norway."[13] Indeed, the well-established custom of bringing sengemat to new mothers dates at least to Viking times.

The popular custom became an integral part of the well-regulated pattern of socializing that characterized rural nineteenth-century Norway. Each farm belonged to an identified group of neighboring farms—the *grannelag*—whose inhabitants from landowner to laborer customarily "attended the funerals, weddings, and the like on all of the bordering farms," says Johan Liverød (born 1887 in Vestfold).[14] The grannelag also determined who brought porridge to a new mother. "When a child came into the world, every woman in the grannelag would come with a large container of *rømmegrøt* [sour cream porridge] so rich it fairly floated in butter," says Knut Eriksen Birkenes (born 1878 in Suldal). The women of the grannelag carried their rømmegrøt or fløtegrøt in an intricately carved or painted *ambar* (wooden container) painstakingly made by their husbands and often including a cleverly locking lid that also served as its carrying handle. Later in the century, fruit soup joined cream porridge as a favored dish neighbors most often brought to new mothers.[15]

 SENGEMAT IN SOUTH DAKOTA

The custom of bringing *sengemat* (bed food) continued well into the 1900s. Frieda Nowland tells of receiving sengemat in Aberdeen, South Dakota, in 1956.

Our first son was born just before Christmas. We were
not home from the hospital long before there was a knock
on the door of our tiny, second-floor apartment, and there
stood Gusta Holum with a gift for the new mother: a jar
of homemade fruit soup. She also gave firm instructions
that it was for me to eat, not for my husband and not for
visiting relatives.

Gusta was tall, stately and old—at least she seemed
old to me. I was in my early twenties. She said in pioneer
times fruit soup was always taken to new mothers.

I thanked her warmly for her thoughtful gift, but it was
several days later before I realized why this was such a
good "new mother" gift. The fruit soup was delicious and
nutritious. And worked as a very good natural laxative—
an excellent remedy before pills were so easily obtainable.

Ella Grunewald (born 1916 in Fergus Falls, Minnesota) notes how
the doctor's orders that a new mother lie in bed eight or nine days
increased the need for the laxative. Known as "*kjæring suppe*" in her
neighborhood, the fruit soup brought to new mothers consisted
of "water, sugar, dried prunes, raisins, apricots, apples, cinnamon
and tapioca." Good nutrition, a needed laxative, and the welcome
warmth of friendship—sengemat provided them all. No wonder
this cozy custom lasted so long.

Letters to the author, 2004 ❧

With the gift of sengemat, women both celebrated and commiserated
with the new mother. Sometimes they also pitched in to do necessary chores,
said Martha Myrvold (born 1886 in Modum, Buskerud), recalling a time
she and her mother went to visit their neighbor who had just given birth to
twin boys: "The churn was standing on the floor with cream in it, so Mother
churned the butter for her. The woman was lying in the small side room off
the main room, and in the main room stood the husband's planing bench on
one side and the loom on the other."[16]

Myrvold's description captures the gender-specific labor of the self-
sufficient, nineteenth-century Norwegian farm. The husband made all the
farm's tools and implements, constructed and repaired the buildings, and

cured the animal skins and hides. His wife, meanwhile, tended the livestock, wove all the clothes and other textiles used on the farm, prepared
the food, and—of course—bore children, who, at an early age, would begin
helping with the chores appropriate to their gender. Work-related activities
dominated the small dwellings.

The porridge that came to these dwellings, said Myrvold, "had to have
a lot of fat, sugar, and cinnamon," for its quality reflected the reputation of
the one who brought it. Originally, only women participated in the sengemat custom; they came in small groups of two or three beginning on the
second or third day after birth.

When immigrants continued the sengemat tradition in America, no
regulated pattern of neighborhood socializing existed. Instead, neighbors
practiced the custom spontaneously. "If a baby was born a mile or so away
over the prairies," wrote Erling Ylvisaker in *Eminent Pioneers*, "Mrs. Ellestad
(born 1841 in Valdres) found both time and means to cook a kettle of nourishing 'rømmegrøt' for the mother."[17]

On the prairie, men occasionally took part in the visit as well, as Roan
once did himself, finding it "a fine custom": "I can remember very well that
in the 1890s when I was a boy, I accompanied mother to a neighbor's place
to carry the basket containing the fløtegrøt. It was a peculiar job for a lad to
do, but it was exhilarating and interesting."[18]

Colliding cultures: The district doctor and sengemat

Roan's positive attitude toward sengemat contrasts with the approach recommended by district doctor Michael Krohn (1822–97) of Ytre Nordhordland
on Norway's west coast near Bergen. "I am truly sorry to have to forbid
the so-called 'konemat' [wife food], which as a rule consists of rømmegrøt,
no less—when available—and which every neighbor woman feels duty-
bound to bring, from the very first day after the delivery," Krohn declared
in an April 1861 lecture on child care.[19] Krohn's social background often put
him at odds with the population of his district. As a product of Bergen's
upper-middle class (his father was a prominent merchant and his uncle the
founder of a bank and steamship line), Krohn found the almue's customs
foreign and backward.

Contemporary conditions influenced Krohn's attitude as well. Diseases
ran unchecked in western Norway at the time he held his post (1855–61),

and doctors were making a concerted effort to control the leprosy that flourished along the coast and to stem shockingly high rates of child and infant mortality. Leprosy would remain mysterious even after Armauer Hansen (born 1841 in Bergen) discovered the leprosy bacillus in 1873, but Krohn and his colleagues thought they knew what caused the high rate of childhood mortality: "peasant carelessness."

Attempting to scold the peasants into reform, Krohn castigated their traditions, not least the beloved sengemat. Instead of eating "too rich" porridge, he chided, new mothers should "at most" eat "sugar rusks, white bread, or pastries (kringler)." (Nutritionists today would hardly see Krohn's choices as a great improvement.) Even these foods, he insisted, she did not need: "In the blood that has nourished the child and of which only a small amount is lost during birth, nature has provided nutrients for the first four to five days. During this time, moreover, the woman's system must be brought back to normal functioning, and all disturbance of it avoided." (The good doctor had clearly never given birth.) "Make a big kettle of porridge!" entreated Kari from Oppdal after delivering her child during the 1850s. "I'm so weak and empty there's hardly anything left of me."[20] Krohn would have denied Kari's request and barred the door to her porridge-bearing neighbors: "Such visits tire, disquiet, and harm the mother for whom as little company as possible is best."

But new mothers welcomed these visits. Some even reciprocated by serving their guests a little brennevin (hard liquor), as Lars Skjeldsø reported from Øvre Gjerstad in Agder: "The new mother would often have a bottle of French cognac ready for her delivery . . . to offer a dram to the hjelpekone [birth helper]—who was, after all, the first to bring her porridge. She would also serve some to the other women who came bearing gifts of porridge a couple of days later."[21]

But Krohn had other ideas: "During the first 4 to 5 days the birthing mother should have only a light drink, such as sour milk mixed with water [known as blande, the daily drink in rural nineteenth-century Norway], barley soup or a little elderberry and chamomile tea." On the fifth day after the birth, the new mother could begin eating more nourishing food, Krohn stipulated, "if she is careful." But never must she change to ordinary food "until she gets up from bed between the eighth and tenth day."

The nine-days-abed routinely prescribed by Krohn and other district doctors may have been possible among the privileged class, but few peasants

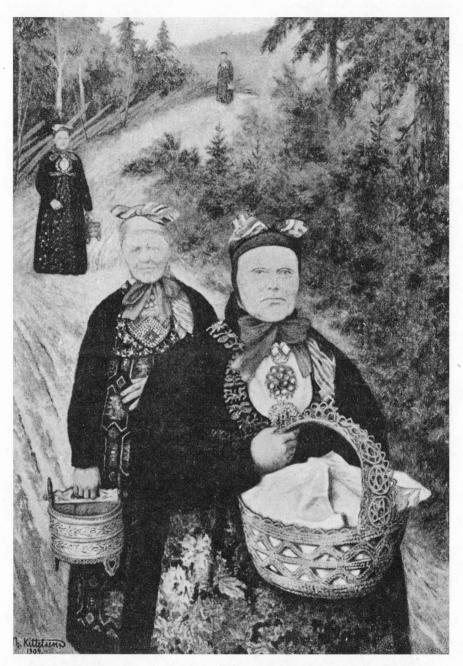

Women dressed in their own local *bunad* (festive clothing) bring *sengemat* (bed food) to a new mother. The first carries a birch-root basket with baked goods, while the others carry carved wooden *ambar* holding porridge in Theodore Kittelsen's *Grautkjerringer* (Porridge ladies).

had the luxury. The chores of farm, forest, and fishing required the work of all hands. In Oppdal, for example, they told of neighbors taking "sengemat to a new mother the third day after she delivered" only to find her "out in the field, spreading manure."[22]

Immigrant mothers followed suit. On the fifth day after Roan's mother bore her second child in 1857, "Beret was up taking care of her household duties." Writing in the 1940s, Roan would have preferred the eight to ten days Krohn prescribed, while today's doctors advocate the peasants' more abbreviated bed rest, if not the manure spreading. "What puts women in an early grave or robs them of their health," Krohn countered, "is getting up from child bed irresponsibly early." What Krohn called irresponsible was the almue's inescapable necessity.

"Above all," continued Krohn, "the mother needs calm after the birth. All the unnecessary and harmful chatter, to which the almue are so inclined, must be strictly forbidden."[23] Unable to take the prescribed nine days of recovery, the almue were *unwilling* to give up the custom of bringing sengemat to new mothers because these visits were ingrained in the culture. Their so-called "unnecessary chatter" afforded the new mother a welcome opportunity to visit with more experienced women who could ease uncertainties about the unsettling—and once terrifying—time between birth and baptism.

Between birth and baptism

Because the short time between birth and baptism was believed to influence a newborn's future, the almue carefully observed rituals to ensure a positive future. The phrase "*Er du ikke riktig navla?* (Wasn't your umbilical cord cut right?)" is still heard in Norway in response to a stupid question or idiotic mistake. Though said in jest, the expression derives from an old belief about the importance of properly cutting the umbilical cord. After a birth, the *hjelpekone* (birth helper) placed the infant between the mother's legs to rest until the pulse in the cord had almost stopped. Then she tied off the cord with thread in two places and cut between the ties at a right angle, never diagonally, for that could make the child "not right" or cause otherwise inexplicable developmental defects.

The afterbirth or placenta required ritual treatment, as well. Before burning or burying it, Norwegian peasants traditionally scored it with a cross to prevent its return as a ghost. When the remnant of the umbilical cord fell off, they burned it, too, to keep it away from the *huldrefolk* (hidden people) or witches who might use it to gain control over the child.

Belief in the huldrefolk slowly waned in the nineteenth century, but it inspired enduring practices such as swaddling. After bathing the newborn child, the birth assistant swaddled it, first by covering it with several small cloths and inserting a large wad of very absorbent, unwashed wool between its legs. Then she wrapped the baby in a larger, thin, homespun cloth, kept in place by winding a long, narrow, handwoven band around the infant several times around. Most infants were similarly *reivet* (swaddled) during the first four to six months of life.

Doctors and pastors decried swaddling as child abuse. They reported seeing steam rising from the soaked cloths when the bands were infrequently untied. They accused parents of tying the swaddling bands so tight that they left permanent marks on the child's skin and impeded proper bone development.

Though these criticisms were not unwarranted, the exquisite care intended by swaddling—and the trembling fear that motivated it—emerge in these directions from Engerdalen, Østerdal: "The swaddling band [*lind*] should be seven *alner* [about fourteen feet] long, neither more nor less, in order to prevent harm from befalling the child. Sew in one end a silver shilling, and a needle in the other. When wrapping the band around the child, be sure to wind it three times below the knees, just one time around the thighs and three times around the waist. Place the child's arms so they lie in a cross and tie the band so it, too, forms a cross over both chest and back."[24] The magical numbers three and seven, protective metal, and the sign of the cross provided a potent arsenal of defense against the huldrefolk, a fortress only reluctantly removed.

When changing the swaddling clothes, parents may have applied a soothing powder to the baby's skin. They made this powder by grinding the bark of fir trees exceedingly fine and adding *makkemjøl*, the absorbent "worm flour" that the almue collected and saved for this purpose.[25]

Norwegians continued to swaddle their babies well into the 1890s, according to Martina Søilen (born 1885 in Voss). By then, though, magic had apparently given way to practicality, for her description no longer includes the ritually protective numbers, crosses, or metal: "First they wrapped the child in some raw sheep's wool held in place with a handwoven band, five-six alen [ten-to-twelve feet] long. They left the infant's bottom outside this wrapping, covering it with a couple of woolen cloths they called *tjeld*. This enabled them to change the infant without taking off the *lind* [woven swaddling band] and redoing all the wrappings."[26] Supernatural protections gradually became less important toward the end of the century, while cleanliness became more important.

Still, swaddling had much to recommend it. Lanolin in the unwashed wool soothed the infant's skin, and the practice eased transport in a landscape too rugged for a baby buggy. "When the mother went somewhere," said Marta Myrvold, "she would tie the firmly packed infant to her back, where it could rest securely as she walked."[27]

Many mothers also thought swaddling would keep their infants from developing bowed legs. They "swaddled their children and tied the bands tight," said Valborg Skåret, whose mother bore her first child in Gudbrandsdal in 1895. But Skåret's mother was "ahead of her time in many ways, and did not follow suit." She remembered, "One day three well-meaning women came to Mother's house and told her that if she didn't swaddle her child, it would be deformed, developing crooked arms and legs. Mother thanked them for their advice and then did as she herself thought best."[28]

While swaddling could not straighten limbs crippled by rickets, it did keep infants from falling out of the cradle. This was no frivolous concern when the cradle was suspended from the ceiling, as Martina Søilen (born 1885) recalled from her neighbors' cabin near Voss. "They had a long birch rod supported by a couple of willow bindings attached to the ceiling. A rope suspended from the rod held an oblong wooden box, where the woman placed her child. Pulling on another rope attached to the box rocked the child to sleep. A rope could also raise and lower the box, which hung in about the middle of the room."[29]

Hanging cradles saved floor space, always at a premium in the one-room cabin. They also made less noise than cradles that rocked on the floor, as district doctor Johannes Gotaas wrote when he recommended them in an 1859 article for *Folkevennen* (The people's friend, a magazine of popular enlightenment).[30]

By day, infants lay in the cradle usually rocked by an older sibling, but at night, says Hans A. Baastad (born 1888 in Trøgstad, Østfold), "the mother felt it safest to have the child with her in bed." This practice, like so many others, derived from the almue's fear of the huldrefolk, but sometimes exacted a dreadful price.[31]

"There are many cases of the child being *ligget i hjel* [slept to death, or suffocated] by the mother" when she rolled over it in her sleep, reported

Gotaas in 1859. Such accidents happened commonly enough to warrant preventative rituals. In Vest-Agder, "they read the Lord's Prayer over the child as soon as it was born so the parents would not 'liggja det ihel' in the bed." Yet despite the danger, many parents refused to leave the child in the cradle at night, the danger of capture by the huldrefolk apparently outweighing possible suffocation.

A similar calculation justified the sheep shears found in many an infant cradle as recently as the childhood of Ludvik A. Hope (born 1879 in Masfjorden). "As soon as a newborn was placed in the cradle, they put either a hymnal or shears under the pillow to keep the child from becoming a *bytting* (changeling), or kidnapped by the huldrefolk and exchanged for one of their own off-spring. I remember well that my grandmother always did this."[32] Any cuts or discomfort the rough, wrought-iron shears might inflict did not measure up to the protection they provided against the huldrefolk.

Fortunately, the postbirth interval of imminent danger passed quickly. "As soon as the child was baptized, the huldrefolk were helpless to cause it harm," said Hope. Parents took their infants to be baptized as soon as possible, "often the day after the child was born." This was no easy matter, because weather, climate, rough terrain, and long distances to parish churches often made for a treacherous journey. Yet these perils, too, paled in comparison to the ultimate protection baptism would provide.

Baptism

"In fear of the child being exchanged and without consideration for season or weather," complained Krohn in his 1856 annual report, "they rush the child to church. For this reason, regrettably, children have frozen to death on the baptismal journey." "Unbelievable carelessness," charged Krohn. Protection from the huldrefolk, belonging to family and community, and an eternal life in heaven, believed the almue.[33]

Risking a final opportunity for the huldrefolk to steal the unbaptized child, the trip to baptism was fraught with hazard. Protecting the infant was the principal function of the baptismal sponsors, usually five or six in number during the nineteenth century. The child's decorative clothing had the same function. Embroidered with crosses and fastened with pewter, the long dress or swaddling clothes might also feature a silver brooch or a pocket to conceal the extra safeguard of a silver coin or darning needle. Before the baptismal party set out for the church, some parents made the sign of a cross with a burning branch over the child and recited the Lord's Prayer.[34]

Uneasiness about the baptismal journey—and even about taking the unbaptized infant outside—long remained part of Norwegian and Norwegian American culture. "I recall how anxious I was about driving from Waterloo, Iowa, to my home church near Black Earth, Wisconsin, to have our first-born baptized in 1951," writes Ann Urnes Gesme, now of Cedar Rapids, Iowa. "It seemed to be a tradition that babies in our family were baptized at about six weeks—and it was critical to have it done as soon as possible 'in case something happened.' At any rate, I felt greatly relieved when Butch was safely baptized. Tradition dies hard among us!"[35] Though Lutheran doctrine stipulated that unbaptized infants who died went directly to heaven, in practice only the completed baptismal ritual made parents feel secure.

Baptismal water, besides removing the danger of kidnapping by the huldrefolk, had medicinal value, some parents believed, and they kept it on hand to treat childhood skin rashes, warts, and even consumption or rickets. Collecting a small quantity of the water after the service was among the duties of the baptismal sponsors. During the ceremony, sponsors accepted responsibility for the child's Christian upbringing, thus joining the strands of folk belief and Christianity in the fabric of traditional lore.[36]

For immigrants who longed to continue these rites in America, it was "a momentous occasion," wrote Roan, when an "ordained pastor with collar and gown in the same style as they had known in Norway arrived in Bergen Township. Pastor Bernt J. Muus organized the Bergen congregation in 1860, riding the 120 miles from Holden parish in Goodhue County to Bergen Township on horseback "over roads as yet scarcely worthy of the name. His coming meant a great deal to the Norwegian settlers anxious over the lack of baptismal opportunities for their children, a considerable number having already been born in the settlement."[37] Among these children were two of Roan's siblings, born in 1857 and 1859, whose baptism was "significantly delayed by the absence of a pastor to perform the rite." Worry about the lack of protection for their children must have weighed heavily on the early settlers, though as the century progressed and old beliefs began to fade, the interval between birth and baptism gradually lengthened among Norwegians on both sides of the Atlantic.

Baptism conferred the child's name, a choice often determined by tradition.

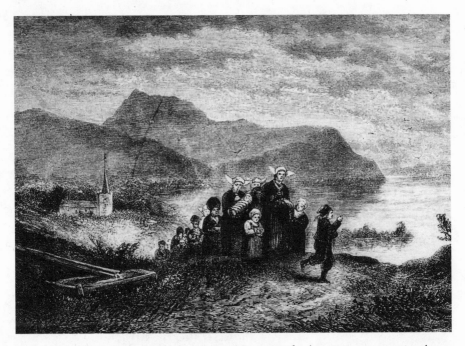

A baptismal procession winds above a west Norwegian fjord in 1879, accompanying the securely swaddled and protected infant.

In the names they chose, Roan saw "evidence of the emigrants' high regard for their parents," perhaps not realizing the powerful folk beliefs that enforced those choices. "*Navnet følger slekten*" (the name follows the family), tradition decreed, and Norwegians had for centuries strictly followed the custom of naming the first son after his *farfar* (father's father), the second son after his *morfar* (mother's father), the first daughter after her *farmor*, and the second daughter after her *mormor*. Many parents continued this custom well into the twentieth century, if only by using the appropriate grandparent's initials.

After grandparents were *oppkalt* (honorifically named), other relatives had to be honored as well. Oppkalling often outweighed other considerations, to the extent that several siblings in one family received the same name, distinguished, for example, as *Store-Ole, Mellom-Ole,* and *Lille-Ole* (Big, Middle, and Little Ole).

The belief that the dead could haunt the living and influence their choice of a name helped to enforce honorific naming. The person wanting to be

oppkalt might appear in a parent's dreams, and going against the appari-
tion's wishes could make a child sicken and even die. Ghost stories enforced
this belief. In Møre, for example, they told about Johanne Ellingsdatter
Roppen, who lived on the coast at Ulstein. Two boats from her neighborhood were lost in a terrible storm during the 1850 winter cod fishing, and
not long afterward a man wearing fisherman's garb appeared in Johanne's
dreams, walking around the cradle of her unbaptized son. Johanne knew
the dream meant she should name her child for one of the lost fishermen,
but she named the baby as she had planned. Soon the child's health began
to fail, "and he was retarded to the end of his days."[38]

Revenge of this sort was considered sufficiently common to warrant
black-book formulas specifically for curing "children who are sick due to the
haunting of a ghost who was going after its name." A formula recorded in
1889 in Nordland advised: "Carve the name the child should have had on a
piece of wood and throw it into the sea if the deceased who wanted to be
oppkalt was lost at sea, or bury it in the churchyard if it is there he lies. It
also helps to carve or write the name on the back of the church altar."[39]

The high mortality rate in nineteenth-century Norway provided plenty
of material for ghost stories and affected naming customs in other ways as
well, since infants customarily received the name of recently deceased siblings.
When the family of Nina Mathieu (born 1908 in Mayville, North Dakota)
continued the honorific naming tradition in America, they met with an un-
anticipated result. Nina's sister, Vivien Lenore (born 1921), died at age two,
when Nina was a teen. Nina writes: "We missed our baby a lot; the house did
not seem the same without her. But that fall, we were blessed with another
little girl. Dad [Ivar K. Johnson, who emigrated in 1889] said when she was
born that he knew they would have another little girl because of a dream he
had after our baby died. In his dream he was told they would get another
girl who would be very healthy and was to have the same name as the baby
who died. So Dad insisted on giving her the same name." The second Vivien
Lenore grew up healthy, writes Mathieu, though she had "difficulty when applying for a Social Security number. They said she was dead!"[40]

Infant mortality

A defective heart claimed the first Vivien, but infectious diseases accounted
for most of what immigrant historian Hjalmar Rued Holand (1872–1963)

called the "frightful and virtually beyond belief" mortality of infants and children in pioneer settlements. "As in the land of Egypt, there was hardly a house in which death did not strike. More than half of all the deaths in the early settlement years were of small children under one year."[41]

The children of the James O. Berdahl family of Sioux Falls, South Dakota, personify the dreadful statistics. Albert Oliver was born on January 31, 1876, "strong and healthy," but, "stricken down with that dreaded croup disease," he died on February 16, 1879. Kari Olina, born on December 10, 1877, "matured to be a strong and healthy child, but at the age of nearly six years old, was taken with that dreadful Diphtheria Croup disease and died December 6, 1883." Anna Torina, born on February 16, 1880, "got along very nicely until the age of three," when she caught the measles and died on March 4, 1883. Alma Constance, born on December 19, 1881, "the Lord in his wisdom selected to take in the early stage of her life to his Heavenly home." And for Anne Mathilde, born January 21, 1892, "providence had similarly destined only a short stay at the parental home," before she died of lung fever on February 5, 1896. Ultimately, only four of the nine children born to the Berdahls survived childhood, and one of the four, Christine, died in pregnancy at age twenty-four. At the time Berdahl wrote his family history in 1941, only two children were still alive, John Edward (born 1883) and Carrie Hellena (born 1887). Berdahl hoped they might be "spared to assist us in our declining years and be with us when our Lord and Savior calls us to his Heavenly home."[42]

As typical as the death rate of Berdahl's children was his view that "providence had destined" their deaths. Physicians on both sides of the Atlantic decried the "irresponsible passivity" of this kind of fatalism because it kept the almue from seeking medical care. Yet, considering the meager means doctors had to fight infectious disease before the 1880s, professional help would likely have done little to forestall these deaths.[43]

The statistics Hjalmar Holand collected in Upper Coon Valley, Wisconsin, show that thirteen of the fifteen deaths recorded in 1874 were of children, and 86 percent (114 of 133) of all deaths between 1861 and 1870 were of children under the age of five. Holand blamed the lack of medical care but also cited the mothers' exhaustion and the tiny homes where "fresh air was a rarity and cleanliness was often unknown." These conditions made preserving food especially difficult. "It was awful hard to keep the milk sweet, with no ice, no nothing," confirmed Helen Olson Halvorsen (born 1863), whose twins, born in Leland, Minnesota, in the late 1880s lived only four months.[44]

Cholera, diarrhea, and typhoid fever, all caused by the contamination of food or water, accounted for most childhood deaths during the early years of settlement. In the later decades of the nineteenth century, epidemics of diphtheria, scarlet fever, and whooping cough often claimed several children at a time. Bearing silent witness to these tragedies, headstones divided into two, three, and even four sections still stand in the churchyards of many old Norwegian American churches, registering multiple deaths that left no time for separate markers.

DIPHTHERIA STRIKES A FRONTIER FAMILY

On June 22, 1876, the *Glencoe* (Minnesota) *Register* reported the death of four siblings:

> We are sorry to learn that Mr. Ole Johnson of Bergen Township has lost two of his children within the last ten days—a boy and a girl, and several others of the family are reported very sick with Diphtheria.
>
> Since writing the above, we have met Mr. Johnson, and learned from him that two more of his children are dead. The ages of the four which have been so suddenly taken from his hitherto unbroken family of eleven children were respectively eleven, five, three, and one year old. All the other children—eight—are now sick with this fearful disease, and two of them we understand are considered dangerously ill. Mr. Johnson is one of Bergen's earliest settlers. Himself and family are very much respected by his neighbors, all of whom deeply sympathize with him and Mrs. Johnson in their great loss.
>
> When diphtheria appears in its malignant form, it is one of the most dangerous of diseases, and demands for its treatment the best-trained medical skill. As soon as its symptoms appear, not a moment should be lost in calling a physician. The symptoms are sore throat, swelling of the glands behind the jaws, fever, headache, rapid pulse,

bad breath, thick yellowish deposits of exudations in the
tonsils and in the throat. Diphtheria is a blood disease, and
not as most people suppose, a merely local inflammation of
the throat. The causes which produce it are generally to be
found about the place where it appears. We fear its spread
in Bergen will not be confined to Mr. Johnson's family.

"The art of healing was groping in the dark," Dr. Carl Roan observed in his 1946 memoir. Less than ten years after Roan's siblings
were suffocated by the membrane that closed the throats of diphtheria victims, however, Edwin Klebs described the bacterium that
caused the disease, and in 1884 Friedrich Loeffler cultivated it, work
that opened the door for the production of an antitoxin that Roan
concluded "saved thousands of children every year."

Carl Roan, *"The Immigrant Wagon"* ⮨

In Norway, child mortality rates were tragically high, too. "Between one
in four and one in seven children die before their first birthday," observed
Krohn in an 1861 lecture on child care. Contaminated food and water fos-
tered the spread of disease, and overcrowding in one-room dwellings made
matters worse. "The child shares its quarters with the entire household,"
wrote district doctor Gotaas in 1859, "in the midst of all manner of cooking,
wet clothing being dried, meals being eaten, and without any satisfactory
measures being taken to provide fresh air or cleanliness."

Krohn blamed these deplorable conditions on the mothers' indifference to
the lives of their children and to ignorance. "They either don't want to aban-
don the customs of their ancestors or they don't know any better." Krohn
naturally felt frustrated by the almue's reluctance to adopt the measures his
training had taught him would save lives. But if he could have viewed the
customs through the eyes of the almue, he might have seen less negligence
than painstaking care defeated by poverty.

Krohn scolded almue parents for feeding their newborns cream and
porridge instead of putting them immediately to the breast. "Thinking they
can never get enough fat into the little one, they stuff the weak infant stomach with thick *fløte* [cream], *rømme* [sour cream] and *rømmegrøt*, when they
possibly can." "Milk soup or milk porridge must wait until the child is about
a year old," Krohn countered, advising that if mother's milk was lacking, it

should be replaced by cow's milk diluted by boiled water with a little sugar added.[45]

Krohn asked why the almue gave infants something so hard to digest as rømmegrøt. Explained an experienced midwife from Valdres, where the custom also prevailed, "It was fine-fine food, celebration fare." Though she herself fed infants as Krohn prescribed, "in earlier times many people would have thought that simply was not suitable, almost like giving the child nothing at all." Far from intending abuse, the almue were welcoming the child with the very best they could manage.[46]

If Norwegian mothers delayed the onset of breast-feeding, in part to test the infant's chance of surviving, they more than made up for it by extending the practice beyond limits now considered customary. Reports from nineteenth-century Sunnhordland and Setesdal tell of children feeding at the breast until age ten, though two or three years was more common. A nationwide study conducted in 1910 showed that breast-feeding for two or three years was still not unusual.[47]

Many believed that prolonged breast-feeding strengthened the child. Yet, as Norwegian American Travis Cleveland of Worth County, Iowa, reported, the custom could have its awkward moments: "Great-grandpa Herbrand Langeberg Olsen, who spent his initial eight years around Flå in Hallingdal before emigrating with his people [in 1853], related later in life his experience with breast-feeding. This, he said, continued until he was quite ambulatory, causing mild embarrassment when visiting friends around Flå. In those instances, his mother would excuse herself and young Herbrand, adjourning to an outbuilding so that he might feed."[48]

Embarrassing as it may have been for the older child, extended breast-feeding valuably augmented the limited food supply. It also provided a measure of birth control when mothers had few if any other means.

Before nursing bottles were available, Norwegian women used rams' horns "hollowed and scraped out thin, and thoroughly cleaned," said Valborg Skåret, describing the practice her grandmother followed in the 1860s. "In the tip of the horn they made a little opening about the diameter of a knitting needle. Then they filled the horn with the milk mixture and stopped up the mouth of the horn with a 'bung' of wood. The child got the tip of the horn with its tiny opening in its mouth and nursed away."[49]

For thicker foods they used nursing horns that had a "larger opening in the tip covered by a thin cloth that was secured by a groove carved a little below the opening." The horn was then filled with thin porridge that the child sucked through the cloth. "They always found *råd for uråd* [solutions for the unsolvable]," wrote Skåret, admiring her grandmother's generation, who Krohn criticized for "filling the horns with thick porridge, liver, fish, and smearing it all with syrup."[50] Parenting skills no doubt varied widely, then as now, but reading the district doctors' reports alone, one would conclude that almue parents were incompetent or cruel.

Krohn surely opposed the custom of "giving the infants *tygge* [chew]" that Martha Myrvold termed "very common." Parents "put food in their own mouths, chewed it well, and then fed it to the child." "Think of the germs!" exclaimed Skåret's mother, born in the 1890s just as germ theory was taking hold. Myrvold (born 1886 in Modum, Buskerud) saw the practice more positively: "The mother chewed ordinary dinner food, then put it into the mouth of the youngster, who shrieking and waving its arms and legs, couldn't take it in fast enough." Feeding the child as she ate her own meal, the mother also gave it a bottle or the breast afterwards, said Myrvold. "It didn't matter which; there was never talk of children not eating, and they grew good and round and healthy."[51]

Breast-feeding remained common on the prairie, where the traditional seating pattern used in Norwegian churches—men on the right side of the center aisle, women on the left—also continued. (In preindustrial Norwegian society, men and women operated largely within their own separate spheres, dividing not only work but also social and religious activities distinctly by gender.) Nina Mathieu links these two seemingly unrelated practices in her description of the Hoff Church in Mayville, North Dakota, in the early 1900s: "Mom told us the reason ladies always sat on one side was because some had to travel quite a ways to go to church and babies would get hungry. With ladies sitting on one side, it gave them more privacy to nurse their babies. Most nursing mothers wore a shawl over their shoulders to cover the baby while nursing."[52]

The poverty that also characterized preindustrial Norway emerges in Dr. Krohn's description of the farms in his district as "small" with "poor pastures" and "rarely suited to efficient implements." The farmers had an exceedingly modest standard of living with "less than nourishing" food, he observed, since "the beef, pork, butter, and cheese they produce goes to Bergen to pay taxes and obtain the bare necessities."[53] Yet if peasants had to forgo nourishing food to make ends meet, they clearly could not afford the professional health care Krohn constantly urged them to obtain. Trained to know the benefits of such care, Krohn nevertheless regarded the peasants' behavior as ill-advised penny-pinching motivated by an "exaggerated concern for the shilling and understated concern for their health."

Resisting Krohn's exhortations in general, the almue especially refused his entreaties to replace their self-trained *hjelpekoner* (birth helpers) with the officially appointed, formally educated *jordmor* (midwife). Even if they could have afforded her services, most rural Norwegians saw no reason to alter the traditional custom of helping each other through childbirth. Nor could the professional midwives cover the enormous districts they were appointed to serve.

Midwives: Self-taught or professionally trained?

The district midwife for Ytre Nordhordland lived in Lindås parish, much too far for most residents to reach in time of need. In 1864 she assisted only twenty-four of the district's 450 births, wrote Michael Krohn's successor, Thomas Collett (1835–88). "The midwife's activity is significantly hindered," Collett added in 1869, "by being summoned only in case of dire emergency and then getting the blame when such difficult births result in lasting debility."[54]

Despite these challenges, more than a thousand Norwegian women trained to be professional midwives during the nineteenth century. Most attended the one-year course offered by the *Fødselsstiftelse* (birth institute) in Christiania after 1818. By 1861 similar training became available at the Fødselsstiftelse in Bergen. Midwifery provided the first professional training available for women, who had to wait until the 1870s to train to become teachers, telegraphists, or nurses.[55]

"Potential pupils must be between twenty and thirty years old," the midwifery school stipulated, "have a testimonial for virtue from their parish pastor, another for physical suitability from their doctor, and no skin rashes or deformity that would arouse fear or disgust in the birthing mother."[56] The school especially encouraged peasant women to apply, offered extra education in reading and writing in the evenings, and made the year-long course available to all women, regardless of their ability to pay. Initially able to admit only twelve pupils a year, the school only slowly filled the district midwifery appointments established in 1810.

During the first years of its existence, the Fødselsstiftelse frequently moved, but it found its final home on Akersgate in 1837. The pupils rented rooms in town, but took turns living at the school, rising at six in the winter and five in the summer to maintain the facilities and tend patients. In 1844, F. C. Faye (1806–90), the institute's founder, wrote its first textbook.

The midwife, he instructed, should carry in her bag a scissors and thread for the umbilical cord, a silver catheter and syringe to empty the mother's bladder and colon before delivery, bloodletting equipment for mothers who were hypertensive or experiencing great pain, Hoffmann's drops to rouse lethargic infants, and a bandage for the birth canal.[57] Once the midwife had arrived at the mother's home, she should secure some oil or fat for her hands to ease the internal examinations she would perform on the mother. She should also find a basin, cold water and vinegar for the syringes and bandages, and hot water for hand washing and bathing the infant.

First, wrote Faye, the jordmor should comfort and encourage the mother. Then the jordmor should examine the mother internally to determine the progress of the birth. When the mother's water broke, the jordmor was to examine her again to see which part of the baby was entering the pelvis and consider calling the doctor if it was not the back of the head (although many midwives learned to manually turn the baby in the womb). During birthing, she should support the skin around the birth canal to keep it from tearing and, when the head emerged, ensure that the umbilical cord was not around the baby's neck and that its mouth and nose were unobstructed.

After cutting the umbilical cord, the jordmor should examine the mother for a second baby, then deliver the placenta, pulling hard on the umbilical cord if necessary to encourage the process. Popular custom allowed the birthing mother a hardy supply of *brennevin* (hard liquor), leading the pastor of Spydeberg, J. N. Wilse, to complain in 1779: "Women in childbirth are given such profuse amounts of brennevin that many a man's proper wife ends up a drunkard." Given the lack of available anesthetics, this practice had understandable appeal, but Faye advised against giving any pain-killing medications.[58]

The professional midwives' refusal to give the mother brennevin ranked among the reasons the almue resisted them, and so did their insistence that the mother deliver in bed. "The almue have the belief that a woman can never give birth in bed, insisting to be on the floor," wrote Krohn in 1856. "The people of this parish share this belief with so many others, that I would have been surprised if they did it any other way." The Norwegian word for "midwife," *jordmor* (earth mother), derives from this practice, as does *liggja á golfui* (lying on the floor), the term the Vikings used for childbirth.[59]

"My grandmother delivered several children on her knees," said a woman from Nissedal in Telemark. "And when a professional midwife first came to the community and wanted her to lie in bed for the birth, she thought it would put an end to her." Helen Olson Halvorsen (born 1863) preferred kneeling, too. She married her husband in Blaire, Wisconsin, in 1884 and moved to the tiny town of Leland, Minnesota, where in 1895 she bore her first child, Clarence. Together with a self-trained midwife, young Clarence soon attended the birth of his sister: "When Clarence was two years old, Henrietta was born. Mrs. Bronsted, an old woman who had lots of children, was taking care of me. I was on my knees by the side of the bed because it goes faster that way, I think. Little Clarence crawled down there out of bed. He looked around and said, 'Hello, Baby!'"[60]

Other nineteenth-century Norwegian women gave birth while sitting in their husbands' laps, according to an observer (born 1865) from Askvoll in Sogn and Fjordane: "Around 1870 or 1875 there were no official midwives here. Grandfather had a sister who acted as a *hjelpekone* (self-trained assistant). She had delivered seventy babies in her time, including me. A woman giving birth had always to sit on the lap of her husband or another man. The hjelpekone sat in front of her on a chair to assist the birth. . . . Until I was about seven years old it was common to see children being born this way. Then the professionally trained midwives came. After that the mother had to lie in bed."[61] Most professional midwives changed the traditional birthing position to one that their training had taught them afforded greater convenience and efficiency.

As late as 1866, Professor Faye observed, professionally trained midwives assisted at only half of all births. That same year authorities divided Norway into more manageable midwifery districts. In towns and cities, upper-class women increasingly used professional midwives as they became available, but in rural areas the jordmor continued to be little used and underpaid. As late as 1883, the professional jordmor in Bygland, Setesdal, for example, still assisted only twelve of the sixty births recorded.[62]

The almue did not want to lose their accustomed practices, nor could they see any advantage in calling the professional jordmor. If the delivery stalled, for example, the jordmor, no less than the self-trained hjelpekone, had to

The classic textbook of obstetrics by F. C. Faye, first published in Christiania in 1844 and reissued several times, was much used by Norwegians on both sides of the Atlantic. *(Photo by Stokker)*

wait for the doctor to arrive with the forceps. In 1862, district doctor Krohn wrote a wrenching account of such an arrested delivery, the most hopeless situation faced by nineteenth-century midwives, whether self-trained or professional: "Two days had passed since the woman's labor had stopped with an audible crunch that left her pale and in a cold sweat. She had a weak pulse, cold extremities, a barely audible voice, and she vomited constantly. The husband had sent the self-trained midwife to get something to induce contractions. Since the woman had previously given birth to four living children by nature's hand alone and was still in her most robust age, the husband felt there was no emergency and they should just give it time." The hjelpekone returned and applied the medicine she had fetched to encourage the contractions, which instead ceased altogether. "Now the husband finally fetched the professionally-trained midwife, who declared the situation hopeless, the child dead, and the delivery possible only with forceps." At this point they fetched Krohn, who thought her condition too fragile to use the forceps but relented when the husband insisted. "With the forceps, I removed a much decayed fetus with great difficulty, due to the swelling caused by the decomposition." The woman died the same day, Krohn reported, "but felt significant relief after the delivery and declared her satisfaction that the doctor had been fetched and agreed to use the forceps."[63]

Only forceps seemed able to help an arrested delivery, but most doctors refused to let professionally trained midwives use them. Aiming to rectify this situation, Dr. Peter Herman Vogt, director of the Bergen midwifery school since 1870, began training professional midwives to use forceps in 1884. Vogt's colleagues debated this move, dividing roughly along town and rural lines, with urban doctors mainly opposed while district doctors, responsible for thousands of women in largely roadless areas, strongly approved.[64]

As the debate raged on, mothers kept dying in childbirth. "It must be the public's duty to get these mothers more timely help," pleaded one district doctor. Few births actually required the forceps, but those that did could put the midwife in unspeakably tragic situations. "All professional midwives should be required to learn to use the forceps and always have them along," argued Nils Christoffersen, who served as a district doctor in Finnmark around 1900. He illustrated this need by telling the story of a highly competent jordmor with twenty-four years of experience. On an April morning she delivered a "living baby boy," the first child of the mother, a trained nurse, thirty-one years old (as the midwife wrote on the required form), and her husband, a teacher. "Since the doctor couldn't be reached during the birth," she noted under the heading of technical delivery assistance, "a hook had to be inserted in the baby's head to accomplish the delivery because the wife's strength was completely depleted." The jordmor wrote no more but said when the district doctor finally arrived, "If only I'd had a forceps."

Two days after the birth had begun, they had realized they needed the doctor's help and sent someone to fetch him across the ice-packed fjord, a journey that took half the day. The return trip lasted even longer, and as the jordmor watched, hour after hour, for the doctor's boat to arrive, the weakened mother went in and out of consciousness. Such a long time had passed since life signs had come from the baby, whose head had been lodged in the opening of the birth canal for twelve hours, that the jordmor had reason to believe it had died. In an effort to remove the baby and save the mother's life, the jordmor had resolutely inserted a fishhook in the infant's head.

The district doctor's report filled in the rest of the details, telling that when he finally arrived with the forceps, the jordmor "presented me with the crying infant whose temple had a large T-shaped wound exposing bone and part of the brain." Though Vogt's course taught professional midwives how to use forceps, the women never formally received the *right* to use them, having instead to abide by the decision of the local district doctor and health commission.[65]

Nor could the professional jordmor boast of greater success than the hjelpekone in saving mothers from childbed fever. In fact, the opposite seemed to be the case. The danger of contracting childbed (puerperal) fever actually grew exponentially when the child was delivered by a jordmor, instead of spontaneously with minimal help. The many internal examinations stipulated in the jordmor's training made it all too easy to infect the mother with bacteria.

Childbed fever (*barselfeber*), wrote Faye in his 1844 textbook, was a mystery that could not be cured. The popularized *Lægebog for hvermand* (1879) described the symptoms accurately enough (debilitating weakness, shivering chills, fever with great thirst, sleeplessness, the abdomen so swollen and tender that the patient can hardly stand to be touched even by the bed coverings, and strong pain around the navel, often accompanied by diarrhea, bad headache, and hallucinations), but identified the cause as "cold, poor diet, and strong emotions."[66] The 1886 edition of Faye's book could finally identify barselfeber as a disease that came from materials introduced into the mother during childbirth that infected her internal organs. As a result, the book urged jordmødre to reduce the number of internal examinations to a minimum.

Despite Pasteur's pioneering work in discovering bacteria and Lister's in applying that knowledge to kill bacteria, years passed before this knowledge influenced daily life in rural Norway. Poverty and tradition delayed hygienic reform, which according to Christian Schou, the district doctor of Førde in 1877, left much to be desired: "Clean water is used very sparingly whether to clean home or body. One rarely sees well-washed faces and hands except on Sunday. If one asks for wash water and towels, the woman of the house has a hard time. First she has to look for a basin, then there's a long search through her trunk for an appropriate piece of cloth. At last, in desperation she tears a less than clean scarf from her throat or head and presents it as a towel."[67]

Under the circumstances, professional midwives had a hard time following antiseptic procedure. "People look with disdain at all the washing and disinfecting we were accustomed to do at the Bergen Midwifery school," observed the Spangereid jordmor in 1907. Nor did the professional midwife herself always get the best training, said N. A. Quisling, a professor of midwifery at the Christiania school. Those who completed the course before 1890, he charged, had not received sufficient training in the antiseptic procedures that were "of the greatest importance in distinguishing between jordmor and hjelpekone." Added Quisling in 1900, "An old jordmor who doesn't know antiseptic procedure is more dangerous than the ignorant self-trained hjelpekone."

Nor did the trained jordmor have a reliable remedy when hemorrhaging during delivery threatened fatality. Under normal circumstances, mothers lose about a pint of blood before contractions stop the blood flow that has sustained the fetus through pregnancy. If the contractions fail to stop this flow, women go into shock and may even die. To treat hemorrhage, self-trained healers sprinkled camphor or pepper around the opening of the birth canal and administered drinks of hot brandy laced with pepper or camphor, occasionally fortifying these remedies with a black-book formula for stopping blood.

Though woefully inadequate, these remdies were not appreciably worse than the applications of cold water and vinegar Dr. Faye recommended in his midwifery text. "When hemorrhage occurs during and after birth," observed Dr. P. M. Dreijer as late as 1907, "the woman dies whether she received help, as in the old days, from a self-trained neighbor or now by a jordmor." No wonder the public finds the jordmor "superfluous," he continued. "The cases she can manage can also be managed by a cheaper hjelpekone, and both must simply look on when the case requires a doctor."[68]

But Dreijer had good news, too. Fewer women were dying in childbirth, less than half the number in 1899 as in 1860, an improvement Dreijer credited to better nutrition. Healthier mothers could better withstand the rigors of childbirth, he noted, adding that gradually improving hygiene was also lowering the risk of childbed fever.[69]

By the end of the century, more infants were surviving difficult births, too. Emerging from such births, the baby's head occasionally retains a fragment of the amniotic sac. Known in Norwegian as a *seierslue* (literally a "victory cap"), this "caul" was widely considered a sign of good fortune (the child had, after all, survived the ordeal), and birth assistants by tradition preserved it for the child to keep as a talisman.

Since the almue had traditionally consulted the district doctor only for difficult births, and then only after all else had failed, doctors typically witnessed only the most extreme cases. This surely gave them a distorted notion of the self-trained midwives' usual techniques. Krohn spoke in an 1858 lecture, for example, of the hjelpekone making the mother "roll around, walk on her knees across the floor, and stand on her head" to adjust the fetal position. "If the baby still wouldn't come, they made the woman jump down from a stool or trunk, or '*veie salt*'" (place her back against the back of a strong woman or man and take turns lifting each other off the floor). "To proceed in this manner," Krohn concluded, "is as morally and legally indefensible, as it is regrettable and sad."[70]

Krohn and other district doctors castigated the "wanton recklessness, foolhardiness, and impudence" of the self-trained hjelpekoner not least as part of their campaign to persuade reluctant health commissions to spend money on the training and hiring of professional midwives. Professional midwives, meanwhile, voiced their own criticism of the "hoard of filthy hjelpekoner who rob us of our meager income," as the Elverum jordmor Lovise Dorthea Hagen put it in 1895. "Only one-fourth of the births in Skjærvo parish fall to my practice," complained a Tromsø midwife in 1896, while the rest are served by "dirty, crooked fingered hjelpekoner."[71]

Balancing the reports of incompetent self-trained hjelpekoner that dominate the historical record is the urging of Mimmi Benjaminsen (born 1894 in Værøy) not to forget the self-trained hjelpekoner: "Though they had no education in midwifery, most of them were enterprising, intelligent, and above all helpful women. Like other women in the community, they had farms, homes, and children to take care of, and like everyone else they had to work hard to make ends meet. Yet when someone came to fetch them to assist at a birth that usually involved travel over impossible terrain or a long boat trip, they went willingly. Unfortunately there was nothing they could do for abnormal births. The doctor was usually difficult to contact and often came too late."[72]

Gradually, as more daughters of cotters and craftsmen took midwifery training, the almue's resistance to professional midwives began to ease. Growing access to education enhanced the almue's appreciation of cleanliness and professional skill, and for this reason, too, they increasingly turned to the officially appointed midwives.[73]

For many years, Faye's textbook advised professional midwives to enlist the help of local hjelpekoner. They thereby continued the age-old tradition by which several women with varying degrees of experience attended neighborhood births, some assisting and others learning techniques for future deliveries. This advice appeared in the original 1844 edition, as well as in its revisions in 1857 and 1872, but when Peter Herman Vogt revised the text in 1886, he discouraged the presence of all but the professional jordmor and one assistant. So it was that by the end of the century, as fewer and fewer women shared in their neighbors' births, midwifery was becoming specialized knowledge possessed by only a few.

In 1898 the *Jordmor lov* (midwifery law) made the movement from untrained assistants to professional midwives official by forbidding hjelpekoner from accepting payment for their work. The number of professionally trained midwives in Norway had grown from less than fifty in 1810 and five hundred in 1860 to one thousand in 1900. "Providing professionally trained help where none had been used before," says Kristina Kjærstad in her 1987 history of Norwegian midwifery, "these women helped Norwegians take the first crucial step toward accepting professional health care in general."[74] Yet we have also seen that in the time before professional medicine had appreciably better results to render, the almue did a remarkably competent job of managing their own care.

AN INADEQUATE ART

Physician Carl Roan observed the "heavy penalty" immigrants often paid for "lack of an adequate art of healing." He described one frontier woman's doomed attempt to deliver Kari Skog's baby in Bergen Township in 1873.

> Kari had struggled and suffered with labor pains for
> several days. Kerstine Torgrimson was at her side until
> the end but could do nothing to hasten the coming of the
> baby or to relieve Kari's pains. There was no physician

within reach of the settlement who knew any more about midwifery than Kerstine Torgrimson did. The women in the neighborhood had gathered to give to this midwife whatever possible aid they could, but to no avail. They knew the cause of the delay; the child came wrong-end first and Kerstin had not been able to turn it right before it was too late. Even the men in the neighborhood gathered and stood in the barn where they heard the cries and moans of the struggling woman who was giving her all to bring a new life into the world. Finally, when the release came, Kari was so exhausted that the sharp hemorrhage that followed sent her into shock and she died. The child was stillborn.

She "died as so many frontier women had died in making their contribution," wrote Roan, "without the aid of modern scientific facilities and knowledge which in such cases can avert disaster."

Roan also recorded a birthing experience in 1865–66, when his mother, Beret Johnson, hired a professionally trained midwife to deliver her sixth child. Her five previous children had been delivered by friends and relatives, but with her husband in the Civil War, the prospect of giving birth worried her for the first time. "She had prepared as much as possible for the event in the early part of the winter by gathering and chopping a considerable quantity of wood, enough to last several months. In the fall, with the aid of [neighbor women] Stava and Thore, she had put up enough wild hay to keep the cows through the winter." She had engaged the trained midwife Kerstine Torgrimson to come in the due season to care for her, the children, and the cattle.

Child care and cattle-care constituted part of the midwife's normal workload. Beret's "war baby," as she came to think of him, was born without complication and got a good start in life before being struck down by diphtheria, the first of four Johnson children to die within days in the 1876 epidemic.

Carl Roan, "The Immigrant Wagon" ꝥ

7

Rickets Remedies and Lore

From changelings to English disease

> "My aunt's great-grandmother had a changeling. He looked like a
> weather-beaten old man and had eyes that glowed in the dark, red
> like an owl's. His head was as long as on a horse and as thick as a
> cabbage. His legs bowed like a sheep's and his skin felt like a spoiled
> sausage. He never did anything but howl and cry, but was hungry
> as an old hound dog and ate everything in sight."
>
> P. C. Asbjørnsen, "En Signekjerring"

A S SCIENCE UNRAVELED THE MYSTERY of infectious diseases, once
the great scourge of early childhood, one pervasive children's disease
continued to elude explanation. The almue called it *svekk* (general debility) or *valken* (for the swelling it caused around the child's joints), and they
blamed the *huldrefolk* (hidden people) for the condition that C. E. Mangor
in his *Lande apothek* termed "very common among both rich and poor."[1]
Since doctors could neither explain nor cure the disease, Norwegians of
all social classes consulted folk healers when their children showed telltale
signs of the affliction.

"When the superstitious almue see a formerly healthy and alert child
gradually sicken, develop an enlarged head, black teeth and constant crying," wrote C. E. Mangor in his *Lande-apothek*, "they call the child a *bytting*
(changeling), for they believe that the huldrefolk have stolen their healthy
child from its cradle and replaced it with this monster." Mangor's description suggests that several maladies underlay the belief in changelings, but in
nineteenth-century Norway the most common by far was rickets.

The delayed onset of rickets made plausible the stories of deformed

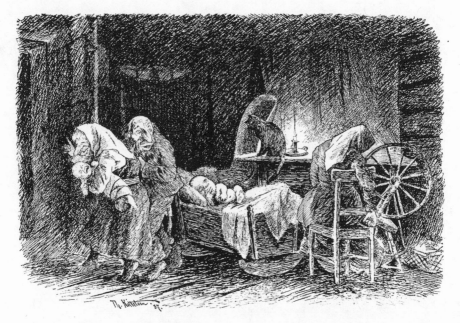

The *huldrefolk* (hidden people) steal a healthy human child, leaving behind one of their own deformed offspring while an exhausted woman sleeps at her spinning wheel.

offspring left behind by the hidden people. A child would be born in seemingly good health but sicken around the age of six months, as improper nutrition began to take a visible toll. The child's bones became soft and pliable, while its wrists and ankles swelled to abnormal size. Finding movement painful, the child with rickets made little attempt to stand or walk, instead lying listlessly in its cradle when not crying inconsolably. So radically had the child changed that it seemed almost inhuman.

"Valken was a fitting name for the disorder," wrote Laurits Løvmo (born 1888 in Hedmark), whose sister had rickets. "The victims grew *valker* [rolls of padding] like rings on a tree."[2] Symptomatic of nutritional deficiency, this thickening revealed the disease's true cause, lack of Vitamin D, which facilitates the body's essential absorption of calcium. As bones softened, the child's increasing weight produced the pigeon breast, bowed legs, and knock-knees typical of the disease. Calcium, in addition to building strong bones, enables brain cells to send electrochemical signals, and deficiency can result in painful spasms of the hands, feet, and larynx, along with difficulty in breathing, nausea, convulsions, and even death.

Known since ancient times and first described in 1650, rickets proliferated under the smoke-filled skies of nineteenth-century England's industrialized cities. Upper-class Norwegians called the illness *"engelsk syke"* (English disease), although it also prevailed in Norway, where the winter sun fails to provide sufficient ultraviolet radiation to penetrate the skin and produce Vitamin D.[3] The association of rickets with sunlight and Vitamin D remained unclear until well into the 1900s.

Although British researcher T. A. Palm had discovered the link between rickets and sunshine by 1892, the next breakthrough had to wait until the discovery of vitamins, a term coined in 1911 for nutrients the body needs in addition to the protein, fat, carbohydrates, and minerals known since the 1870s. By 1921, Sir Edward Mellanby had shown that cod-liver oil could cure rickets, but he credited the cure to the just-discovered Vitamin A. The curative component in cod-liver oil was identified as Vitamin D in 1922, and in 1928 Adolf Windaus discovered its molecular structure, promptly winning the Nobel Prize in chemistry.[4]

While these scientists understood that sunlight produced Vitamin D in the skin, they could not explain how the process occurred or how Vitamin D functioned. These questions went unanswered until the 1960s and 1970s, when scientists at the University of Wisconsin reclassified "Vitamin" D as a hormone, i.e., a regulator of nutrients, rather than a nutrient itself. These researchers also determined the three steps that enabled Vitamin D to control the body's absorption of calcium (and phosphorus), finding that after the sun produces Vitamin D in the skin, two chemical reactions—one in the liver and another in the kidneys—are required to activate it.

No wonder nineteenth-century Norwegians found rickets perplexing. Lacking an explanation, the disease seemed frightening and mysterious, curable—many believed—only by magical means.

Ritual remedies for rickets

In 1891 Laurits Løvmo watched his sister undergo a magical procedure known as "threading" (*smøyg*), ritually scraping away disease by passing the patient through a small opening. The *"trollkone"* (magical healer) had told Løvmo's mother that the procedure must be performed where the fences of three properties met. Having made suitable holes in the fences, Løvmo's mother, directed by the trollkone and assisted by one of her neighbors, passed her daughter through these openings, head first and facing the sky.

"I had to stand a respectable distance away," Løvmo recalled, while the women repeated the entire process three times, the "trollkone reading a formula so softly that it was impossible to make out the words." Secrecy and the number three (three participants, three fences, three performances of the ritual) traditionally enhanced the magic of rituals.

Unimpressed by the magic, Løvmo said the procedure "did not help the child, of course," but he recognized that it brought "reassurance" to his mother. "When the formalities were finished, they had coffee. By then the bundle that the trollkone carried in her hands had grown considerably," he concluded. Completing the ritual with a cup of coffee was as commonplace as seeing the trollkone as greedy, an image that dogged even the most altruistic of folk healers.

Anne Marie Djupedalen (1841–1945) recalled threading treatments from her childhood in Heidalen. Sick people could be "threaded" through all manner of small openings—holes in the ground, between branches of trees, through windows, under bridges. A folk healer in nearby Vågå, Gudbrandsdal, she said, used threading especially to treat children suffering from *liksvekk* (corpse svekk), a gradual sickening believed to be caused by the longing for the child by the dead.[5]

Also known as *dødsvalken* (death swelling), this ailment was considered the most serious form of wasting disease. The Vågå folk healer based her treatment on "sympathetic magic," the fundamental principle of folk medicine. Often expressed as "like cures like," it stipulates among other things that the cause of a disease can also cure it. Believing that the dead caused dødsvalken, the Vågå folk healer cured it by threading the afflicted child under a corpse, a practice facilitated by the high mortality and constant presence of death in nineteenth-century Norway. People usually died at home, where they lay in repose for several days before the funeral, which also took place at home. Parents customarily brought their children to view the deceased, not only to pay respects, but also to gain the health benefits traditional lore attributed to touching a corpse.[6]

After the Vågå folk healer threaded the sick child under the corpse, says Djupedalen, she would do a "measuring" to determine the "distance between the child's joints." Known in Norwegian as *måling*, this procedure, too, was deeply rooted in European folk medicine, though few agreed exactly how it was to be done. Some measured the length of the child's arms and legs, others between the bones of the spine, and still others the distance from temple to foot. The values thus obtained could indicate the precise form of the disease that afflicted the child or the number of weeks it had lasted.

Many folk healers used ritual measuring as a cure in itself. They took the requisite measurements three times, then wrapped the measuring thread around the sick child's wrist, and left it there for three days. When they removed the thread ring, they spit through it three times and threw it into the fire. When the fire had consumed the thread, the disease was considered cured.

Immigrant O. S. Johnson (born 1842) experienced måling as a child in Ringerike and described it in his 1920 account of Spring Grove, Minnesota: "Grandma often measured me for *mosot* [general debility] when I was ten or twelve years old. With a wool thread she measured both arms and legs, length and thickness, and then wound wool thread into a little ball that I was to throw behind me over my head. She read a prayer over a piece of flatbread or waffle spread with sour cream that I was to eat."[7] Throwing the wound-up thread behind the child, like tossing it into the fire, symbolically discarded the disease. Johnson readily admitted that he "liked being measured often, as I got such good food when she finished measuring." The nourishing food, along with the fact that children need less calcium as they grow older, probably accounted for the child's improvement, but magical measuring often got the credit.

Like smøyg, ritual measuring brought a welcome sense of assurance. "Symbolically, measuring may be understood as a way of preventing the ravages of the disease from extending beyond a certain area," explained American folklorist Wayland D. Hand. "Once the limits of the disease were thereby demarcated and the disease confined, it could then be removed symbolically by transferring it to another site."[8] Måling set limits for the disease and allowed it to be transferred to the thread. Once the thread was destroyed, the disease was gone.

Besides threading and measuring, the Vågå folk healer treated rickets using *jordfaststeiner* (earth-fixed stones). Stones firmly anchored in the soil, especially those marking the boundary line between properties, have since prehistoric times been believed to possess special power. Norwegian farmers knew only too well the enormous energy required to remove such stones from their fields, and magically harnessing that force lies at the heart of this remedy. "Take three jordfaststeiner, dig them down into the coals and keep them there through the night. In the morning put one of the stones into the child's wash water. By then, it is 'strong' enough to make the water steam. Afterwards replace all three stones in their original holes." The Vågå folk healer's cure augments the precaution that almue parents routinely took to "consecrate" their unbaptized infants' wash water with hot coals. The coals lessened the infants' vulnerablity to witches and huldrefolk who might gain control over them by means of bits of their skin or hair left behind in the wash water. Using the difficult-to-move jordfaststeiner emphasized the challenge of treating valken, while the steaming wash water gave visible proof that the necessary power had been transferred from the hot stone.[9]

Like fire, metal could also disarm the huldrefolk, so the Vågå folk healer advised parents to "rock the child with a *bismer* [a scale consisting of an iron rod and hook] inherited through three generations." This remedy augmented the common custom of putting metal into infants' cradles to protect them from supernatural harm. Any metal would do, but *arvesølv* (inherited silver) handed down in the family held the greatest power. Folk healers consequently asked for family keepsakes such as brooches or coins to enhance the magic of their cures. Though unscrupulous healers doubtless used this belief to steal precious heirlooms, the folk healer's request for arvesølv was not in itself a demand for payment, as outside observers often claimed.

In addition to metal and fire, Christian symbols could also keep huldrefolk and witches at bay. Parents carved crosses into their children's cradles or placed a Bible or hymnal in the child's bedding for extra security. Metal filings from church bells provided particularly potent protection, combining the power of metal and Christianity. Scrapings of this sort played a role in a mysterious incident that took place around 1870 in Garmo, Gudbrandsdal. On the night before Christmas, says Ingebjørg Henningsdatter, her grandmother was helping the cotters' wives finish the holiday baking when she needed to fetch something from one of the outbuildings. The clock was approaching midnight as she stepped outside "into the clear moonlight of the night." Then, "she espied a little child's shirt, hanging ghostlike, displayed and glittering in the pale rays of the moon in the steeple of Garmo Stave Church [now at Lillehammer's Maihaugen Museum]. Just at that moment she also heard a scraping sound from the church bells." Said Ingebjørg, "Grandma instantly knew the meaning of this process. . . . Someone was seeking 'remedy' for the formidable *rachitis* [rickets]. . . . Some tiny grains from the church bell were to cure her little child, whose tiny shirt hung displayed in the church steeple. But Grandma said ever afterwards that she never understood how anybody had got inside the church."[10]

Scraping metal from the church bell to treat rickets did not puzzle Ingebjørg's grandmother in the least because it was a common "cure." How

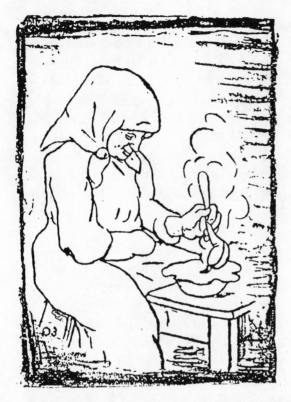

A folk healer performs a "casting" to diagnose *svekk* (rickets), pouring molten lead into cold water through a hole in a piece of flatbread. The shape of the hardened metal will disclose what form of svekk is making the child sick.

the person had managed to get inside the church so late at night was the mystery. The event's timing, Christmas Eve at midnight, added to the power of the church metal because at "the seam of the year," when the old year ended and a new one began, a myriad of normally hidden forces haunted the human world and added extra potency to ritual remedies of all kinds.

The "church metal" folk healers used to treat svekk might also be scraped from the leaded church windows. With these filings, folk healers made "castings" to diagnose the child's svekk, using a process known as *støyping*. The folk healer melted the lead, poured it into cold water, and then interpreted the shape the metal assumed to determine which supernatural being had caused the disease. With this information, she could devise an appropriate cure.

A story of witchcraft

The melted-lead method of diagnosis figures prominently in Norway's classic story of healing and witchcraft, "En Signekjerring," a word that means both "healer" and "witch." Written in 1845 by Norway's most famous collector of folklore, P. C. Asbjørnsen, the story portrays the healer Gubjør and her efforts to treat the mysteriously ill child of the cotter's wife, Marit Rognehagen.[11]

In the account, Gubjør fills an ale bowl with cold water, covers it with a piece of barley flatbread pierced with a needle, and slowly pours molten lead through the hole into the water. Marit meanwhile recounts all the precautions she has taken to keep her child well: "In his cradle I have, of course, put *bevergjel* [a foul-smelling beaver secretion thought capable of warding off evil]; I have burned candles and consecrated his wash water with hot coals; I have also made the sign of the cross and pinned a *sølje* [silver brooch, often inherited] on his shirt, and placed a knife above the door, so I don't know how they managed to exchange him."[12]

Studying the shape of the congealed lead in the water, Gubjør concludes the child has "corpse svekk," cast upon him by the spirits of the dead when Marit failed to say *"i Jesu navn"* (in Jesus' name) as they passed the churchyard. Gubjør decides to trick the spirits into thinking that they already have the child by making a doll to bury in the churchyard. The Vågå folk healer similarly advised making "three dolls from the child's clothing" to put into the cradle so the "huldrefolk will take one of them instead of the child." In 1856, district doctor Michael Krohn described the identical procedure still being practiced in Ytre Nordhordland. The almue make "a doll with rags of the sick child's clothes," he wrote, "and bury it in the churchyard to fool the dead into believing the longed-for child has entered their realm."[13]

Clearly, Asbjørnsen drew upon authentic tradition in writing his story. He altered it to suit his own purposes, however, when he has Gubjør ask for Marit's inherited silver to put with the doll to lure the spirits to take it. This contradicts the widely accepted folk belief that metal would ward off the spirits.

Why did Asbjørnsen, an otherwise astute observer of folk practices, insist on adding the inherited silver to Gubjør's cure? His unflattering description of the healer suggests an answer, for he takes great pains to undermine her credibility: "Grey hair stuck out from under the scarf, which surrounded a dark face with bushy eyebrows and a long irregular nose. The dim-wittedness suggested by the low forehead and the width of her cheekbones contrasted with the unmistakable cunning of her small, shining eyes, while the wrinkles and play of the muscles in her face masked her inborn shrewdness. Her clothing showed that she came from a village farther north; her entire being suggested the wise woman could be impudent and brazen or humble and ingratiating, just as the circumstances warranted." Asbjørnsen's Gubjør is greedy and cunning, an ethnic and social outsider, and thus the very image of a witch. By portraying Gubjør this way, Asbjørnsen reflected the negative view that his kondisjonerte contemporaries shared about self-trained healers.

Asbjørnsen's story appeared during Norway's period of national self-awareness that followed adoption of the 1814 constitution. Celebrating their distinctiveness as a people, Norwegians were also attempting to define their identity as a nation. To personify the national spirit, the political elite had chosen the peasant farmer. Now the elite began a concerted effort to reform the peasant class, whose practices they found repulsive, to fit the constructed ideal.

Though Asbjørnsen avidly collected peasant lore, he revealed in a March 15, 1874, newspaper article titled "Om overtroens væsen og betydning" (About the nature and significance of superstition) that his goal was to debunk the peasants' archaic folk beliefs: "The superstitious almue, from the cradle to the grave, try to acquire a greater power and increase their own welfare or attempt to hurt and hinder others' welfare through the utilization of an almost unbelievable number of precautions, remedies and occult tricks which are tied in every conceivable way to a person's entire family life, his possessions and activities."[14] The beliefs that ruled the peasants' lives had to be exposed, believed Asbjørnsen and others in the cultural elite. Only then could the almue take their place as full citizens in an enlightened Norway.

Asbjørnsen accordingly contrasts the primitive Gubjør with Marit's more enlightened cotter husband, who, the story reveals, disapproves of folk healers and has even offered to take the sick child to the doctor. Having neither Gubjør's low forehead or narrow eyes, Asbjørnsen's cotter is alert, hardworking, and respectable. He might return before the healer leaves, Marit worries, and the 1845 version of the story shows why, as he threatens to put Gubjør in jail and beat Marit for seeking the healer's advice. Though Asbjørnsen removed these details from the 1859 and 1870 editions, the point was made and the story was well on its way to becoming a classic.[15]

The cotter's offer to consult professional medical care surely found favor with Asbjørnsen's kondisjonerte readers, though the expense, distance, and cultural differences made it unlikely. Nor would it have proved fruitful, since Norwegian doctors had no scientific understanding of rickets for several decades to come.

The pioneering description of rickets in Norway appeared in 1886. Written by Dr. N. A. Quisling, it showed that the disease was widespread among Norwegian children, a finding most of Quisling's colleagues at first viewed with skepticism. The very next year Dr. Edvard Schønberg agreed with Quisling's findings and declared that Norwegian doctors simply didn't recognize rickets when they saw it. They confused its symptoms with other diseases and failed to diagnose rickets before serious skeletal damage had occurred, he observed, while "the almue can usually diagnose the disease quite accurately." Rickets escapes the attention of doctors, he argued, because "the almue have not seen it as part of the doctor's realm, and even believe they should hide it from doctors and pastors. . . . They therefore have sought and still seek the advice of their wise women . . . an activity that continues here in the capital city even among mothers of the upper class because doctors overwhelmingly persist in regarding the disease as rare."[16]

Five years later Schønberg once again urged doctors to treat rickets as a serious problem. He repeated his observation that doctors had not sufficiently opened their eyes to the connection, while folk healers in Kristiania and the almue themselves "use the terms *svekk* and *Engelsk syke* interchangeably!" Asbjørnsen's classic witchcraft story appeared decades before this improved understanding of rickets and the valuable role folk healers had played in treating it.[17]

While Asbjørnsen's story described the graying and wily healer fabricating falsehoods to trick the cotter's wife into retaining her services, the healer's comment that "doctors do not understand how to treat svekk because it is not in their books" is simply stating a matter of fact. Nevertheless, arising in the context of doctors' frustrations with the public's trust in folk healers and amid patriotic efforts at national reform, Asbjørnsen's widely read classic helped shape and perpetuate the image of the folk healer as a witch.

 ## TRUE STORY OF A GYPSY FOLK HEALER

Gypsies reputedly knew supernatural cures for mysterious wasting diseases like rickets. Around 1900, one of these healers treated the sister of Elias Toralv Huse (born 1891 in Harøy [Møre og Romsdal]).

My sister Petra got an illness that Doctor Rambech did not understand. He examined her several times, but had

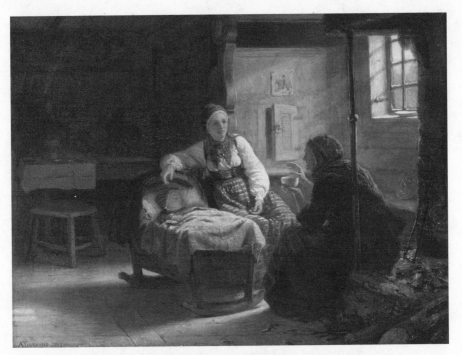

Adolph Tidemand portrayed this *signekjerring* (magical healer) doing a *støyping* (casting) to discover the nature of a baby's illness.

no cure. And the last time he saw her said she would not live much longer. About this time the "Johan family" came for the summer. Boat-gypsies, they spent each summer in Bakkan around the time I was ten years old. Soon, Johan's wife, Josefina, a *klok kone* (wise woman or folk healer) came to our farm to trade, as she always did these summers. She exchanged sewing needles, knitting needles and many other small things for pork and beef—and usually got some fish thrown into the bargain.

When Josefina heard about my sister, she asked to see her and, after examining her, asked if my mother would like her to cure the child. My mother hesitated: Should she believe more in this gypsy than in Doctor Rambech? "That would be my dearest wish," she finally answered.

Josefina said the illness came from sitting too long on

the ground early in the springtime, and the next day she returned with the medicine. Evidently it involved some magic, for she had taken along nail clippings from my little sister's thumb and little finger, as well as some hair from both sides of the child's head.

After taking the Josefina-medicine several times, Petra began to improve. Josefina dropped in several more times to check on her patient before the family left at the end of the summer. "Rest assured," she told my mother when she came to say goodbye, "your child will recover completely." And so she did.

Elias Toralv Huse, quoted in
Møre og Romsdal i manns minne

Since doctors had no cure for rickets, parents continued to consult folk healers for magical cures. Visiting a *signekone* (folk healer) in the capital city in 1911, the journalist Inga Bjørnson found the traditional rituals of *støyping* and *måling* still very much in use. "The sign on the door read 'Rickets Treated,'" she wrote in 1911, "and one Wednesday afternoon, I went in. The healer said, 'Now you must take off your hat and I will measure you with a woolen thread; then I can tell what is wrong with you.' Over on the sideboard lay a rolled-up piece of gray woolen thread all by itself."[18]

Intrigued, Inga Bjørnson returned to Konow Street the following Thursday, the healer's busiest day (another tradition upheld). Bjørnson's article leaves no doubt about the terror that rickets could still arouse: "The place was so full of people, it was hard to get inside, and still many women were waiting out in the yard, too, holding children in their arms, ranging in age from a few months to ten, even twelve years. [The children] looked miserable, several had enlarged heads—and legs that dangled like rags."

The signekone then leaned over one decrepit little boy who lay on his stomach in his mother's lap as she "*målte*" between the child's vertebrae with her fingers, counting out loud—ten, eleven, twelve. The anxiety in the mother's eyes grew with the numbers. "Fourteen," the healer concluded, straightening as she indicated that the mother could dress the child. "For fourteen months the child has had *svekk*," the healer declared as she beckoned the mother to bring him into the støyping room. Bjørnson could hear lead hissing out in the kitchen.

To Inga Bjørnson, the scene that now unfolded bore an unholy resemblance to a Christian baptism: "A big, white cloth was draped over the child, with one edge raised to reveal his head. A tray on a small table held three white cups filled with water. The signekone disappeared into the kitchen and returned with the molten lead in a long casting ladle. Holding the tray of cups over the child, so the cup covered by a bread crust stood directly over the child's head, she began the ceremony.

"'What is the child's name?' 'Emil Hansen.' 'Emil Hansen (the lead hissed into the bread), I heal you in the name of God the father, God the son, and God the holy ghost for nine kinds of svekk and nine kinds of English disease.' This she repeated three times, each time pouring the lead into a new cup with the words, 'Peace be with you. *I Jesu Navn*, Amen.'" The signekone made the sign of the cross in the cloth covering the child, and the ceremony ended.

"And this happened in Kristiania in the year 1911 in broad daylight and with the windows open!" concluded Inga Bjørnson, aghast. But rather than a desecration of Christianity, might not the healer's ceremony reflect the profound belief in the healing power of Christian ritual that has characterized Norwegian folk belief since medieval times?

No matter how we choose to see these magical rituals and the women who performed them, some folk healers had devised purely rational remedies for rickets. It was Anne Brandfjeld's uncanny ability to treat rickets that made her famous, and no less renowned in her own part of Norway was the folk healer known as Mor Frøisland.

The case of Mor Frøisland (1829–99)

Born in the forest-covered mountains of Nordre Land near Lillehammer, Anne Marie Frøisland was well educated, wealthy, and rumored to be the granddaughter of a Polish nobleman. The Pole had sought refuge in Norway, built a log cabin near Torpa, and lived there with his wife and child until he and his wife mysteriously disappeared. A local couple, Marie and Ole Vestrom, subsequently raised the little girl, Ingeborg, as their own.[19]

At age sixteen, Ingeborg went into service at Nord-Kinn, one of the area's largest farms, where owner Ola Kinn took a liking to her and eventually proposed. Their only child, Anne Marie, inherited the sizeable farm. As the community's best marriage prospect, Anne Marie caught the eye of Nils Frøisland, who had a large farm of his own. So Anne Marie became known as Mor Frøisland.

Anne Marie and Nils ran both farms, honoring the traditional *føderåd* contracts each had made to provide food, clothing, and living quarters for their retired parents. This was a demanding effort since the farms lay almost five miles apart, a considerable distance in a rugged landscape with primitive transportation. Like all landowners' wives, Anne Marie had to supply clothing and food for everyone who lived on each farm (as many as thirty or forty people) and tend to their illnesses and injuries, as well. She must have gained a great deal of medical experience from this activity, but, according to oral tradition, it was a problem with her own health that transformed her into a renowned folk healer.

Ingeborg Sæther, whose parents lived in Torpa during this time, said that complications of childbirth sent Anne Marie to Kristiania's Rikshospital for extended treatment. During those long, painful days and nights, Anne Marie realized how much she could help people in Torpa if only she knew more about medicine. As her condition improved, she read medical books supplied by her doctor, who also helped her gain admittance to student lectures at the hospital. When Anne Marie returned home, her neighbors eagerly came to her for advice on how to treat their ailments. When word spread that she could provide effective treatments, even more patients arrived.

"They came all the way from Oslo and other cities," said Sæther, "even foreigners made the trip to the Frøisland farm and received the medical advice and assistance that the doctors they had previously consulted couldn't provide." Among those seeking Mor Frøisland's help were many parents whose children had rickets.

Anne Marie Frøisland could devote herself to healing because at an early age she had become a *kårkone* (landowner retired from running a farm but supported, usually, by their oldest son or daughter, who has taken over daily operations). As a healer Mor Frøisland specialized in tending deep wounds, eye ailments, and broken bones, but it was her understanding of rickets, wrote David Seierstad in 1943, that made her "one of the most famous women in Norway of the past 100 years." He continued, "She could heal this disease in all its various stages more than a generation before medical science had begun to understand it." Her recommendations included healthy food, especially vegetables, and exercise outdoors. Sunshine activated the Vitamin D that ensured the body's proper absorption of the calcium and phosphorous in the food, but who knew that then?

Those who recovered under Mor Frøisland's care did not question why her regimen worked. Like Erik Åsdokken, whom she treated in the 1870s, they were simply happy that it *did*. The eighty-year-old Åsdokken told his story to another of her patients, Gunnar Skrutvold:

> I was supposed to start school, but couldn't walk that far. So that spring, my father hoisted me up onto his shoulders and carried me all the way to Torpa to see Mor Frøisland. She invited me to live on her farm and I stayed the whole summer. What a good time I had! Before long, she had me outside, running errands and helping with various small chores. In the fall I was healthy enough to go home when my father came to get me. This time I could walk the whole way on my own two legs. The next summer I herded sheep on the Frøisland farm and after that had no trouble with my health for the rest of my childhood.[20]

David Seierstad, too, came to know Mor Frøisland's healing firsthand, when he contracted a kidney disease in his early twenties. He consulted doctors in both Toten and Gjøvik, and even a couple in Kristiania, considered among the best. Then, as a last resort, he tried Mor Frøisland. Arriving at the Frøisland farm in 1888, he found her at the spinning wheel in the large kitchen, "corpulent, and powerful, dressed in her homeweave skirt and jacket of blended wool and linen." He accepted her invitation to come inside, submitted to her examination, faithfully took the medicine she prescribed, and returned six weeks later as instructed. When Mor Frøisland pronounced him "already much improved," he "realized she was right."

The power of personality no doubt contributed significantly to the success of Mor Frøisland's remedies. "She had the ability to see through both people and circumstances clearer than anyone else," recalled Ingeborg Sæther. "I know of no one in the community whose words held greater sway." At the same time, she could console and comfort as no one else could. She used "not just empty words" Sæther insisted, but words that "sprang from the rich experience of her soul and the warm heart that never held back in time of trouble."

Sæther, a victim of *giktfeber* (rheumatic fever), had also experienced Mor Frøisland's treatments and especially remembered the healer's eyes watching over her bed. "It was the warmest, most loving look I have ever received. Her eyes seemed to penetrate both body and soul, but it felt good to be under that gaze."

Hospitality constituted another important element of Mor Frøisland's care. Everyone who came for medical help received coffee and food, and if they had come a long distance, they stayed overnight. All this she did free of charge, and for one young woman in service to Mor Frøisland, it seemed a bit much. "She held office hours all day long," the woman later told Sæther, readily recalling her annoyance about the constant making of coffee, not to mention the additional chores her employer's doctoring duties added to her own responsibilities.

But a sense of pride in the healer's work also comes through the serving girl's account of Mor Frøisland's methods, a combination of reading doctor books and relying on her own intuition. Only "the experienced eye," Mor Frøisland once said, can determine the appropriate treatment, and "such a thing cannot be taught."

> When it was an especially difficult case, Mor Frøisland went into the large, formal parlor and sat there alone to think. If I came in to ask about dinner, she'd wave me off saying, "You know just as well as I do," and I'd have to tend to it myself as best as I could. But when she had sat there a while and gotten a clear idea of what she should use to help the patient, she came out so happy, and those good, wise eyes of hers would shine like the sun. Then she'd find the appropriate medications and give them to the person saying, "With God's help, I think these will do the job."

Despite Mor Frøisland's goodwill, conscientious efforts, and usually successful results, one healing went horribly wrong. Karen Gulbrandsdatter (born 1862 in Nordsinni and in service at Grøtåsen in Torpa) began to feel pain and stiffness in her leg in 1880. Dr. Nils Aal Kolbjørnsen (1834–1912) advised that she go to the Rikshospital in Kristiania, but both Karen and her parents, to whom she had by now returned, were deathly afraid of hospitals.

Instead, Karen's parents went to Mor Frøisland and begged her to take the case. She refused and urged them to follow the doctor's advice. When Karen's parents returned to Frøisland later in the month, Karen could hardly walk. Seeing that the girl would otherwise receive no care at all, the healer agreed to treat her in May and June.

Karen's pain again worsened in August, and her mother remembered that Mor Frøisland (who was away traveling) had mentioned that bloodletting might help. She then contacted Ole Andreas Andersen Jørgenstuen, a local "cupper" or blood-letter, who apparently used contaminated instruments and infected the wound. When Dr. Kolbjørnsen examined the girl's knee again, he became furious that Mor Frøisland had advised the bleeding and immediately sent the patient to Rikshospital with the suggestion that the hospital's director of surgery, Julius Kristen Nicolaysen (1831–1909), join him in bringing suit against Mor Frøisland.[21]

When word of the trial spread in the spring of 1881, more than 150 letters (many signed with "assisted pen" by patients who did not know how to write) arrived emphasizing Mor Frøisland's self-sacrificing care and the effectiveness of her treatments. The writers clearly feared losing their "doctor," who, in addition to being inexpensive, had qualities they valued, such as a strong Christian faith. "She was inexpensive and a good source of support for the poor," wrote one, who added, "Her medicines might cost a little, but they were free to the destitute. . . . I feared the doctors' bill would be too high for our family, since we would still be unsure of a cure." Another observed, "Tending the sick and at their deathbed both at our place and elsewhere, she has greatly helped by bringing them consoling words of God and referring them to Jesus Christ, the true healer of the soul, while praying for them aloud and in silence, which I believe really means a lot to them." Concluded yet another, "If we'd gone to the doctor, the price would have been considerably different and we would neither have been served both food and drink nor received in addition a treat to take home."[22]

The trial commenced on the Finni farm with Drs. Kolbjørnsen and Nicolaysen confronting Mor Frøisland in person. Entering the courtroom in her finest silk dress, black-beaded shawl, and stiffly starched white headdress, she bowed to the court with a calm dignity that, according to Ingeborg Sæther, "even a queen would envy." Nicolaysen leapt to his feet to return the bow, then scurried to find the best chair in the chamber to offer her.

Then came testimonials from "droves" of patients, who came forward spontaneously after hearing about the trial. A lumberjack told of accidentally sawing off some of his fingers; Mor Frøisland had gone into the woods, found the bloody digits in the snow, and kept them cold until she sewed them successfully back on to his hand. But the biggest impression on the court was made by the many parents of children that Mor Frøisland cured of rickets. No physician in all of Norway or Europe could have managed this task as well, said Sæther, and the doctors knew it.

Mor Frøisland testified that she had employed only simple, harmless treatments (cold compresses, massage with the oil and spirits of camphor, and tinctures of iron and valerian taken internally) and that she had taken no payment. The doctors agreed that the treatments had themselves caused no harm but had delayed more effective professional care.[23]

When the court found Mor Frøisland guilty, her patients joined together to pay the fee, using the money left over to buy her a "gift of silver" whose inscription expressed their sympathy and gratitude. For Ingeborg Sæther, "the most amazing thing of all" happened at the conclusion of the trial, when the court granted Mor Frøisland permission to practice freely in the future "without fear of prosecution."[24]

Ultimately, the trial strengthened Mor Frøisland's position among prospective patients. "Anyone who had not heard of her before the trial, knew about her now," said Sæther, and among these was the wife of Dr. Kolbjørnsen. The couple's four-year-old daughter was suffering from rickets and had never learned to walk. It must have been "a sour apple for Dr. Kolbjørnsen to bite into," Sæther observes, when his wife informed him that she intended to take the child to Mor Frøisland. Mor Frøisland did not welcome the case either, but when Mrs. Kolbjørnsen pleaded with Mor Frøisland to put her own feelings aside for the sake of the child, the healer relented, agreeing to keep the girl at her farm for two weeks. When Mrs. Kolbjørnsen returned to see her daughter, Mor Frøisland placed the child on the floor and told her to walk to her mother. The little girl did so, and the mother wept with gratitude. After five more weeks in Mor Frøisland's care, the Kolbjørnsens' daughter returned home and made a full recovery.

Cod-liver oil across the Atlantic

Did Mor Frøisland owe her success in curing rickets to cod-liver oil? No records remain to say, but we do know that healer Anne Brandfjeld, who enjoyed similar success, used "cod-liver oil fortified with tincture of iron" to supplement the sunlight and fresh air, herbs, and egg shells (a good source of calcium) that characterized her regimen.[25]

By the 1400s Norway was exporting cod-liver oil for use in lamps and treating leather to Lübeck and other cities of the Hanseatic League, a medieval trading consortium with its Norwegian headquarters in Bergen. Gradually, "Bergen tran," as it was known, also developed a reputation as a salve for rheumatism and other muscular aches and pains. Dr. Samuel Kay used cod-liver oil as a treatment for rheumatism in Manchester, England, in the 1820s, when it also became a popular cure for rheumatism and rickets in Germany, and in the 1840s, Norwegian physicans were using it to relieve pain. The pattern repeated itself, according to one researcher; individual doctors discovered cod-liver oil being used as a home remedy and then passed that knowledge along to other doctors. Still, by the turn of the twentieth century, most regarded the oil only as an "easily digested and easily assimilated fat," essentially a solvent for other ingredients they considered more active.[26]

"A fattening tonic, easily absorbed by the body and useful in all chronic illnesses where nurtrition has suffered," said Norway's popular *Veileder i Sundhed og Sygdom. Lægebog for norske Hjem* (Advisor in health and sickness. Doctor book for Norwegian homes), published in 1903. Though its author, the director of the national hospital, regarded tran as "especially useful in children suffering from English Disease," he also strongly recommended "a lot of sweet milk and a daily bath in warm, salty water" for curing rickets. Coming closer to the truth, the 1905 district doctor's report from Ål in Hallingdal observed that rickets "develops when children eat too little fish fat." But not until Mellanby's work in the early 1920s would anyone begin to understand why cod-liver oil works.[27]

The "miracle" described in Jessie Hanson Johnson's memoir of life in Hanska, Minnesota, was surely brought about by cod-liver oil. Johnson's maternal grandparents had emigrated from Lom, Gudbrandsdal, in 1880, and both of her parents were born in Hanska. When Jessie was born in 1905, her father had just been appointed head butter-maker at the creamery. Jessie's sister Myrtle followed two years later, but she "was not the strong healthy baby I had been," wrote Jessie. She cried and fussed a great deal, and the "doctor seemed unable to help her, though he had diagnosed her illness as rickets."[28]

Since the doctor had no cure, Jessie's mother "in desperation" sought help from folk healer Marit Tofteli (born 1844 in Dovre, Gudbrandsdal), "who was said to have secret, powerful medicines for all kinds of illnesses." Marit "reluctantly agreed" to help Myrtle under the promise of the "greatest secrecy" and only with "assurance that Mother would follow her instructions to the letter." Then the folk healer "went into her tiny kitchen and behind the closed door mixed her potions." When she finally reappeared, according

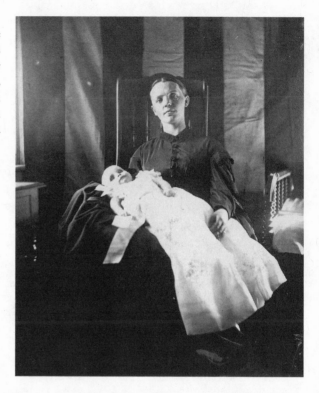

Cherstin Mattson, wife of Minnesotan Hans Mattson, holding her child who has died, about 1865. Infant death was a common sorrow in the nineteenth century.

to Johnson, she "gave mother a paste to put on Myrtle's sore eyes, and some medicine to be given regularly. Soon a miracle happened, and Myrtle became a happy, healthy baby. No one ever knew what had been in the 'magic potions' which Marit had given Mother, but suffice it to say, they saved Myrtle's life!"

Easily absorbed cod-liver oil probably constituted a major component of the paste Myrtle's mother applied to the child's eyelids, whose thin membranes would have assured its rapid transfer into the bloodstream. Strengthening the guess that cod-liver oil was Marit Tofteli's miracle medicine is the visit by Clara Becken (1895–1992) that yielded an "amber liquid" (described by Doug Becken in Chapter 4).

Advocating the virtues of cod-liver oil in Norway, the 1903 *Veileder i Sundhed og Sygdom* recommended downing it by the spoonful: "Keep it to the very front of the mouth," the book helpfully advised, "then gulp it down with cold water, beer, coffee, or sweet wine." The terrible taste of tran made it the bane of Norwegian children on this side of the Atlantic, too. Claire

Kristensen, born in Brooklyn in 1933 to an immigrant mother from Karmøy on Norway's southwest coast, called it "the one horrible memory all of us first-generation Norwegian kids have." She continued, "The fish stores always carried 'ekte [genuine] Norwegian cod-liver oil,' and my mother never let me go to school without a tablespoon of it in one hand and a glass of orange juice in the other to wash it down."[29]

Bad taste and all, the secret of cod-liver oil was circulating on both sides of the Atlantic by the 1930s.[30] To people in turn-of-the-century Hanska, however, the medicine remained mystical. "Marit's father had brought this mysterious knowledge with him from Norway, and passed it on to his daughter," believed Johnson, and "The 'magic' died with her."

Perhaps not surprisingly, Marit's "mysterious knowledge" had marked her as a witch—in the eyes of children, at least. "How we youngsters hurried by her little house in fear and trembling!" wrote Johnson. "These transplanted Norwegians in Hanska still carried with them many of the old superstitions about witches, ghosts and trolls from the old country." Like so many other folk healers, Marit had a skill her neighbors desperately needed and appreciated, but they envied and even feared her for it. These conflicting attitudes, along with the cultured class's disdain for self-trained caregivers, sustained the image of the folk healer as a witch. Although Sarah Oelberg, a recent pastor of Hanska's Nora Unitarian Universalist Church, wrote that some parishioners recalled being "spooked by her house and hurrying past it on the opposite side of the street," she added that there was "also generally great admiration for her gifts."[31]

Other Hanska residents provided ample evidence of both attitudes during the author's visit in 2004. One recalled how Marit had healed an aunt whose fingers were crippled from childhood rickets, and another remembered waiting as a little boy in Marit's house while she went upstairs to mix the medicine that ultimately cured his sister's ringworm. But Marit had also been "controversial," rarely mixing with others and keeping an overgrown yard that "we children went out of our way to avoid," recalled a man in his seventies.[32]

Tofteli's obituary in the August 10, 1934, *Hanska Herald* makes no mention of her medicines. Referring to her as "one of the oldest pioneer women of our village," it notes only that "Miss Mary Tolfteli" was "a good and kind-hearted woman, lived a quiet life alone, and did washing etc. for the local people." Sidestepping Marit's activity as a folk healer entirely, the obituary correctly predicted that "her memory will linger long with the old time residents of our village."[33]

"Most of the town went to [Marit's] funeral," wrote Oelberg. "It was held in the [Zion] Lutheran church, and Clara Becken went, too. She said afterward that Rev. [V. F.] Larson gave the best sermon she had ever heard," perhaps, Clara opined, out of "fear for *Marit's* powers!" "It is too bad that folks did not get to know her better," Oelberg continued. "In those days, however, a single woman living alone and reclusive was often shunned and considered evil. I am not sure it was her healing gifts that gave her the reputation of a witch as much as her lifestyle." Considering that folk healers frequently acquired reputations for witchcraft, Marit's special talents—and, of course, her possession of the black book—doubtless contributed to her image.

By the time Marit Tofteli died in 1934, most people knew about how rickets related to Vitamin D, sunshine and cod-liver oil. Yet, as late as 1933, Leif Salomonsen could write in the popular health book *Vår helse* that "a great deal of superstition still clings to the English disease, 'svekk,' as seen in the large portion of the public who still regard it as belonging to the domain of the 'kloke koner.'"[34] By the time the 1949 edition of the same book appeared, he no longer felt the need to emphasize "you don't need a klok kone to cure rickets." But even at that late date, the supernatural legacy of the disease had by no means been forgotten. While "formerly extremely common, misunderstood, and believed curable only by kloke koner," Salomonsen observed in 1949, "rickets is now cured quickly and certainly by giving the child a teaspoon of tran three times a day and taking it outside into the fresh air and sunshine."

The advice manifested itself in a practice that subsequently became common in Norway. On cold but sunny winter days, mothers park their carriages outside in the yard, where babies, nestled in a fluffy *dyne* (feather comforter), can absorb the sun's rays. Though the huldrefolk have long since vanished, the need to supplement Norway's pale sunshine lives on. "Tran is part of *den norske folkesjel* (the soul of the Norwigian people)," proclaims Raymond Dalen in a recent article titled, "Tran, the Artic Vitamin Bomb." He advises Norwegians for whom cod-liver oil is only a "gruesome memory from childhood" to "renew their acquaintance" with modern tran, now available in orange and strawberry flavors.[35]

8

Alcohol as Medicine and Scourge

From "water of life" to "Devil's yoke"

"People firmly believed that alcohol could cure all ills. Good for
colds and other internal ailments, it could also heal external injuries. It provided relief from exhaustion, warmth in cold weather,
and refreshment from the heat. Women in childbirth had to have
brennevin [hard liquor] from the time they delivered until they
regained their strength. Brennevin was a 'must' at baptisms and
funerals, too, but most of all at weddings, where its absence would
have been an unthinkable disgrace."

Erling Bækkestad, describing Ål in Hallingdal in the early 1800s

MOST NORWEGIANS BEGAN the nineteenth century believing that
alcohol benefited the body and regarding *brennevin* (hard liquor) as
essential to every celebration. Fifty years later, many could be found campaign-
ing furiously against *drikkeondet* (the evil of drink). This dichotomy prevailed on both sides of the Atlantic, as some people drank to tragic excess,
while others "went to their graves without a drop of hard liquor having ever
moistened their lips," as Eugene Boe described his grandparents, Osten Bø
and Caroline Soliah, homesteaders near Fergus Falls, Minnesota, in the 1870s.
"If a doctor had prescribed whiskey to alleviate some pain or affliction," Boe
insisted, "they would have ignored the prescription and suffered in silence."[1]

A great many other Norwegian Americans did as Shirley Olsen Sorensen's grandparents, who kept "a bottle of whisky for medicinal purposes, but
no other liquor" in their Eau Claire, Wisconsin, home. Since alcohol had
traditionally been considered a medicine, it often retained this use even as
people increasingly saw drinking as a health and social scourge.[2]

Evaporating fermented liquids over a flame with a distillation device produces a more highly concentrated alcohol. Vapors cool as they pass through the barrel of cold water and condense.

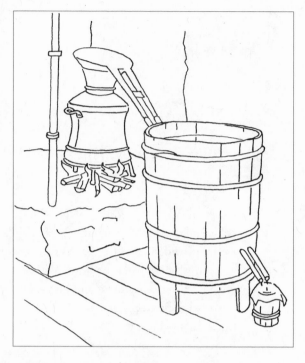

Fermentation, the chemical action of yeast on the sugars of fruit, malted barley, or potatoes, is the basis of all alcoholic beverages, and the process was known as early as 6000 BC. The process of "distillation" (heating fermented alcohol and condensing its vapors) to produce an alcohol of higher concentration dates to about 800 BC, when it was practiced in India and China. Distillation did not arrive in Europe until 1100 AD, when it was performed at the renowned medical school of Salerno, Italy. By the 1300s, European monks had learned to distill herb-flavored alcohols to derive spirits they called *aqua vitae* (the water of life), to which they attributed miraculous medicinal properties. This process eventually gave rise to the still-popular Benedictine liqueur, first produced in France around 1510, and its lesser-known Norwegian counterpart, St. Halvard.[3]

Monks who cultivated medicinal herbs in Norway's medieval cloisters probably used alcohol to extract and concentrate the herbs' active ingredients, but the first documented evidence of *brennevin* (literally, "distilled wine") in Norway appears in a letter dated 1531 sent by Danish nobleman Eske Bille from his castle in Bergen to Archbishop Olav Engelbrektsson in Nidaros (now Trondheim). The letter accompanied a gift of "some water that is called Aqua vitae, and helps all manner of internal illness a person may have."[4]

Apparently finding the "water" effective, the archbishop founded the industry that in subsequent years circulated bottles of these spirits all around Norway with the label, "*Medisinen for alt* [The medicine for everything]." The word *dram*, still used in Norwegian for a "shot" of alcohol, derives from this medicinal past, being the old Greek word *drachm* that apothecaries used as a measuring unit. A Danish doctor book in 1555 cited brennevin as an effective remedy for the then-common conditions of "syphilis, apoplexy, sore eyes, and fever."[5]

Norwegian beer traditions

While hard liquor came relatively late to Norway, beer occupied a central position in the country's culture long before the Viking era (ca. 800–1000 AD). Celebrating their rituals with beer brewed from sprouted and fermented barley, the Vikings cultivated ritual drunkenness as a way of cementing social relations and facilitating communication with the gods.[6]

Rather than abolishing these deeply rooted drinking customs, the early Christian church incorporated them. Norwegians continued to drink midwinter toasts to ensure fertility and a good harvest as the Vikings had done, but they offered their toasts on December 25 rather than in mid-January and drank to Christ and the Virgin Mary instead of Odin, Thor, and Frey.

Early Christian law required that landowners brew beer to share with their neighbors during Christmas and at other times of celebration, threatening the noncompliant with stiff fines and the loss of their land. For centuries, beer (*øl*) remained the essential drink for observing the yuletide (known as *å drikke jul*, or "drinking Christmas"), as well as betrothals (*festerøl*, engagement beers), christenings (*barnsøl*, child-beers), and funerals (*gravøl*, grave beers).

The brew that accompanied these celebrations had to be strong. It stood out from the weak beer made for daily consumption by recycling the malt first used to make the festive brew. Norwegians looked forward to celebrating the milestones of life and the yearly cycle as a welcome break in their otherwise dreary, work-filled lives, and they drank on these occasions with the aim of getting drunk. A good host made sure that they did. Noise, fighting, and drunkenness signified a successful gathering that would enhance the host's reputation. *"Velkommen grande i mit hus"* (Welcome neighbor to my house), reads the inscription on an 1843 ale bowl from Todalen in Møre og Romsdal, *"Sæt dig ned og drik en rus"* (sit yourself down and get soused). "People thought drinking made them happy," observed Armauer Hansen in his 1910 memoir, "a misunderstanding that can be fitting for Norwegians who are otherwise too inhibited to let themselves go."[7]

ALE BOWL INSCRIPTION FROM 1780

"Smag paa det, jeg haver inde,
Drikk saa ud det, hver en taar.
Se saa, om du dør kan finde,
Naar du ud af huset gaar."

(Taste what I have inside,
Drink it all, to the last drop.
Then see if you the door can find
when out of the house you go.)

Valdres Samband, *March 1913*

Brennevin: From medicine to scourge

Beer remained the dominant drink in Norway during the 1600s and 1700s. Years of crop failures kept grain in short supply, and the available brennevin tasted like bad moonshine after the monastic tradition of herbal-flavored distillates largely disappeared in the wake of the Lutheran Reformation of 1537.

Most early-nineteenth-century Norwegians nevertheless had a healthy regard for brennevin, which they associated with good health. A civil official complained about the blockade that kept necessary goods from reaching Norway during the Napoleonic wars, noting that the "lack of brennevin and tobacco throughout the realm was having a damaging effect on people's health." Friends and relatives customarily brought brennevin to patients at Norway's Rikshospital (national hospital) to expedite their recovery.[8]

Foreign visitors commented on the "unbelievable quantities of brennevin" that Norwegians consumed. When Englishman Deervent Conway met a seventy-four-year-old farmer in Øvre Telemark during the 1820s, for example, he noted that the farmer attributed his good health to brennevin, while the German traveler Treschow Hanson remarked that Norwegian peasants drank brennevin to "strengthen their marrow and bone." A traveler to Hallingdal in 1829 observed that overnight guests received a bedtime dram to improve their sleep and that the host returned the next morning with a brennevin bottle in hand to pour them another.[9]

The surge in brennevin drinking these travelers observed resulted from new legislation passed in the wake of Norway's 1814 constitution. Exercising freedom from the Danes, an 1816 law granted all Norwegian landowners the right to distill spirits freely from their own harvest. Greeted with "widespread joy throughout the land," this right, it was believed, would advance agriculture and promote the interests of the Norwegian farmer over that of urban officials.[10]

Brennevin quickly became Norway's most important industry, especially as the easier-to-grow potato replaced grain as the raw material. "It was the custom in those days for every farm to distill spirits," wrote a woman born in 1807 on the Sneve farm in Opdal, Trøndelag. As a girl, she closely "watched the large copper cauldrons used for *hjemmebrenning*" (home distillation) both day and night, from the time the fire was lit under them until the last drop had run out. The process took several days, and "the first drops that emerged from the long and painstaking process were put into bottles and used only for medicine."[11]

Having spent her first seventy-three years on the farm in Opdal, this woman lived the last twenty-four on a South Dakota homestead, where in the 1880s she regaled her grandchildren with tales of her life in Norway. When they asked if there had been "a lot of drinking and drunkenness," she told them that "people used the brennevin very sparingly. You needed the best grain to make it, and a whole barrel of grain yielded only a small amount of brennevin. So brennevin was only used at Christmas, weddings, and other celebrations."

Consumption of brennevin, once limited to special occasions, rose rapidly in the years after the 1816 law and soon became a problem. The drinking of copious amounts of strong beer had traditionally been confined to ritual occasions, but brennevin, with its perceived health benefits, became a daily necessity for many. Alcohol consumption soared from 3.5 liters per person per year in 1815 to 7.0 liters per year by 1837. (Easy access to alcohol and good economic times encouraged drinking in the rest of Northern Europe and North America in this period, as well.)[12]

By the 1830s and 1840s, brennevin accounted for as much as ninety percent of Norway's total alcohol consumption, with every adult drinking an annual average of thirteen liters of alcohol, mostly brennevin. "No one wants good, strengthening beer anymore," observed Bishop J. S. Munch in 1827. "Now only brennevin will do."[13]

The pioneering Norwegian sociologist Eilert Sundt, whose classic study of alcoholism (*Om ædruelighetstilstanden i Norge*) appeared in 1857, observed that the 250 guests at a traditional three-day wedding held at Haram in Møre og Romsdal drank approximately 240 liters of brennevin and 800 liters of øl. That amounted to almost one liter (nearly a quart) of brennevin and three liters of øl per person, he figured, but since women and children drank considerably less, each male was drinking more. During Christmas, many residents were "half drunk during the entire [twelve-day] holiday."[14]

The social consequences of drinking so heavily could not be ignored. Gatherings ended in fights with drunken combatants stabbing each other or biting off each other's fingers and noses. The clergy drank, too, some in considerable quantity. Pastor Christian Fredrik Hvidt, the parish minister at Nordal from 1821 to 1840, was hardly alone in his reputation for staying to the very end of the three-day wedding celebrations and imbibing no less than the other guests. Though most ministers drank more moderately, few shunned alcohol, and many produced their own. The renowned pietistic reformer Hans Nielsen Hauge (1771–1824) made aquavit on his Jarlsberg estate, for example, and Caja Munch, the wife of pastor Johan Storm Munch (1827–1908), cheerfully wrote from their parsonage in Wiota, Wisconsin, that she prepared Christmas ale and wine. Minister's son Christopher Hammer (1720–1804) published in 1776 the best Norwegian textbook on home distillation, a volume that not only described in detail how to make and flavor brennevin but pointed out: "When a laborer has to get up at 2 o'clock and even earlier and go to work in the woods or barn, he needs brennevin and a slice of bread to keep him going. Whether cutting trees, burning charcoal, hauling wood from the forest, or performing other cold-weather work, brennevin is both healthy and good if used in moderation."[15]

SOMETHING STRONG FOR THE PASTOR

"My Norwegian grandparents were stalwart Norwegian Synod Lutherans," wrote John Christianson, professor emeritus at Luther College, in 2003. "Grandmother was a teetotaler, but she gathered wild grapes along the fence-rows of the family farm and made wine from them. One of my uncles teased her for this and asked, 'Why do you make wine if you don't drink it?' Grandmother replied, with a certain irritation for having to say the obvious, 'I have to have *something* to serve the pastor when he visits at Christmas time.'"

But attitudes toward alcohol were beginning to change. Prompted by injuries, killings, drownings, and other accidents that ensued as drinking went from ritual observance to daily habit and as hard liquor replaced beer as the drink of choice, authorities passed new legislation in 1848 to reverse the liberal law of 1816. *Hjemmebrenning* (distilling alcohol at home) was now declared illegal.[16]

Even before the 1848 legislation, more and more of the population had begun to doubt the merits of brennevin. While Judge Hans Møller promoted temperance in 1828, he accepted that brennevin had its place among the workers, "especially in a country like Norway, where cold, snow and ice generally prevail during eight months of the year" and where the "farmer trudges to the mountains amid blowing snow and frost or toils in the raw wind and rain to do hard labor that drains his bodily resources." Citing similar challenges faced by the fisherman and soldier, Møller concluded that "in such circumstances, a drink of brennevin is useful for providing warmth and refreshment." Surprising new evidence cited by Henrik Wergeland in an 1831 article in *Folkebladet* (Magazine of popular enlightenment), however, indicated that stopping drinking did *not* endanger health and that those who stopped drinking actually became healthier.[17]

During the 1840s, temperance groups initiated by the upper class formed and spread rapidly. By 1846, the parish minister in Nissedal, Telemark, could report "much abstinence," in stark contrast to district doctor Krabbe's 1839 annual report from the same parish noting such "overwhelming brennevin drinking" by both men and women that "delirium tremens" were "not un-common."[18]

Some people even resorted to black-book formulas to "make an alcoholic put aside his ways," including this formula from Nord Rustad: "Take three baby mice. Place them in 1/2 quart of brennevin for fourteen days. Then let the person drink the brennevin." Aslak Bergland (born 1862 in Morgedal, Telemark) wrote: "Seeing older people drink so much that they became confused was quite common in my early years, but the younger generation never over-indulged," an acknowledgment that change was taking place.

By the mid-1850s, the first temperance movements peaked across the country, boasting 25,000 members who opposed any use of brennevin except as a medicine, but tolerated beer and wine drinking. By this time, brennevin consumption had dropped to half what it had been in 1835, while annual coffee consumption had grown from less than one pound per person in the 1820s to over four pounds per person in 1845, especially in rural areas.[19]

Coffee quickly replaced both the "morning dram" downed by workers be-fore their earliest morning chores and *blanda*, the daily beverage of water and whey formerly favored by adults and children. Coffee also replaced brenne-vin as the drink received by women in childbirth. But its rapid rise rested in part on a misunderstanding. German scientists had asserted that since both coffee and meat contain nitrogen, coffee had the same nutritional value as meat. Based on this assertion, district doctor Michael Krohn advised in an 1859 lecture that coffee could also replace milk, and P. C. Asbjørnsen repeated both of these assertions in his popular 1864 cookbook, *Fornuftig madstel* (Common sense cooking).[20]

The changeover to coffee went hand in hand with the revival of religion, and most Norwegians came to regard drunkenness as "ungodly." So it was, writes Norwegian food historian Astrid Riddervold, that "a thousand-year-old tradition of drinking alcohol to honor the gods and communicate with the divine by means of drunkenness went into reverse. Suddenly drinking had become sinful and drunkenness a disgrace."[21]

While Norway's earliest temperance movements were initiated by the professional class and promoted moderation, the movements that followed, begun among the lower classes, called for total abstinence. These move-ments started slowly among the grass roots in the 1860s but gained remark-able political power in the 1870s, increasing from eleven unions with 1,700 members in 1870, to forty-five unions with 6,500 members in 1873. As an indication of their power, the number of places where brennevin could be served declined between 1847 and 1870 from 1,128 to 501.[22]

Alcoholism among the immigrants

During the mid-1800s, many Norwegians emigrated from the parishes that most intensively practiced home distillation. They brought their drinking habits to the New Land, where they found plenty of saloons, or retail businesses selling beer and whiskey by the glass, ready to indulge them.

Norwegians in the Long Prairie settlement near Capron, Illinois, complained Pastor J. W. C. Dietrichson, continued their "penchant for drunkenness." "The men would go to Capron in the morning to deliver milk to the creamery, then be tempted to drop in at the saloon, where they could always find someone they knew," said Alfred C. Stimes (born 1922), who heard about conditions from his grandfather, Ole O. Stimes (1838–1936), an 1851 emigrant from Vik in Sogn. "Some ended up sitting in the saloon all day and came home drunk to their wife and children."[23]

Long Prairie was far from the only Norwegian settlement whose residents wrestled with the consequences of this "family secret." In Mekinock, North Dakota, not far from Grand Forks, Ole Anderson Skjækermo (born 1854 near Verdal, North Trøndelag) "had a history of alcohol abuse," wrote Carol Hanson Schwinkendorf. Ole's grandfather had been a landowner, but high taxes and an exploding population left nothing for Ole to inherit. Seeing no future in Norway, he emigrated at age seventeen to America, where he soon met Jorend Olson. The couple married on December 8, 1872, and moved to Mekinock in 1877. By 1886, they had seven children. One was still an infant the year that Ole went to the river with his shotgun and took his own life.[24]

Describing the tragedy, Rev. Olav Houkom, the pastor of Ole's church, wrote in a February 1, 1886, letter to his sister in Minneapolis: "A man who lived about three miles from here on the Sunday between Christmas and New Year at high mass time committed suicide by firing a rifle against his forehead. His wife is left with seven small children in poor circumstances, although people have done not so little to help her."

Rev. Houkom officiated at Ole's burial in the Middle Grove churchyard.

"When mother visited that church," said Schwinkendorf, "she recalled his grave being 'outside' of the fence, a place reserved for parishioners they considered had committed very grave sins." The Norwegians had transplanted to the New Land their long-standing custom of excluding suicides from a proper burial, adding distress to already troubled and grieving families. "So powerful was Ole's act," Schwinkendorf asserted, "that the family reflex was to behave by silence. Little was understood about the disease [of alcoholism]. Families suffered in silence to preserve the facade of normalcy, and many tragedies occurred." Her great-grandfather's act influenced "every relationship in the family for generations," Schwinkendorf observed. "One hundred and fifty years have passed since this happened, and even today there remains a silence, a hurt, and more important a feeling of protection for Ole."

With seven children to raise in a time before government asistance, Jorend needed the support of a husband. Three years later, she remarried, but her new husband also had a drinking problem. "Life again became difficult for Jorend," who by then had four more children. Her oldest son, Andrew (Schwinkendorf's grandfather), had been twelve years old when his father committed suicide, and finding unbearable "the pressure of living in an alcoholic household as one of eleven children," he left home in his early teens and "grew to manhood separated from his family and with an ache in his heart." While Andrew eventually married and raised a family, the shock of his father's act remained, and the pain it inflicted became a driving force in Schwinkendorf's family history.

Generations removed, Carol Schwinkendorf provided no details of daily life in her grandfather's "alcoholic households," but Aagot Raaen's autobiographical novel, *Grass of the Earth*, written in 1950, gives a child's-eye view of how drinking undermined a family's financial foundation: "Far [father] took the family's best milk cow and sold it in Grand Forks for needed supplies, but a neighbor subsequently saw him drinking up the money at one of the town's many saloons." An entire month passed before he returned home— with neither money nor the salt lick, halter rope, ax, pitchfork, and spade he had gone to buy. Perhaps financial woes also motivated Ole Skjækermo's desperate act.[25]

While "in the shadows" (as Aagot Raaen referred to her father's drinking bouts), he signed a mortgage that committed his family to constant struggle for economic survival despite their diligent hard work. Physical violence may have been the hardest to bear. Raaen omitted this aspect of her father Thomas's drinking from the novel, but revealed it in a brief piece about her parents found among her papers in Hatton, North Dakota.[26]

Thomas was a periodic drinker, but once started, the orgy would often last for weeks. In order to shorten the time of these orgies, Ragnhild [his wife] hit upon the plan of hiding some of the liquor. When she told Thomas, it almost cost her her life, since from that time on when his supply of whisky was gone, he suspected and accused her of concealing it. Then in a drunken fury he abused her. Once she fled to the stable where the children were doing chores, blood streaming from her face and two of her teeth knocked out. Another time she was hit on the head with a heavy pewter dipper, a blow which caused a permanent scar and for years induced severe head pains. On another occasion, her three little girls awoke to hear their father in a drunken frenzy shout: "Put the baby away so I can kill you." Speechless with fright they watched their mother with the baby in her arms edge slowly toward the bed and secure a blanket then gradually move backward toward the door, all the time holding the frenzied man with her eyes, as he stalked her, knife in hand, his face distorted by drink.

Thomas Raaen, born on a large farm in Hol, did not start life with difficulty. He was the son of a well-to-do schoolmaster, who counted bank officials, judges, teachers, and army officers among his ancestors. The famous poet Ivar Aasen frequently visited his home, and the museum in Oslo had many articles bearing the Raaen name. Thomas emigrated from Hallingdal in 1869 at age forty-two, having already sacrificed his military career to excessive drinking, however. While spoiled as a child after his father's death, he grew into manhood with a keen sense of humor, ready wit, and jolly personality that made him a natural leader. Engaged to his beautiful, patrician cousin until his excessive drinking caused her to break off their relationship, Thomas subsequently squandered his inheritance, lost his position, and was persuaded by his brother to emigrate to America to live with their sister, Birgit Mark, in Worth County, Iowa.

Skilled as a wood turner, he brought his lathe to America, and during the three years he lived with Birgit, he worked "like a Trojan," wrote Aagot, making beautiful furniture and tasting no liquor. Then, a favorite nephew's unfortunate choice of a marriage partner sent Thomas off on an extended drinking spree. Wishing to be rid of him, his sister and her husband manipulated a marriage for him to Ragnhild Rødningen in 1873.

Ragnhild came from peasant stock. Her parents had emigrated from Etnedalen, Valdres, in 1860, leaving Ragnhild behind to continue supporting herself as a servant girl. She followed them to Worth County, Iowa. By 1875 Ragnhild and Thomas had settled with three children in a 16-by-14 foot, one-room log cabin near what is now Hillsboro, North Dakota. Of the five children Ragnhild eventually bore in her marriage, four survived, but Ragnhild also had another daughter, born in 1871, two years before she married Thomas.

Ragnhild may have been pregnant when she left Norway. Peasant culture accepted premarital sexual relations that couples typically initiated after they became engaged. Pregnancy usually marked the time to plan the wedding, but as over-population and a difficult economy dramatically reduced resources, fewer couples could afford to marry and set up housekeeping, and the number of out-of-wedlock births soared. Unwed mothers with no marriage prospects were shut out of the peasant society and condemned by the church and professional classes. Many women chose to emigrate to America instead.

Like most cotters' daughters, Ragnhild had supported herself since confirmation by working for board and room on a prosperous farm. Young women in service often shared sleeping quarters with the farm's male servants. Whether it was a broken engagement or more casual sexual relations that led to Ragnhild's first pregnancy, records do not say, but she apparently felt a persistent guilt about her background that may have kept her from leaving Thomas.

Ragnhild had considered divorce and even spoke about it occasionally with her children, writes historian Barbara Handy-Marchello, and though divorce among Norwegian pioneers was rare, it was not unthinkable. But Ragnhild had no money to file papers, and plans to divorce Thomas faded before a "sense that her troubles were punishment for her transgressions."[27]

Besides, Thomas Raaen had a good side. "When not drinking," Aagot wrote, he was "a man of remarkably fine moral character, scrupulously honest, a man who despite the misfortune and misery occasioned by his weakness for alcohol found opportunity to do many kind acts."[28] He had helped organize the Goose River Church, the congregation that excluded him from membership because of his drinking. Aagot found this an "arbitrary decision," because others "known to be dishonest in their business dealings and immoral in their acts" still were "church members in good standing." The punishment, "drastic in its effects," ultimately did more harm than good, since it failed to end the drinking but "altered the man immeasurably. He shunned everybody after that, and very rarely did he ever enter a neighbor's house." He became silent and moody even with members of his family.

Ragnhild often felt like an outsider too. Her husband's drinking and the desperate poverty it inflicted on her family kept her from associating with the others on an equal footing. On the morning of January 10, 1890, however, she did join the neighbor women, and together they marched into the nearby town of Hatton to take matters into their own hands.[29]

Resentment against the local saloon had long been brewing. "Every time Far went away," wrote Aagot in her novel, "some women from near Hatton visited Mor." One of them was Olaug Aasen, who "preached like a minister." Hatton had one general store, one post office, two grain elevators, and six saloons. The saloon keepers were poor when they arrived, but had grown rich, Mrs. Aasen railed, by keeping their saloons "warm and cozy so the farmers will want to come in." "I have often seen the saloon keepers in the streets begging the men to come in for a hot drink before starting the long, cold drive home—only to keep them there until their money is gone."[30]

On the morning of January 10, 1890, Ragnhild tied her best kerchief on her head, wrapped her red plaid shawl snugly around her shoulders, and pulled on her wool mittens for the march into Hatton. A mob of women gathered on the outskirts of town, some armed with hatchets, some with hammers, and some with long sticks. The women rushed into the saloon and madly chopped, smashed, and raked down liquor bottles so that the whole floor was quickly soaking wet. They took chairs and benches, lifted them and hurled them at the shelves full of bottles, at windows, and at big mirrors. The crowds in the streets cheered.

Then the women went down into the cellar, where kegs and barrels were kept; they chopped spigots until streams of liquor flowed and their shoes and long skirts were wet. That night the women went home rejoicing in their achievement.

In the excitement, however, an old drunk had his hand slashed. He did not keep the wound clean, developed blood poisoning, and died. In May, the sheriff of Traill County served papers on Aagot's mother to appear at a trial; the women were implicated in the man's death.

For the trial, Mor had to go to Caledonia, the county seat, for more than a week. While the children were glad when she returned, Mor enjoyed the experience. "We had good food and slept on good beds," and the women had "such a good time listening to all the funny things the witnesses said and the speeches of the lawyers and the judge." On May 20, the verdict came in, and the women were judged not culpable for the man's death. "The saloon keepers learned a lesson." Alcohol was neither harmless nor healthy.

ALMKLOV AND ALCOHOL

In 1877 Severin Almklov took a call to become the Lutheran minister in Benson, Minnesota, a town of 300 inhabitants with no fewer than five of the "infamous American saloons." The impoverished settlers lived in sod huts, and the saloons were their only public gathering spaces. So, in establishments named *Lille Helvete* (Little Hell), *Sodoma*, and *Gomorrah*, they sat and argued the political, social, and religious issues of the day.

"So-called church people" sat there night and day discussing the *kirkestrid* (the bitter church battle that divided the Norwegian Lutheran church during the late 1800s), said Almklov, peppering their debate with cursing and swearing that they alone had the pure doctrine and that the others were just heretics. "They slammed their glasses down on the bar so hard they shattered, cutting themselves in the process so the blood ran red." Others fought for the "pure doctrine with such holy zeal that the police had to pull them apart."

To oppose this "outrageous behavior," Almklov organized *avholdstaler* (temperance talks) and singing organizations. He soon learned that "keeping the Mississippi River from flowing to the sea" would have been easier than getting people to listen. So it was with little regret that he left his ministry in Benson to open the drugstore in

Cooperstown, North Dakota, where he felt he did a "thousand times more good in a single year than in the twelve long ones in Benson." Earning a thousand times more, he also felt a thousand times more appreciated.

Severin Almklov's memoir, Nord-Norge, 1931

Patent medicines on the prairie

As temperance movements took hold, the sale of patent medicines soared, not least because of their high alcohol content. Gaining in popularity since the 1840s, aided by newspaper advertisements (not least in the immigrant

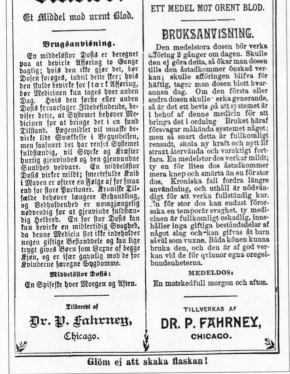

Fourteen percent alcohol by volume, Kuriko was the patent medicine of choice among Norwegian Americans. Directions for use in four languages covered the sides of the square bottle—Norwegian and German in gothic script, Swedish and English in modern type. The top and bottom lines remind users, "Shake the bottle well."

press) and low postal rates, these concoctions were patented in name only. The competing brands usually differed little from each other in content and consisted largely of herbal extracts laced with ample doses of alcohol, sometimes further fortified by morphine, opium, or cocaine.[31]

Each ethnic group seemed to have a favorite patent medicine, and among the Norwegians it was Kuriko. "Kuriko could be found in every home," says Oscar Overby, who emigrated from Norway in 1882 and settled with his wife near Cooperstown, North Dakota. Devoted to their patent medicine, many Norwegians even saved the empty bottles, which mothers used a thousand different ways in their pantries and children filled with drinking water to carry to school. In 1890, North Dakota immigrant Edward Hauge reportedly used a Kuriko bottle to make his "poor man's Christmas dram," mixing brennevin, sugar, water, and caraway to imitate aquavit.[32]

No law required patent medicine manufacturers to disclose their ingredients prior to the Pure Food and Drug Act of 1906, so Kuriko's 14-percent alcohol content probably caught many consumers unaware. Even stalwart teetotalers like Torkel Torkelson Fuglestad (born 1856 in Bjerkreim, Sogn) swore by Kuriko. "Kuriko was the only known medicine until after World War I" in their Cooperstown home, according to descendent Swanhild Algaard, even though Torkel and his wife, Abigael (who emigrated in 1883 from Stavanger, the heart of the Norwegian temperance movement), were "avidly in favor of total abstinence." They "welcomed temperance speakers into their home," and their "sobering speeches" made a "deep impression."[33]

Among the many who believed in Kuriko, no one was more ardent than Mathia Stene of Crookston, Minnesota. Mathia married Ole Torkelson in 1889 and bore nine children. During a birth in 1899, she fell desperately ill. Neighbors diagnosed her condition as jaundice, recognizing the telltale yellowing of her fingernails and eyes (caused by a failure to excrete bile, perhaps because her pregnancy blocked the duct). Seeing the symptoms that typically accompany jaundice—indigestion, sluggishness, fatigue, constipation, chills, vomiting, and fever—Mathia's neighbors "didn't know if she would make it or not," wrote her son, Melvin Olaf Torkelson (1899–1983), in his memoir. There was "no doctor nearer than Crookston [forty miles from their farm] and he wouldn't go out unless you had a good fast team."[34]

Convinced that "if she could get some Dr. Peter's Kuriko she might survive," Torkelsen's father "hit the trail on a dogtrot." He aimed to get to St.

Hilaire about six miles away by daybreak, but finding no Kuriko in St. Hilaire, he jogged on to Crookston, which then had a "rudimentary" drugstore. Through it all, neighbors came to visit, though "they had little faith in seeing her alive again," wrote Torkelsen. "But Mother was a strong woman, and she had faith in God, and also in the Kuriko."

The Fuglestads, too, tended their ills by "fusing a generous amount of prayer with whatever other measure they took," wrote Swanhild Algaard. Though they would not have welcomed the comparison, this combination of faith and medicine harkened back to the Catholic prayers that the seventeenth-century folk healer Lisbet Nypan read over the salt she massaged into her rheumatic neighbors' limbs until the authorities condemned her to burn at the stake. Just as faith benefited Nypan's patients, it apparently helped Mathia Stene Torkelsen, for she made a full recovery and lived on their homestead another forty years.

The miracle medicine that "saved" Mathia was a laxative. "Two evacuations daily," promised the multilingual label on Kuriko's square bottle. "A remedy that purifies the blood, cures illness," declared the Kuriko advertisement printed in the October 1, 1907, *Ungdommens Ven* (Young people's companion). Stating the fundamental principle of nineteenth-century medicine, the ad proclaimed, "Nine out of ten common illnesses derive from impure blood.... Peter's Kuriko has yet to meet its match in cleaning the blood and fortifying the system. It has been in use for over one hundred years, long enough to prove its value time and again, and contains nothing that is not good for you."

In German and Norwegian gothic script, as well as English and Swedish typescript, one panel on each of the bottle's four sides, the label advised that "if the first or second dose sickens you, it is proof that your system needs this medicine as a corrective." Cautioning that while "it may weaken you while you are using it, when it has thoroughly renovated the system, your return to strength and vigor will be rapid, safe and permanent. An overdose can only result in temporary weakness, as this medicine contains no poison whatever and may as safely be given to infants as adults, to either sex, and is beneficial in disorders peculiar to females." Seemingly calculated to promote maximum consumption of the product, the directions further advised that a tablespoonful taken both morning and evening constituted a "medium dose." [35]

As a stimulant, Kuriko may indeed have helped restore the normal flow of

Mathia's bile. Kuriko tasted good, too, perhaps explaining why it remained Torkel Fuglestad's "favorite remedy for everything" through the late 1920s, said Algaard. "When his grandchildren came to visit, they often developed mysterious ailments, and Torkel would invariably come with a tablespoon and the Kuriko bottle." By that time, law required that the label clearly indicate its contents, which included numerous invigorating herbs such as senna, fennel, peppermint, spearmint, mountain mint, horse mint, sarsaparilla, sassafras, hyssop, blessed thistle, dittany, ground ivy, St. John's wort, lemon balm, sage, spikenard, and yarrow—and 14 percent alcohol.[36]

Brennevin, the universal cure

The Fuglestads may well have known about the alcohol in Kuriko, for Norwegians and Norwegian Americans often found no conflict between their temperance convictions and their medicinal use of hard liquor (brennevin): "As a Christian, she was a teetotaler," wrote Nancy Stout about her mother, Sara Berg (born 1892 in Climax, Minnesota), but she often used "hot sweetened brandy to help break up our colds and fevers. To this day the smell of brandy brings back visions of sore throats." The makers of American bitters, or herb-flavored alcohol such as Angostura bitters (45 percent alcohol) used in Old-fashioned and Manhattan cocktails, encouraged this perception, while agreeing that "distilled liquors richly deserve the stigma that has been cast on them by friends of health and temperance." Alcohol was claimed to be essential to preserving the medicinal properties of vegetable extracts in a fluid state: "Only by a diffusible stimulant [could] the medicinal constituents . . . be conveyed discretely to their destination," explained the Hostetter Bitters Almanac in 1869. With the endless list of symptoms that "bitters" drinks claimed to cure, people readily found reasons to take them, and their warmth and exhilaration seemed convincing proof of their value.[37]

In Norway at century's end, "old folks had an unshakable faith in brennevin as a medicine," said Marcellus Helleland (born 1884 in Etne, Hordaland), and "most households kept a bottle of brennevin on hand in case of illness." Hot beer and cognac was an "excellent" cure for colds," concurred Ludvig N. Holstad (born 1885 in Hareid, Møre og Romsdal). People "cook[ed] up a mixture of milk, pepper, and syrup to pour down their throats boiling hot; I saw my dad do this many a time." Nineteenth-century Norwegians also continued the tradition of flavoring their medicinal brennevin with herbs, especially perikum (St. John's wort) and malurt (wormwood), a practice whose roots date to the Middle Ages.[38]

The five-petalled, yellow blossoms of St. John's wort imparted a distinctive scent along with a surprising red color to the *perikum brennevin* that many Norwegians kept on hand to treat stomachache and heartburn. "The perikum blossoms were dried and crushed and put in a bottle and covered with genuine cognac," says Margit J. Samulsen (born 1892 in Tyristad, Ringerike), whose grandmother regarded this mixture as a *universalmiddel* (cure-all). As a little girl, Margit "got many tablespoons full of it, and whether it was the belief or whatever—it did help!"[39]

With its bright yellow flowers that produced a red juice when crushed, perikum naturally attracted attention. In Telemark, people said that perikum had grown beneath the cross at Golgotha, where Christ's blood imparted the flowers' red juice and their miraculous ability to heal. Seeing perikum reliably bloom each year at the summer solstice, the Vikings consecrated the herb to Balder, the Norse god of light. Christians named it St. John's wort to honor John the Baptist, whose saint's day the early church fathers celebrated on the summer solstice, June 24.[40] Norwegians still know Midsummer's Eve as St. Hans or *jonsok*, St. John's wake, and their medieval ancestors stayed awake all night to celebrate the saint.

For centuries the so-called "doctrine of signatures" taught that the red color of crushed perikum signaled its ability to treat disorders of the blood, while its yellow flowers meant it could cure jaundice. Norwegians used perikum brennevin for both those ailments, as well as for relieving pain, easing digestion, and treating colds and other respiratory infections. Modern research has indicated that St. John's wort includes an essential oil, polyphenols, and tannin that produce its astringent qualities and soothing effects, though its red dye (hypercin) can result in over-sensitivity to light.[41]

Today's Norwegians know hypericum as *prikkperikum*, referring to the apparent "pricks" visible when holding leaves up to the sun. These specks that seem to perforate the plant's leaves are oil glands and account for the plant's Latin name (*Hypericum perforatum*). Legend says Satan pierced perikum leaves in vengeful jealousy of the herb's potency, which outstripped even his own diabolical power. Believing in its strength, people around the world and through the ages have worn protective amulets of St. John's wort.[42]

So commonly did Norwegians once rely on perikum brennevin that St.

John's wort became known as *brennevinsgras* (liquor grass), but that was before herbal remedies fell into obscurity. "We found a carafe of perikum brennevin in the closet among my grandmother's medicines," wrote Karen Holtet (born 1885, Rakkestad), but, not knowing how she used it, "we poured it down the drain when she died."[43]

Karen Holtet found *malurt* in her grandmother's closet, too, but this herb she readily recognized from the yard of her childhood home. Picking the tiny, light yellow flowers from their downy, silver-gray stems, Holtet's mother would dry them to make the bitter-tasting malurt brennevin, then a popular cure for digestive problems. "If we had a stomachache," echoed Harald Anderson (born 1889 in Ullensaker), "we got a dram of *malurt brennevin*, made by mixing malurt with cognac." Known as wormwood in English, *malurt* (*Artemisia absinthium*) added to white wine makes vermouth, a drink consumed as medicine long before it flavored the classic martini. Hippocrates held wormwood in high esteem, claiming it alleviated disorders of the brain, and for centuries afterward people used it for sedation and to ease stomach pain. Despite these medicinal benefits, wormwood retains a menacing image. The Bible coupled wormwood with calamity, affliction, and remorse (Deuteronomy 29:18, Proverbs 5:4, Jeremiah 9:15, and Amos 5:7), associations that apparently derived from the ancient custom of preserving corpses with wormwood before burial (a practice that continued in Norway well into the 1800s).[44]

Wormwood's sinister reputation did not improve when it became the flavoring in absinthe, the 136-proof, emerald-green aperitif that addicted so many late nineteenth-century artists and intellectuals. Hauntingly portraying its nerve-damaging effect, Edvard Degas's 1876 painting *L'absinth* shows two hollow-eyed addicts, oblivious to everything around them. Some say it was under the influence of absinthe that Van Gogh famously cut off his ear in 1889, also in France, the country that produced most of the world's absinthe. France also consumed two-thirds of this supply before it joined other Western countries in the early 1900s in banning it.

The volatile oils of wormwood that produce the characteristic taste and fragrance of absinthe contain thujone, a consciousness-altering compound said to resemble the TCH in marijuana. While thujone is concentrated in absinthe, it is destroyed in other concoctions of wormwood such as vermouth, whose tannins and aromatic compounds promote digestion by stimulating the secretion of saliva.[45]

The Vikings mixed malurt with mead (honey wine) to prevent seasickness, a remedy that recurs in many medieval books of herbal remedies. Most nineteenth-century Norwegians used malurt to kill intestinal worms, a use Hans Jacob Wille noted in his classic *Beskrivelse over Sillejord Præstegjeld* (Description of Seljord parish) from 1786. Caja Munch mentioned this standard cure in an August 12, 1857, letter to her mother, thanking her for the homemade jam she had sent to the Munches' parsonage in Wiota, Wisconsin. Mrs. Munch wrote of having delightedly "sampled and tasted" the jam "so often that now I feel the worm is getting lively in my stomach, so I very likely will have to swallow the bitter pill and take some essence of wormwood," which her thoughtfully packed crate also contained.[46]

Flavored Spirits: Old Country medicine in the New Land

In making wormwood brennevin, Caja Munch carried on the Old Country tradition of herbally flavored alcohols. She may have even known Christopher Hammer's classic 1776 book describing the process.

The dandelion wine commonly made by many Norwegian immigrants descends from the same tradition. "For colds and flu, dandelion wine was helpful, especially for youngsters," writes Ella Grunewald (born 1916, Fergus Falls, Minnesota) in a February 6, 2001, letter. "While I was in country school during the day, mother would pick the flower tops from dandelion plants," adds Marion Oman (born 1917 in Kenyon, Minnesota): "I don't have her recipe but remember that she used oranges, lemons, sugar, and water. The mixture was kept in a crock behind the cooler side of the wood-burning kitchen range, where the heat would make the wine ferment. When it was ready to bottle, out came the board that Dad used for capping his home-brewed beer. . . . Some of our guests enjoyed a small wine glass of the brew," adds Oman, "but I hated it because when we were ill, dandelion wine was used as a medicine. It really seemed to help in some cases, though, perhaps because it was a relaxing remedy."[47]

The recipe used by Oman's mother probably resembled the one handed down in Ella Grunewald's family: "To 1 gal. boiling water add two quarts of dandelion blossoms, let stand from 24 to 48 hours (in a stone crock). Strain the above through cheese cloth. Add 4 lbs sugar, 3 lemons, 4 oranges (sliced unpeeled) and 1/2 package dry yeast. Mix well and let stand for 6 weeks in basement. Fruit can be removed sooner if desired. Strain and bottle."

While herbs enhanced the medicinal effect of some alcohol-based remedies, camphor and various chemicals fortified others. "*Kamfer* was bought
dry and brennevin was poured over it to produce *kamfer dråper*," says Karen
Holtet. "Camphor drops were a 'must' in everyone's home. They healed everything," echoes Frances Anderson Haase. These drops once ranked as the
single most widely used medicine among Norwegians on both sides of the
Atlantic and long remained in vogue. In Norway, "I grew up with camphor
drops," Haase continues, and when the family emigrated to Staten Island
in 1936, her mother brought along "all her medicines, which basically consisted of—camphor drops." But when she ran out of them and went to the
American drugstore to renew her supply, she could only get "camphor cakes."
She put these small squares into a pouch and pinned them on Haase's un-
dershirt, but "these did not help the cramps in the stomach the way camphor drops did."[48]

Though camphor drops long remained a "universal cure," no one savored
its taste. "A terrible drink," declared an elder in Sogn during the summer of
1996, "but it helped!" The 1915 *People's Home Medical Book*, however, listed
camphor as a poison and warned against its use, recommending antidotes
in case it was ingested by accident. Camphor's phenomenal popularity as a
medicine among nineteenth-century and early-twentieth-century Norwegian
immigrants thus speaks tellingly of making do with available treatments.[49]

In some families the camphor bottle became an indelible memory. "In
1861 when my great-grandmother Hæge Evenson and her four children left
Rauland in Telemark, they brought along a little bottle made at Hadeland
Glass Factory," writes Olga Edseth (born 1914) of Mt. Horeb, Wisconsin.
"In this bottle they had camphor and brennevin to bring along to America.
We have this camphor bottle still, for it became a little *klenodium* [treasure]
in our family."[50]

The crate that came to Caja Munch in August 1857 also contained camphor drops. Caja's friend Sophie Pehson had carefully labeled vials of the
drops, along with several other medicinal substances she thought they would
need. One of the vials had broken and spilled its contents, making the instructions illegible, but Caja reassured her friend that she knew exactly how
to use the camphor.

In other letters Caja told of her husband's severe case of laryngitis that
"lasted for several weeks and bothered him tremendously." Unable to sleep

or even lie down, "he could neither eat nor hardly swallow liquid food," she wrote on January 5, 1857. They tried all manner of poultices and gargles, "but nothing helped and there was no doctor we dared ask." Finally, they "made some brandy and salt, and after having gargled this several times, he improved. I suppose something in his throat broke, and in the course of one day, he was relieved of pain, but the swelling did not go down until a long time after." Brandy and salt came to the Munches' rescue again later that year when their infant daughter Else became seriously ill with a high fever and vomiting.[51]

"Brennevin og salt" had become exceedingly popular in Norway with the 1842 translation of the British pamphlet, *Brandy and salt, invented by William Lee, Esquire.* Promising that the mixture would "cure rheumatism, asthma, consumption, and other evils," the booklet instructed users to place six ounces of salt (completely dry and finely crushed) in a bottle together with a pint of the best French cognac and shake the mixture for ten minutes before setting it aside for another twenty minutes to allow all the salt to dissolve. "*Brennevin og salt hjelper mot alt*" (Brandy and salt cures all) became the Norwegian version of the British motto, "Brandy and salt, the medicine for gout," an affliction suffered mainly by the kondisjonerte class, the intended market for this cure.[52]

Brandy og salt, like camphor drops, apparently helped. "The patient usually recovered quickly," wrote Peter A. Munch, "if for no other reason than to avoid having to swallow another dose of the stuff." As an added bonus, the horrible taste of these elixirs removed all doubt that the brandy was being consumed strictly for medicinal purposes.

Meanwhile, and with nary a thought of medicinal benefit, some Norwegians on both sides of the Atlantic were slipping brennevin into the newly respectable coffee, to make "*kaffedoktor*" (coffee doctor, also known as *karsk*). So popular did this concoction become among Norwegian immigrants that Knut Teigen (1854–1914) dubbed Wisconsin's Koshkonong settlement, "*Karskelandet.*"[53] Characterizing the old Koshkonong settlers as "good Lutherans in their way," he wrote in 1907 that they "took pleasure with those who were happy, enjoyed the things that brought joy, and loved their women—along with wine and song." And, though they "might lose their inhibitions on especially festive occasions, it was seldom more than was good for them or beyond what they could handle." He continued, "There was no talk of temperance then, and øl (beer) and *brennevin* were available year round. . . . When the beer ran out, they brewed some more. For Christmas they brewed in especially great quantity and extra strong; they laid in a good supply of hard liquor then, too. Each of us boys received a bottle of brennevin so we could serve each other and otherwise imitate the drinking habits of our elders. . . . That's just the way it was in those days."

9

The Letting and Staunching of Blood

Traditional remedies newly relevant

"I have bled myself so I feel a little better, but my body seems
so weighed down that I can't seem to get much done."

Hans Halvorsen Vadder, schoolteacher
and church deacon, Telemark, 1862

NINETEENTH-CENTURY NORWEGIANS of all classes believed in the
therapeutic effects of bloodletting. Some did it annually as a spring
tonic; others engaged in the practice more often. If toxins in the blood
caused disease, they reasoned, getting rid of the "bad blood" would invigo-
rate them and make them well. Doctors relied on bloodletting, too, making it the single most widely used therapy on both sides of the Atlantic for
much of the nineteenth century. Already extensively employed by the time
of Hippocrates, bleeding, or phlebotomy, may have initially been inspired
by the natural cleansing process of menstruation. Imitating nature, the first
doctors who bled patients may have noticed that the procedure reduced
fever and relieved pain.[1]

Bloodletting continued as an important therapy in the Middle Ages. European barbers advertised this specialty with the still-familiar striped poles: red
for letting blood and white for staunching its flow. Nineteenth-century dentists also practiced bloodletting through the use of blood-sucking leeches. For
most Norwegians, bleeding was as trusted and popular a cure-all as aspirin is
today.[2]

Bloodletting

Bloodletting had its most enthusiastic advocate in Dr. Benjamin Rush (1746–1813), whose name appears on the Declaration of Independence just above that of his friend Benjamin Franklin. One of the most admired teachers of medicine in Philadelphia, then the medical center of America, Rush taught more than 3,000 medical students during his career. They carried his influence to every corner of the growing nation and honored him by founding the medical college in Chicago that still bears his name.

Believing that "excitation of the blood vessels" caused disease, Rush urged copious bleeding to cure it. Rush attributed redness, heat, and swelling— now recognized as the body's attempt to counteract infection—to congestion in the circulatory system. Citing nosebleeds as evidence of the body's need for bloodletting, Rush advised that twenty of the body's twenty-five pounds of blood could safely be drained.

Unfortunately for some of his contemporaries, we now know that the body holds less than half the amount he estimated, usually around ten pounds, just over ten pints or about 160 fluid ounces (about 7 or 8 percent of a person's body weight). When a pint of blood is withdrawn from a healthy individual, the body largely replaces it within an hour or so (although weeks may pass before the hemoglobin content returns to normal). If blood loss exceeds 10 percent of the body's total volume, blood pressure drops precipitously as a protective mechanism to aid blood clotting. If less than 30 or 40 percent of the total volume is lost, blood pressure rises again after approximately thirty minutes, but removing a larger volume can result in death if the loss is not promptly replaced.[3]

Rush had no way of knowing these details, and he managed to engender enormous enthusiasm for bloodletting among his students. One of them, Dr. William Montgomery, subsequently wrote to his mentor about treating a South Carolina legislator, saying that over the course of five days, he had relieved the patient of 165 ounces of blood. "He died," Montgomery observed, "but had we taken a still greater quantity, the event might perhaps have been more fortunate."[4]

America's first president fared no better. Suffering a severe throat infection following a ride on his Mt. Vernon farm in December 1799, Washington insisted that his doctors bleed him. After being drained of nine pints of blood within twenty-four hours, he, too, expired.

In response to such excesses, the pendulum began to swing in the opposite direction. By 1881 Dr. Austin Flint could write that bloodletting "is now considered by many as seldom, if ever, called for."[5]

As bloodletting fell from favor, many condemned it as misguided and even barbaric, but more recent headlines, "Phlebotomy: An Ancient Procedure Turning Modern" (1963) and "New Medical and Scientific Uses of the Leech" (1986), have signaled a possible return for this therapy. Perhaps there is some good in the procedures favored by nineteenth-century Norwegians and legions of others.[6]

Two types of bloodletting once prevailed, general and local. General phlebotomy involves cutting a vein (venesection) and allowing the blood to flow freely. Doctors still use this type of bleeding to treat two disorders in particular: polycythemia vera (characterized by an enormous increase in the number of red blood cells) and hemochromatosis (characterized by excessive stores of iron in the blood). Local phlebotomy, rather than allowing blood to flow freely from a vein, involves sucking blood from small incisions in the skin. This could be accomplished by means of leeches or by gourds, devices eventually replaced by animal horns or small dome-shaped glasses, in a process known as "cupping."[7]

Årelating: Bloodletting Norwegian-style

In whatever form it was practiced, bleeding created indelible childhood memories in the Old and New Lands. Halvor Orset (born 1878) remembered watching his grandfather, a fisherman on the island of Otrøy in Møre og Romsdal, open a vein:

> One day *Bestefar* [Grandfather] was going to mend the fishing nets, but was feeling a little poorly and decided to bleed himself. He had an apparatus he called a *sneppert* [spring-loaded lancet] that he used to make a hole in the main vein on the underside of his right leg. The blood spurted out, and I got scared. . . .
>
> He put his foot down in a pail of lukewarm water, and the blood ran into the pail. The next thing I knew, Bestefar had fallen over in a faint. Now *Bestemor* [Grandma] went into action. She put a silver coin on the wound and wrapped a bandage around it. Soon Bestefar regained consciousness and he felt much better.

Falling in a faint was the intended effect of venesection. "Bleed in an upright posture to fainting," Benjamin Rush advised. In other ways, too, the procedure Orset describes matches the general phlebotomy of his time, especially his cutting a vein in the foot and letting it bleed out into warm water. The silver coin Orset's grandmother used to apply pressure to the wound harkens back to the belief that metal could ward off the huldrefolk, although if asked, she would have probably just called it customary.[8]

The sneppert that Orset's grandfather used for the incision probably came from the local blacksmith. Three or four inches long and fitting the hand comfortably, the sneppert had a sharp blade looking like a miniature hatchet and held back by a spring. Touching the sneppert's trigger snapped the blade into the vein. Once considered the leading edge of technology, the sneppert replaced the lancet, a sharp, two-edged knife.

Handling the traditional lancet took some skill to avoid severing a nerve or tendon. It also took courage. Then a late-seventeenth-century Viennese inventor produced a spring-loaded lancet that "snapped" into the vein. The descriptive German word *Schnapper* became *sneppert* in Norwegian, while in English the device went by the less poetic "phleam" or "fleam."

The "proven" Old Country practice of bloodletting naturally accompanied immigrants to the New Land. Vesterheim Museum in Decorah, Iowa, owns several bloodletting devices, including an especially fine sneppert. Measuring three inches long and one inch wide, it fits snugly into a wooden case carved precisely to fit it and topped with a sliding cover.

 ## INSTRUCTIONS FOR LETTING BLOOD

> Bloodletting is commonly done inside the bend of the elbow. No more blood than the equivalent of four small teacups should ever be let. To perform a bloodletting, tie a bandage tightly around the upper arm to compress the blood vessels, but avoid closing off the deeper-lying pulse artery. No blood will come out during the bleeding if the artery is closed off, but as long as a pulse can be felt at the wrist, circulation is continuing unhindered. After the vein is opened and the required quantity of blood has run out, press the vein to-

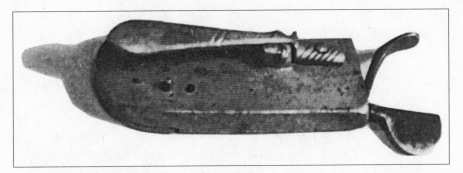

With its hatchet-like blade that snapped into the vein, the sneppert represented a real advance in bloodletting technology when it appeared in the 1600s. The prized instrument was usually kept in a special case.

gether above the wound, loosen the bandage, treat the wound with a folded compress and cover it with a bandage.

Lægebog for hvermand (Chicago, 1879)

Handsome cases often housed the sneppert, clearly a prized instrument. This particular set belonged to Nels Nelson Kjome, who at age sixteen emigrated with his parents and four siblings from Rollag, Numedal, in 1853. The family settled on the Waterloo Ridge in Highland Township near Decorah. Nels taught himself medicine by reading medical manuals and became a sought-after doctor for horses, who also were bled with a sneppert. Nels made his own medicines, too, his "Dr. N. N. Kjome's Liniment" once being in great demand.[9]

Not all who wielded the sneppert had the specialized skill of Nels Kjome, but anyone needing instructions could readily find them in doctor books. The 1879 *Lægebog for hvermand* (Doctor book for everyone) advised bloodletting "only be done under the direction of a doctor (except in the case of apoplexy when a doctor can not quickly be consulted)." It also objected to the "bad habit" of having oneself bled every spring, "as many customarily do." Such warnings notwithstanding, amateur bloodletting continued well into the 1900s among Norwegians.[10]

A Child's-Eye View of Bloodletting

Bloodletting was commonly practiced in the Racine, Wisconsin, household of Helen Olson Halvorsen (born 1863). As a little girl, she found it only natural to bleed her doll: "My doll had porcelain hands and head. The arms and legs were filled with bran, as was the rest of the body, I guess. Father often bled people for rheumatism or other aches and pains. He used to open their veins. So I cut open my doll's arm about where I thought she ought to bleed, and sure enough, all the bran ran out!"[11]

Leeching

Leeching was often a better choice than bloodletting because it provided more gradual relief and less irritation than opening a vein. "Leeches are preferably used for small children instead of general bleeding," advised the 1803 edition of Mangor's *Lande-apothek*, which instructed placement of a leech inside the bend of the elbow. Less painful and more reliable in removing a predetermined amount of blood, leeching was especially useful when bleeding parts of the body hard to reach by lancet or sneppert.[12]

Brita J. Seim (born 1873 in Sogn og Fjordane) recalled a time that leeching relieved her pain when nothing else would: "I was once out spreading manure and got such a pain in my left side that they just about had to carry me out of the field. I couldn't move and could hardly stand to be touched. They heated some stones and grain and put them on me [a common technique for treating pain], but nothing helped. Then my grandmother said, 'I'll get *Store-Mari* [Big Mari], she has leeches.' She came and placed the leeches on me, and believe it or not, before they had sucked themselves full, I could stand on my own two feet again."[13]

Leeches derive their name from the Anglo Saxon *loece*, meaning "to heal," and they were successfully used, as Seim's story suggests, to reduce pain, usually by decreasing pressure. Removing stagnant blood directly from the affected tissues, leeches effectively treated bruises and swellings, too.

Working with leeches could be tricky, though. They crawled out of reach and did not always bite. "Put them in a small empty glass and turn it upside down on the place where they are supposed to bite," counseled the 1879 *Lægebog for hvermand.* "To get the leech to bite for an extended period of time, cover the area with a warm oatmeal compress."[14]

Leeches became widely popular in continental Europe during the first half of the 1800s. France alone imported 41.5 million in 1833 (up from only 3 million in 1824), and collectors drove them almost to the point of extinction. Especially in demand, "Swedish" leeches could draw the most blood (about one ounce). Since Norway and Sweden were united in a single kingdom from 1814 until 1905, so-called Swedish leeches imported by France and other countries including the United States (at the price of $5.00 per hundred in the late 1800s) probably also came from Norway.[15]

Leeches attached themselves to the skin by means of three sharp teeth. Their three-pronged bite resembled the Mercedes-Benz trademark. They injected an anticoagulant to keep the blood flowing and then sucked themselves full, causing the patient no pain because of the local anesthetic in their saliva. Unlike the black leeches commonly found in lakes and ponds, the drab olive-green, medicinal leech *Hirudo medicinalis* falls off when full.

This "inexpensive and practical remedy," said Johan T. Bjerkem (born 1888 in Henning, Trøndelag), could be bought at apothecary shops. "As long as you made sure to change water in the bottle occasionally," they could be kept for years, ready for use as needed. Signs proliferated advertising *"Igler og kopping"* (leeches and cupping), recalled Kristian Linnerud (born 1891), who noted that one local place provided one-stop shopping for two indispensible services: "Leeching and Cupping Performed; Brides Dressed for Weddings."[16]

More frugal Norwegians caught their own leeches. The mother of Knut Larsen Holt (born 1883 in Agder) gathered hers in a nearby grassy marsh. Wrapping a white cloth around an oar blade, she stuck it under the turf. "Suddenly there were plenty of *igler,*" which she stored through the winter in clear bottles covered with a thin white cloth so they could get air. The water had to be changed a few times during the winter, Holt recalled, using water from a pond or marsh since ordinary well water did not provide the necessary nutrients. Making leeches last also required getting them to expel the blood they had ingested. Holt said his mother dipped their noses in salt or ashes. "If this wasn't done thoroughly enough, they died." Holt's mother used the leeches to treat the severe rheumatism that she and her husband, like so many nineteenth-century Norwegians, developed as they grew older.[17]

Though leeches provided an effective and inexpensive cure, many Norweians found their use *nifst* (creepy), the word used by six-year-old Martina Søilen (born 1885 in Voss) to describe the leech lady's treatment of her mother's varicose veins: "The woman came and had a large glass jar of leeches. Mother lay down on the bed. The woman took her socks off, fished up some leeches, and placed them on her feet. With some small picks made of cow horn she pierced holes in the skin to help the leeches get at the blood. I sat watching all this, but found it so *nifst*, I rolled over in a faint. Eventually the leeches rolled off, too, swollen from the blood they sucked." Relieved of excess pressure, "Mother's feet really did improve for a while," says Søilen.[18]

Recently, leeching has again been recognized as having healing value. In particular, they have proven uniquely helpful to plastic surgeons in reducing post-operation swelling. Leeches facilitate the circulation of blood through transplanted tissues in a way that is unequalled and often impossible by other means. The anticoagulant in their saliva keeps the blood from clotting, while other components dilate the blood vessels and provide antibiotic and anesthetic effects.[19]

Daring dentistry

Some patients "struggle with the 'psychological ramifications' of leeching," observes John Colapinto in his July 25, 2005, *New Yorker* article about cultivating leeches to meet today's growing medical need.[20] How could anyone think of putting such disgusting creatures into their mouths? As it happens, many late-nineteenth-century Norwegians did—to treat toothaches.

Ingeborg Knutsen Fjelly (born 1880) and her sister grew up in Skedsmo, today less than an hour's drive from Norway's capital city. In the 1880s, however, the town had no dentist, so when Ingeborg's sister got a toothache, the girls went to Gjertrude, the local *iglekone* (leech lady): "She invited us in and told us to sit down. Then out came the leeches that she kept in a glass of water. She fished up one of them, a really big one, told the patient to open wide, and put the leech on the painful tooth. Now the leech sucked blood until it was completely round. Then it fell out, well satisfied."[21]

"I don't recall if it cured my sister's toothache," said Ingeborg, more impressed by the treatment than its result. The leeches may have brought some relief by stimulating blood circulation in the gums and removing infected matter (and painful pressure) from abscessed teeth, a common affliction in the woeful world of nineteenth-century dental care.

While Ingeborg and her sister seem to have taken their visit to the iglekone in stride, by 1913 Karen Holtet (born 1885 in Rakkestad) found the use of leeches considerably more objectionable, reflecting the changing attitude toward the practice. "She wanted to put the leeches in my mouth," says the horrified Holtet, "but I wouldn't let her. . . . So she put them on my jaw, two of them. Then she came with a mirror and wanted me to take a look, but I closed my eyes. She held a glass underneath for them to fall into when they were full. Then she put them on a plate and sprinkled salt on them to expel all the blood and pus. *Fy!* It was such a creepy experience, I'll never do it again."[22]

By the time of Karen Holtet's visit to the leech lady, Norway by no means lacked dentists, the first having arrived from abroad as early as 1850. Rural Norwegians in the early twentieth century rarely had the means or opportunity to visit them, but in larger towns and cities, dental offices were quite common by the turn of the century. Usually located in private homes and furnished with plush Victorian furniture, these offices and the procedures performed there provided lasting memories. (Tourists today may visit the preserved dental offices at Oslo's Norwegian Folk Museum at Bygdøy or Lillehammer's Maihaugen Museum. The latter—complete with dark mahogany desk, red plush dental chair, and vintage instruments—once belonged to the museum's founder, Anders Sandvig (1862–1950). Sandvig received his dental degree in 1882 in Kristiania and practiced in Lillehammer from 1885 until 1949.)

Professional views of dental disease and treatment have changed a great deal since Sandvig's time, and especially from the reigning folk belief that worms caused toothaches. Home remedies typically sought to expel the worms by "smoking" the aching tooth with the highly poisonous herb known as *bulmerot* (henbane), chewing tobacco, or placing strong-smelling plants directly on the tooth.

Desperate to stop the excruciating pain, people even put hot coals on the offending tooth or tried to burn its throbbing pain out with a red-hot knitting needle. Caja Munch received a similar treatment. "The toothache finally disappeared after I had applied many remedies," she wrote in a January 22, 1856, letter. Dietrichson [J. W. C. Dietrichson (1815–83), the pioneer pastor at Luther Valley, near Janesville, Wisconsin] even burned me with a wire, and since then I have felt exceptionally well."[23] Since toothache sometimes comes and goes, people often believed in remedies that actually had little effect or even caused harm.

Desperation drove some toothache sufferers to the black book, where they did not look in vain. Formulas "*mot tannverk*" (against toothache) outnumber those for any other single ailment. A typical one comes from Fron in Gudbrandsdal (1830):

> *Jeg har orm i mine Tænder hvad heller*
> *de er røde eller hvide eller grå*
> *de skal da saa viselig dø*
> *som Jesus er fød af en Jomfru mø,*
> *I Navn Gud Fader Sønn og Hellig Ånd. Amen.*

> (I have worms in my teeth,
> whether they be red, white, or grey
> they shall as surely die and go away
> as Jesus was born of the Virgin Mary
> In the name of God the Father, Son and Holy Spirit. Amen.)[24]

While that formula sought its power in Christianity, others relied on pure magic, like this popular charm from the Rustad black book:

> Ratalibus+
> Ratalibu+
> Ratalib+
> Ratali+
> Ratal+
> Rata+
> Rat+
> Ra+
> R++.

Do this writing over the course of eight days, and on the ninth day burn the one that remains.

(On the first day, the toothache victim wrote "Ratalibus+" on a strip of paper and placed it on the bad tooth. Writing each day thereafter the word with one less letter and placing it on the tooth, the victim burned the strip reading "R++" on the ninth day, allegedly feeling less pain as the word got smaller.)[25]

A particularly popular toothache remedy involved poking the tooth with a small piece of wood until it bled, and then concealing the sliver under floorboards or in a tree in order to "read" the ache to that place. The mysterious notched sticks found during the early 1980s while renovating the medieval church at Bø, Telemark, may have derived from just such transference rituals, their users relying on the church to enhance the potency of the magic.[26]

Those who believed "bad blood" caused toothache, of course, bled themselves to cure the pain by cutting a vein under the tongue, as several eighteenth- and nineteenth-century medical books recommended. (In comparison, the use of leeches seems almost gentle and rational.)

When home remedies failed to work and the leech lady had no cure, the tooth had to come out. Every community had someone who pulled teeth. The blacksmith often did it, being able to make the necessary equipment himself. Sandvig once gave a graphic description of the blacksmith's ministrations, perhaps in an effort to make those of his own Lillehammer office seem more civilized: "Placing the patient on the floor with his head propped up on a log, he held the patient's head between his knees as in a vise, and using a so-called nøkkel (key), tried to pry out the tooth. If it worked, it worked. If not, he sat the patient on a stool, took a hammer and a wooden chisel, and aimed a mighty blow at the tooth. Whether the tooth was driven out or broken off didn't matter; in any case the purpose was served."[27]

The tannnøkkel (tooth key) resembled the outsized keys then in use, having a five- or six-inch-long shaft with a piece of metal about an inch square attached to one end. This metal piece had an opening for grabbing the tooth, which, as the shaft was rotated, could be wrenched from its socket. Unfortunately, the blacksmith's less-than-precise methods could leave remnants of the tooth behind to cause further problems. This often led people simply to endure the toothache.

Unquestionably painful for the patient, tooth pulling could also be disconcerting to the blacksmith. "People came complaining of toothache in the middle of the night," said Hans Bye (born 1887), the son of a blacksmith in Eidsvoll: "Dad had to get up and warm the *tang* (plier-like tongs) over the lamp glass. Then, *vips*, the tooth was suddenly out, with no anesthetic. He made the tang himself, and it was quite a fine piece of work. Mother told Dad to stop doing this job, though. 'You might break someone's jaw,' she said. He got no payment for this work. He did it because he wanted to help."

Communities devised various ways to make tooth pulling accessible, but self-trained practitioners remained the rule. In Trøndelag, parishioners of the Kvam church looked for Jørgan Vikan after the Sunday service. Vikan had taught himself to pull teeth, and on those Sundays when the pastor conducted services, he held office hours at the Ernst Kvam farm right across from the church. "Anyone suffering from toothache," said Johan J. Bjerkem (born 1888), "could just drop by and get the troublesome tooth pulled."[28]

In Haltdalen, another remote Trøndelag community without a dentist, the almue similarly relied on one of their neighbors. The *prestefolk* (minister's family), however, went to the district doctor, recalled Rasmus Christian Mohr (1850–1938), whose father served as the pastor of Haltdalen in the late 1800s: "One of the local strong men usually took care of pulling teeth, but we preferred to go to the train station when the district doctor came through. During the few minutes the train stood in the station, tooth pulling took place in the waiting room before a sizeable audience!"[29]

The district doctor's dentistry may have provided entertainment, but he certainly afforded no medical advantage over the "local strong man." He simply "pulled a well-used and bloody tang out of his case," says Mohr, "pulled the tooth, and then put it right back in the case once he had completed the job." Germ theory gained adherents only gradually, even among doctors.

Sometimes the minister himself attended to the parishioners' dental needs. Pastor Høgh, who served in Nissedal from 1885 to 1896, learned how to pull teeth from a cousin who was a professionally trained dentist. The pastor kept several *tanntenger* (teeth tongs) in a "lined and beautifully embroidered" black velvet bag for use in both the Nissedal and Skodje parishes, said his daughter: "Father's treatment consisted of a glass of cold water that may have briefly numbed the pain. With a special pocketknife he loosened the gum around the tooth. Then with his left arm he took a good hold around the patient's head and told him to open wide! It cannot be said that the pulling always proceeded silently. Boiling the tongs afterwards rarely occurred. Rinsing them first in cold water, then washing them in soapy water did the job."[30]

WILLING TO TRY ANYTHING

At the turn of the century, a young Norwegian woman (born 1890) went through the full range of available dental remedies before she finally found relief:

> In 1901 we lived about eighteen miles from the nearest town. I was eleven years old, had a terrible toothache, and there was no dentist. Following the advice of the local *klok kone*, I kept a big lump of *skråtobakk* (chewing tobacco) in my mouth for several days. When that didn't help, mother bought a clay pipe and filled *it* with skråtobakk, and I smoked it until I staggered and threw up. Now there was no way around it: I had to go to the doctor and get the tooth pulled.

Settling in remote frontier locations far from professionally trained doctors encouraged settlers to rely on local healers. (*Photo by Templeman*)

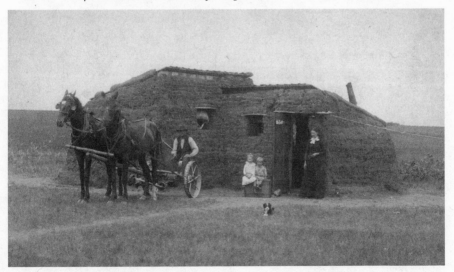

Inside his private parlor, which also served as his office, the doctor, in formal attire, smoked a two-foot long-
stemmed pipe, and a generous selection of similar pipes
filled the shelf above his desk. Otherwise the room had
plush upholstered chairs with upright backs and small
seats, and he placed me on one of these. After examining
the tooth, he opened a door to the next room and called to
the cook, "Petra, you must come here and hold a little girl
for me." Petra came, big and strong, dressed in a white bib
apron. Taking her place behind my chair and bending my
head over its back and into her ample bosom, she wrapped
two solid arms around me and held me like a vise. She had
done this before!

The doctor looked into his drawer and found the
tongs. They seemed to be the only pair he had. When he
pushed them far down into my jaw, both blood and tears
followed. No one could call the treatment painless, and
for all he jiggled and pulled, the tooth refused to come
out. "That tooth is so tough," he said at last, "you'll have to
tell your mother to take you into the city tomorrow to see
the dentist there." I ran home, crying all the way, and told
my mother everything. "Well, now, first you need to go to
bed and try to sleep," she said, and I slept straight through
to the next morning. Then, since I had a large lump in my
mouth and no more toothache, nothing came of the trip
to the city. A train ticket cost .90 *kroner* for adults and .45
for children, "and such an amount can't be thrown away
casually," my mother said.

Five years passed, and by then I had a job working for
an elderly lady. When my tooth began to hurt again, I was
earning six kroner a month and feeling flush. So I traveled
to the dentist in Kristiania and when this dentist took a
look into my mouth he said, "What's this?" Before I knew
it, he had the tooth out with a quick cut in my gum, where
it had been hanging loose for five years.

Anonymous woman quoted in
Oslo og Aksershus i manns minne

Leeching in America

Immigrants in nineteenth-century America continued to use leeches to treat toothache and a legion of other disorders including headache, earache, conjunctivitis, and hemorrhoids. They placed leeches in the throat for bronchitis and laryngitis and in the vagina for uterine complaints. Swedish and Norwegian leeches remained in great demand, since American leeches made a smaller, shallower incision and drew only a quarter of the blood. This led to the announcement in 1835 of a $500 award to anyone who could breed European leeches in the United States. The Americans' additional demand on the international leech market led Germans to complain in 1880 about the exhausted supply of this "irreplaceable medical apparatus."[31]

A reader identified as "J. E." wrote in the April 1894 issue of the popular magazine *Kvinden og hjemmet* (The woman and the home), "I have never yet met anyone who knows of a medication to treat neuralgia, but I am almost certain that if a person had leeches and knew how to place them, they would help." Responding to a reader's request for a remedy to treat neuralgia (nerve pain), she told the following anecdote to illustrate the value of bleeding:

> This winter my husband has been suffering terribly from neuralgia that extended from his cheeks down to his throat. Nothing helped. No matter what he took for it, he could not sleep for the pain. On top of that, he had a decayed tooth that occasionally sent shooting pains of its own. I advised him to have the tooth pulled, thinking the resulting blood loss would chase away the pains. And it did, too, quite incomparably. The pain has not bothered him since. On the previous day, before the tooth came out, he had such terrible pains in his temples that several times that day he had to bathe his head in cold water, the only thing that seemed to help a little.

So strongly did J. E. believe in the therapeutic effects of bloodletting that she credited the blood loss for her husband's recovery, instead of recognizing the role played by pulling the decayed tooth.[32]

Though physicians largely became disenchanted with leeching by 1900, pharmacists serving certain immigrant sections of New York and Boston continued to provide leeches at least through the 1920s. More recently, in anticipation of a renaissance in medical leeching, American biologist Roy Sawyer abandoned an academic career to found Biopharm, a company that produces most of the leeches used in medicine today. In addition to breeding and farming the leeches themselves, the laboratories, located in Wales, are also working to develop new drugs based on the active ingredients in leech saliva.[33]

Cupping

"If leeches could not be had," says Knut Larsen (born 1883 in Agder, Norway), "*kopping* did the same job." Cupping had ancient roots and developed as another form of topical or skin-deep phlebotomy. "Certain individuals went around and 'cupped' people using a self-made apparatus for this purpose," Larsen continued. "First they made a cut in the skin and placed the *koppehorn* (cupping horn) over it. Then they sucked on the horn or created a vacuum within it by burning up a scrap of wool dipped in alcohol." Vesterheim Museum has several cupping horns made from scrupulously scraped and cleaned cow horns.[34]

The tip of the horn was removed to form a hollow funnel. About a half inch below the opening of the tip, a groove was incised to anchor a cloth or other thin membrane (often sheep intestine) that would be tied over the horn's narrow end. Tarjei Heimdal (born 1882 in Nissedal, Telemark) told of watching his father suck the air out of the horn through small needle holes in the membrane, having first placed the wide end of the horn on the patient's skin. The sucking "raised the skin under the horn into a ball," which was then pierced with the sneppert. "I saw father do this many times," said Heimdal. "The spring clicked and the knife dug in and the blood flowed.... When enough liquid had come out, he started sucking through the membrane he had made [to cover the small end of the horn] from a sheep intestine set aside during the fall slaughter. Dad kept the *koppe* on the patient's skin until it finished sucking and fell off by itself." The amount of liquid it held came to about a cup, the reason, some said, that the process was called "*kopping*."[35]

While the name more likely derives from the cup-shaped gourds used for bleeding in ancient times, Heimdal correctly assessed the value of the procedure in a time with few medical alternatives. "I remember one person

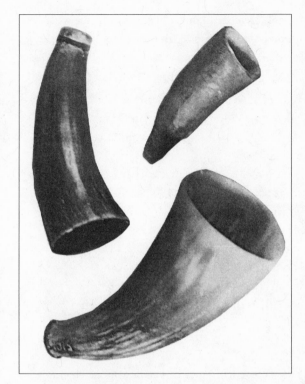

Thoroughly cleaned and scraped, these cow horns have had their tips removed to enable a bloodletter to suck the blood to the surface of the patient's skin.

who was cupped at the back of his neck. He had such a terribly sore throat and headache, and there were no *dråper* [medicines] for such things in those days." The far easier and less risky aspirin, first manufactured in 1899, quickly replaced bleeding.[36]

 ## CUPPING IN 1920S MINNESOTA

One kopping set of sneppert and cow horn came to rural Spring Grove, Minnesota, in 1865. Berte Johansdatter Jansen Veslehagen (born 1847), the grandmother of Bertmarie Melbostad, brought it when she emigrated from Gran, Hadeland. She kept this "piece of unique artistry" (as Melbostad calls it) in a small black box lined with red velvet and subsequently handed it down to Melbostad's mother, who put it to use in 1924. Melbostad was very young at the

time, she says, "so only simple facts stand out in memory," yet she
provided a vivid description of the process in the January 18, 1997,
Spring Grove *Herald*:

> Grandmother was being plagued by backache. She came
> one day and asked Mom to use the Koppe treatment on
> her in hopes of alleviating or lessening the pain. Mom, not
> too enthused over using this method, finally consented to
> do this for Grandma.
>
> Preparations were made, everything cleansed, and
> Grandma's back was bared. Mom then pointed the knife
> to the designated spot, and pulled the "trigger" which
> plunged the blade into the flesh. The hollow horn was
> quickly placed over the wound, and Mom placed her
> mouth over the horn and sharply drew in her breath,
> exhaling outside the horn; this procedure continued
> until enough blood had been drawn to hopefully relieve
> Grandmother's back pains.

In isolated areas and among those with no access to new medicines, cupping continued to be practiced by individuals such as Olena Solberg, the
"Old Cupping Lady" of Arkdale, Wisconsin. Settled by transplants from
the Koshkonong settlement, Arkdale boasted the first church in Adams
County. The congregation was organized in 1853 by H. A. Preus, who continued to serve it as part of his circuit until 1865, two years after he became
president of the Norwegian Synod.[37]

Olena had learned to do cupping in Norway and continued the procedure in Arkdale to help her neighbors. In the summer of 1901, her twelve-
year-old granddaughter, Palma Grahn (1889–1972), observed these sessions
with wide-eyed wonder. Only "a sprinkling of people" came for the procedure, mostly elderly couples that suffered from *Gikt* (rheumatism), *Bronkit*
(bronchitis), night sweats, incessant expectoration, fatigue, and "a long line
of other ills, real or imagined." A few "came with a diagnosis from their family doctor and with his consent, while some of them had figured out a diagnosis on their own. Some hoped to be cured, others asked nothing more
than to be temporarily relieved from their many aches and pains. There

would be a mild flurry of excitement as symptoms were discussed while preparations were made. I watched grandma as she cleansed the area destined for the cupping operation with soap, water and alcohol."

Olena's equipment included a scarificator, a more sophisticated version of the sneppert. With six, nine, or twelve sharp steel blades inside a tiny brass cube, it had a trigger on the side that snapped the knives through an equal number of slits in the bottom of the cube and into the patient's skin. Clever blacksmiths once made these cubes that later became commercially available in both Norway and America. (The scarificator at Vesterheim Museum measures about two inches on each side. It also has a screw on top to adjust the cutting depth of the blades.)

When Palma's grandmother "deftly applied" the scarificator, "blood began to ooze from the surface cuts." Then she put a scrap of cotton saturated with alcohol into a cupping glass (about three inches tall and shaped similarly to the gourds used in ancient times). Then "Olena lit the cotton with a match and quickly inverted the heated glass over the wound, where it adhered because of the partial vacuum caused by the cooling air." Young Palma "stood by, resolutely watching the glass slowly fill with blood." She wrote, "I no longer remember whether Grandma or the patient decided when enough blood had been 'let.' It finally did come to an end. As the patient sank back in his chair, with an eloquent sigh of relief, Grandma applied a clean dressing over the wound." After "profuse expressions of gratitude," monetary payment came to about fifty cents. Sometimes patients brought along other friends to be "cupped."

Palma Grahn suggests that the social reasons for visiting the cupping lady may have equalled the medical ones:

> When the bloodletting was over, there would be a shuffling of chairs, adjusting of garments, and a suggestion of leave-taking. '*Men kjære dig!*' [but my dear], Grandma would exclaim, oozing hospitality. 'Sit down and visit a while. I'm going to put on the coffee pot right now.' And so she did.
>
> Soon the aroma of freshly made coffee filled the room, and in short order we were seated at the kitchen table, with the company tablecloth on it. . . . Thick slices of fresh bread, and thin slices of tasty, brown Primost [carmalized whey, a popular treat], fruit soup,

generous slices of frosted cake and a big pat of freshly churned butter in the covered glass butter dish.

These refreshments blended the food ways of Old Country and New Land,
and they featured the hospitality that has been valued in Norwegian tradition since Viking times. "There went the profit!" writes Grahn, "but that did
not matter. Neighborliness and friendship meant more to Grandma than
money."

Therapeutic in more ways than one, cupping apparently provided Olena
and her customers a way to cultivate cultural ties with fellow immigrants:
"There we sat, Grandma, the patients and I, enjoying all the good food set
before us, and talking about this and that. When the last cup of coffee was
finished we all got up and shook hands with Grandma and said, "*Mange
takk for maten* [many thanks for the food]."

"It's good to have the 'bad blood' taken out," the guests reassured themselves as they left; "it makes me feel so much better." Though Grahn felt the
visitors had a need to "reassure themselves" of the treatment's efficacy, her
description leaves no doubt that they all had benefited.

Staunching blood

If blood flowed too freely after a cupping session, a compress steeped in
vinegar, brandy, or other styptic could usually stop it. Serious injuries and
hemorrhages, however, required more powerful means. In these situations,
many nineteenth-century Norwegians looked to magic and tried to find
someone who "had the black book."

Staunching the flow of blood, even from minor wounds, had traditionally seemed mysterious and sometimes demanded the skill of a talented
folk healer. The overwhelming number of black-book formulas devoted to
stopping blood flow confirms the Norwegians' long standing fascination
with this vital process. Most of these formulas resemble the one collected
in 1821 at Kinsarvik, Hardanger, and they typically invoke the miraculous
pause in the River Jordan's flow that honored Christ's baptism (Matthew
3:13–17)[38]: "*Stat Blo so vatne sto i Jordan Flo*" (Stand still, blood, as the water
in Jordan stood). Other blood-staunching formulas invoke Moses's parting
of the Red Sea (Exodus 14).

Similarly grounded in Scripture, this formula from the Rustad black book refers to the binding of Satan in Hell (Revelations 20:1–2).

Stadt stille Blod paa N.N.
lige som den grume Satan udi Helvede fast staar.
Jesu haver hanem fanget og bunden
i 3 Navn, saa Fader vor.

(Stand still, the blood of N. N. [patient's name],
like the despicable Satan stands snared in Hell,
where Jesus has trapped and bound him well,
in the name of 3 [Father, Son and Holy Spirit].
Then recite the Lord's Prayer.)

The overwhelming number and variety of blood-stopping formulas suggest their widespread need. The sharp blades of axe and scythe cut deep, inflicting serious injury on exhausted, sometimes intoxicated, workers as they toiled in harsh weather and difficult terrain. In a time before infection could reliably be checked, even the simplest task could suddenly end in an accident that threatened life or limb. Consider the worker on the Nygård farm in Jæren who was trying to clear some tall grass away from the barn wall in the 1850s when "a swing of the scythe gashed his thigh, and the injury bled so profusely, they feared for his life. The closest doctor was miles away in Stavanger, so someone ran for help to Johanne Stangeland [known for her skill at staunching blood]. Johanne picked up a book and read something in it, then she told the man who had come running to fetch her that he could now walk more slowly home for the bleeding had stopped. When the man got back to Nygård, he found the injured worker lying in bed. He was pale, but the bleeding had stopped, just as Johanne said."[39] Folk healers had formulas so powerful, many believed, that they could stop the bleeding without even seeing the afflicted. Though we might object that Johanne got the credit for a natural process, the belief that someone could stop bleeding by magic brought nineteenth-century Norwegians much-needed comfort.

In less extreme situations, people tried rational remedies first. Elise Moe, who grew up in the midnineteenth century in the mountains near Mo i Rana (North Norway), recalled that when her father cut his foot with an axe, his family used "beehives that hung from the tree limbs and peeled the sheets off" to stop the bleeding. Many eighteenth- and nineteenth-century Norwegians kept beehives or wasp nests on hand for just such an emergency. "They always brought a nest back from the woods in the fall after the wasps had left it," said Hanna Henriksen Tollaanes (1822–93). "They cut off the branch it was hanging from and stuck it into a crack in the wall in a corner of the log house." In addition to absorbing the blood, the paper-like nesting material helped it to clot.[40]

Spiderwebs did the same job. "If someone was injured by a knife or axe, they put cobwebs in the wound to stop the bleeding," says Ludvik A. Hope (born 1870), who used this remedy himself. As recently as the 1960s, when Alf Sverre Hvidbergskår was collecting folklore in Agder, several men told him of "rubbing their shaving cuts with *spindelvev* [spider webs]."[41]

Spiderwebs and Staunching Blood

Stopping blood with cobwebs was so common that children learned to apply this remedy themselves, says Hilda Kongsberg (born 1899 in Rolvsøy, East Norway): "When we children were playing we sometimes fell and got hurt. Even for deep wounds or a badly pinched finger, we would find cobwebs [*kingelvev*, in her dialect]. Sprinkling finely shaved sugar in the wound first, we would stuff it with kingelvev and wrap a rag around it. Soon it would heal."

Tostein Skjelanger (born 1889 in Herdla, West Norway) echoes this experience: "When someone got cut, we immediately ran around the house searching for cobwebs to put into the wound and stop the bleeding. Cobwebs were applied and a rag wrapped around. As a young boy I was told this by my friends and they got me to do it, too."[42]

Even hospitals used spiderwebs to stop bleeding, applying multiple layers for serious hemorrhages. The staff "used to run around the corridors and attic to collect cobwebs to put on a wound," observed a doctor who worked at Oslo's Rikshospital in the 1840s.[43]

Nineteenth-century Norwegians also relied on herbs to stop bleeding. *Ryllik* (yarrow, *Achillea millefolium*) has been known since ancient times for its blood-staunching effect. Invaluable as a surgical dressing during the American Civil War, yarrow could be found in

the First Aid kits carried by soliders during World War I. Equally
reliable was *kjuke* (tinder bracket, *Fomes fomentarius*), the fungus
that extends in plate-like form from the trunks of birch and other
deciduous trees.[44]

Most commonly, however, Norwegians used *lyng* (heather,
Calluna vulgaris), an evergreen shrub with tiny purple flowers that
is abundant in Norway but rare in the United States. "The almue
use lyng when they injure themselves with an axe," wrote Pastor
Hans Jacob Wille in his 1786 description of Seljord, Telemark. Wille
surmised that the almue had learned this trick from "bears that roll
around in the heather when they are wounded." Whether animal or
human, those who used lyng, yarrow, and tinder bracket found the
relief they sought because the plants' tannins and resins constricted
blood vessels to help stop their flow.[45]

Magical blood-stopping in modern Norway

In Norway today, a land rich in advanced technology, magical blood-
stopping continues. Jakob Enoksen (born 1923 in Tromsø, north of the
Arctic Circle) receives calls from Norwegians from all over the country
begging him to use magical incantations to stop their bleeding. Aware he
had this talent even as a boy, Enoksen said it runs in his family. Interviewed
in 1997 for *Nordlys* (Northern light), Tromsø's newspaper, he had worked
as a city gardener and helped landscape several churches and cemeteries.[46]

Though Enoksen grew up in urban Tromsø, his roots are *Sami* (the in-
digenous people of northern Scandinavia, formerly known as Lapps). Norway's majority population has long associated Samis with the occult. (Until
the 1970s, the Samis were the only ethnic minority with a significant presence in Norway.) The supernatural abilities ascribed to them—as shamans,
prophetic seers, and healers, able to send their souls on journeys outside
their bodies—derive in part from their own ancient lore. But the notion of
the Samis' magical prowess is further reinforced by the human tendency to
attribute unusual capabilities to unfamiliar ethnic groups. (This tendency is
also seen in the European settlers' notion of American Indians as gifted healers, perhaps most notable in the marketing of the patent medicines manufactured by the Kickapoo Indian Company.)[47]

To gain understanding of Enoksen's ability, journalist Linda Vaeng Sæbbe interviewed Professor Arne Nordøy, a blood specialist at Tromsø's Rikshospital. "I don't think blood-stoppers can suppress large hemorrhages or very forceful ones," Nordøy told her, "but I do believe they can stop superficial bleeding." When a hemorrhage occurs, the blood vessels automatically constrict and begin to slow the flow of blood. Then blood platelets form a plug over the wound, which gradually grows denser as a netting forms over it. At several steps in this process, suggestion could operate, whereby "someone could influence the bleeder to produce the bodily substances that inhibit blood flow." Nordøy concluded, "Faith can move mountains—and faith can to a certain extent stop or regulate bleeding." Secret formulas "are just part of the overall setting that creates the mood" making this possible.

Faith in folk healers played a significant role in the stopping of bleeding among nineteenth-century Norwegians, and it apparently also underlies its continuing practice in North Norway, which is surprisingly ubiquitous. "I've never met a Nordlending (native of North Norway) who didn't know something about blood-stopping," asserted Roald Kristiansen, a researcher at the District College in Finnmark. Kristiansen was studying blood-stopping as a religious phenomenon when Sæbbe interviewed him for her article. He identified silence and secrecy—"a wall of silence" and "not knowing the formula being read"—as elements fundamental to the process. Though blood-stopping remains "very much alive and widespread" in North Norway, says Kristiansen, it has almost disappeared from the rest of the country. He admitted that he could not yet explain the mystery of the process, but emphasized having "found no reason to doubt its reality" either.[48]

Journalist Sæbbe, finally, interviewed Odd Nilsen, a professor of social medicine at the University of Tromsø. Blood-stopping "conflicts with the way we doctors have learned to understand these things," Nilsen observed as he emphasized the lack of a valid medical explanation for the phenomenon. Yet, like most Nordlendinger, he admitted having heard over the years "the most remarkable stories of bleeding being stopped by incantations."

"Shock and fear can in some cases cause wounds to stop bleeding," Nilsen offered, "and there may be links between such conditions and the mental state that a blood-stopper induces in the bleeder. In most cases, though, bleeding simply stops by itself and the blood-stopper probably gets a lot of credit for what is actually being done by the patient's own body." The similarity between today's blood-stoppers and nineteenth-century folk healers is striking, notably in the way their methods were aided by silence and secrecy, but most of all by the patient's faith in a positive outcome.

The role of feelings and beliefs in healing

An even more intriguing aspect of modern blood-stoppers is their demonstration of the role that feelings and beliefs play in healing. The ancient idea of keeping the four bodily humors in balance and relating these humors to mood (blood with sanguinity, phlegm with phlegmatic behavior, yellow bile [choler] with a melancholic nature, and black bile with a bilious or choleric one) shows an age-old awareness of this mind-body connection. But the nineteenth-century revolution in medicine pushed aside the emotional aspect of illness in favor of the physical one. Writes Esther Sternberg, M. D., in a recent examination of the topic, "We simply did not have the tools capable of demonstrating the physical and molecular underpinning of both emotions and disease." Now that technology is developing ways to measure the role of feelings in healing, science is "learning to take seriously the emotional component of illness and healing."[49]

"New studies support the reasonable hypothesis that the emotional state of the patient makes a major contribution to recovery," echoes Jerome Groopman, M.D., in a recent study. Patients who are hopeful—whether because of religious faith or trust in the physican—have higher rates of survival, he continues. Belief, expectation, and desire, scientists now agree, activate brain circuits that cause the release of endorphines and enkephalins—chemicals that mimic morphine.[50]

Hope has both a thinking and a feeling component, according to one expert on the biology of positive emotion, Dr. Richard Davidsen. These two components consist of the patient mentally altering the vision of his or her condition and then feeling the result of that altered vision. The act of generating a more positive vision of the condition leads, Davidsen asserts, to feeling better.[51]

These recent findings relate to the way that nineteenth-century Norwegian folk healers like Mor Sæther (whose patients' "hopes awakened" upon hearing of her reputation) and Mor Frøisland (who "greatly helped by bringing them consoling words of God and praying for them aloud and in silence") inspired faith and trust. In researching the placebo effect at Harvard Medical School, Dr. Ted Kaptchuk has found the role of "ancient shamans" pertinent. Noting the way the words and gestures of a trusted authority figure reinforce the patient's belief in the medicine's power and solidify the expectations of recovery, Kaptchuk has furthermore found that the change in mind-set can actually alter the nerve chemistry in the patient's mind in a way that benefits recovery.[52]

Roald Kristiansen's studies of the role played by suggestion in the healing art of North Norwegian blood-stoppers and their ability to influence the body to inhibit blood flow clearly relate to these findings. New insights on this emotional component may also help explain the beneficial effects of bloodletting beyond its ability to relieve pain. "Hope tempers pain," says Groopman, "and as we sense less pain, hope expands and reduces pain further." With the reduction of pain, he continues, a significant obstacle to enduring a harsh but necessary therapy is removed.

The feeling of well-being conferred on nineteenth-century Norwegians by brennevin certainly had a similar effect; so did the black-book formulas and other traditions that brought the solace of ritual, or as Sternberg would say, the "constancy that reduces anxiety." The mind-body connection lies at the heart of many of the therapies this book has described, and the work of the folk healers we have encountered both illustrates and supports the emotional component of healing that scientists are rediscovering today.[53]

10

Remembered Remedies

"I remember my mother saying that when her grandmother was sick, it made her feel better simply to have Dr. Quisling come over and speak Norwegian with her. Apparently he couldn't really do anything for her medically, but the conversation alone helped."

David Cahoon, Middleton, Wisconsin

WHILE RESEARCHING THIS BOOK, I asked Norwegian Americans to send me home remedies their families had used. The responses are presented here by key ingredient or by ailment. Remedies gathered by students in my 1983 folklore class at Luther College in Decorah, Iowa, are also included. These folk cures offer fascinating glimpses into the past and resonate with the nineteenth-century remedies discussed above.

First, a longer recollection from Howard Amundson sets the stage. Born in 1935 in Nimrod (near Wadena), Minnesota, Amundson addresses the conditions that led some families to retain traditional attitudes toward doctors and the home remedies that supplanted professional care.[1]

Growing up on a small dairy farm in Northern Minnesota was a hand-to-mouth existence, and because of the cost, visits to the doctor were few and far between, so we relied very heavily on home remedies. My first memory of a home remedy was about age three. Our father worked on W.P.A. to supplement our income. There was no money to purchase a thermos bottle. As a substitute, boiling coffee was poured into a quart fruit jar and wrapped in newspaper until it fit into an oatmeal box. It would remain warm at least until lunchtime. Mother filled the jar and as she carried it to the table to wrap it, the bottom broke out just as it passed over me as I sat having breakfast, scalding my right hip. I was immediately undressed and the largest potato was chosen, sliced thinly and arranged over the burn. The wet, cold potato slices relieved the pain and as they dried out, they were replaced until the pain was gone.

There were always coughs that accompanied winter colds. A large onion was chosen, peeled, and finely chopped. The onion was placed in a large water glass and almost a cup of sugar was added. The glass was given a good shaking and inverted on a deep saucer. As the sugar absorbed the moisture from the onion and dissolved, it produced syrup that would seep out into the saucer. A teaspoon of onion syrup did nothing for your breath, but seemed to quell the coughing.

There were always wounds that would become infected, too. Households nearly always had some kind of brown soap. I remember P&G and Fels-Naptha, which were used to wash clothes. The soap was nearly always soft from the moisture of the soap dish. A small amount of the soft soap was scraped from the bar and placed on a bandage, mixed with a bit of sugar, and placed over the wound. I believe doctors now say it was the combination of the moisture from the soap, the sugar, and the heat from your body that killed the infection.

When I was about eight years old, I got a piece of the beard from a head of barley in my eye. Barley beards have very fine barbs on them and once it was in my eye, it was there to stay. Before I went to bed that night, Dad pulled down my eyelid and dropped a flax seed into my eye. Flaxseed is very smooth and although I could feel it in my eye, it was not as irritating as the barley beard. The next morning they pulled down the eyelid and the foreign body had a coating on it so it could be wiped out with the corner of a handkerchief.

Ingredients

ASAFETIDA

Because my grandparents lived on a very limited income, father converted a garage on our farm into a cozy little cottage for them. I was about eight years old, and it was my job to deliver fresh milk nearly every evening after the milking had been done. Very often I would stay for about an hour before I returned to our house. It was during this time that I learned a great deal about their earlier lives and hardships.

Grandma would take out a small, soft leather bag with a very long drawstring in the top. She would open it up and take out a strange lump of waxy material about the size of a small egg. It looked like brown bee's wax. We were never allowed to touch it, but were able to sniff its strong smell, which was completely foreign to us. She would walk over to the wood stove that furnished the heat and draw the lump across the hot stove. There would be a small puff of smoke and the room would fill with the strong and unpleasant odor. It was asafetida and guaranteed to repel all airborne sickness including the flu, which everyone of that age remembered so clearly. (Howard Amundson; Minnetonka, Minnesota, 2006)[2]

Due to the early death of their mother, my mother and her sister were raised by their grandparents, immigrants from Hallingdal, in Worth County, Iowa. When the young girls began to attend school and especially in the winter, Grandma Ragnhild Mikkelson Olsen (born 1841) would place amulets laced with asafetida (a gum resin having an obnoxious odor, also known as "Devil's Dung") around their necks. She held that this would ward off evil spirits and contagious diseases. In reflecting years later, my mother allowed that the preventative measure had worked, "for we smelled so bad that no one would come near us." (Travis Cleveland; Dorchester, Iowa, 2000)

BEETS

One summer when I was quite young I was out climbing around in the barn and I got a rusty nail in my foot. My Norwegian-born grandmother took a raw beet, put it on some soft cloth and bound my foot. This was thought to cure or prevent blood poisoning. Somehow it drew the poisoning out of my foot and everything was alright. (Stella Kirby, born 1895 near Decorah, Iowa; reported by Kari Hermeier, 1983)

CAMPHOR

When my mom was a kid, she had to wear a camphor ball hung around her neck to prevent a cold. She didn't know if it worked or not but she wasn't too thrilled about it! (Janice Doering, whose grandparents emigrated from Norway in 1912; Chicago, 2000)

CARBOLIC ACID

Mother poured carbolic acid into a deep wound when I was bitten by a dog as a child. The treatment was very painful, but it healed. (Ulga Swenson, born 1889 in Windom, Minnesota; reported by Mark Hostager, 1983)

COD-LIVER OIL

My father, Olaus H. Olson (1878–1940), told me of the time he had tuberculosis when he was young and his mother made him go out and lie in the sun on both sides for a half an hour, and every time he came into the house he had to take a tablespoon of the cod-liver oil she kept on the porch. Apparently it worked. No one in the family tested positive. (Bonnie Olson Crandall; Mauston, Wisconsin, 2000)

GOOSE GREASE

Mother saved goose grease in mason jars and when one of us had a cold, it was heated and rubbed on our chest. A sleeveless flannel shirt [with front and back the same, and ties at the waist] made by mom was then put over this before going to bed. And it really felt good and seemed to help. (Dolores Mathies, born 1926; Green Bay, Wisconsin, 2000)

HOPS

When I was a child seventy years ago, I would quite often have an earache. My mother would gather hops from her vines growing on the porch. She put them in a small cloth bag, warmed them in the oven, and put them on my ears. (Verna Ellefson, born 1905, Windom, Minnesota; reported by Mark Hostager, 1983)

KEROSENE

Dipping a lump of sugar in kerosene and sucking on it to "cure" a cold or sore throat. The sugar lumps we used were not the neat, precise little cubes of today; they were larger and irregularly shaped cubes. This was primarily introduced in our family by my father, whose grandfather left the Hemsedal/Hallingdal area of Norway in about 1850. (Orville Bakka, raised in Minnesota during the 1920s; Rancho Bernardo, California, 1999)[3]

Lead

E. W. Everson was born in East Toten, Norway, on April 29, 1857. He emigrated to the USA with his father Andrew Everson in 1866 when he was nine years of age. . . . Grandpa Everson studied a great deal about medicine and had books on veterinary medicine and household remedies. He actually made both "Salve" and "Liniment." My understanding is that the salve was a German recipe and had a heavy lead content. That means when lead was banned in the U.S., you could no longer make the salve. I do have a small container that has printed on top: "Everson Salve." Grandpa's son, Edwin, carried on the tradition and made the salve and liniment for many years after Grandpa was gone. Grandpa Everson as well as his son were really unlicensed veterinarians in their day, and they treated many horses and cattle in the region. . . .

The salve was for any infection. If you stepped on a nail or had a bee sting or some other infection, just put on a small portion of Grandpa's Salve and the next day the infection would be gone. The liniment was for bruises or burns, etc. I remember that my sister Violet was perhaps five or six years old at the time she fell in the bonfire at a family picnic down along the Bald Hill Creek near Walum, North Dakota. Her wrist and arm were severely burned. Her treatment was Grandpa's liniment, day after day, wrapped with clean cloths, and she recovered with only minor scars. (Rev. D. B. "Doc" Gilbertson; reported by Carol Gilbertson, Decorah, Iowa, 2003)[4]

Manure

One of the cures I remember as a child listening to parents and grandparents was Grandma Wilhelmine Nettum's cure for "blood poisoning," as they called infections from wounds and the like. She would make a bag out of oilcloth and fill it with hot cow manure, catching the cow in action to make sure it was fresh and hot. The wound, hand or foot, would be dipped right into the hot stew and soaked to draw out the poison. If necessary, there would be fresh hot refills as needed. I heard many stories of her miracle cures with names and times given. Wilhelmine was born May 21, 1868, in Vestre Toten, Oppland, Norway, emigrated in the 1880s and "practiced" in rural Kindred, North Dakota, in the late 1800s and early 1900s. (Dick Vangerud; Waite Park, Minnesota, 2002)

MUSTARD PLASTER

For bronchitis or pneumonia we used warm mustard plasters on the chest. Mixing dry mustard with flour and warm water to make a thick paste, spreading it on a cloth and putting it on the chest. It had to be watched closely so it would not burn or blister the skin, but it did ease congestion. (Verna Ellefson, born 1905, whose mother was from Lillehammer; reported by Mark Hostager, 1983)

ONIONS

Mother had a favorite cough remedy of simmered onions and sugar she would keep on the back of the range during cold seasons—it really did the trick. I have tried to duplicate that syrup since, but it is not really the same done on an electric stove. (Hilda Thompson Quickstad, in Peterson, Minnesota, ca. 1900; Norwegian American Historical Association [P1317], 1982)

If a person lost his voice: take a big onion, cut it up and put it in a mason jar. Add about 1 cup of honey. Let sit over night (at least ten hours). Pour out the honey and take a teaspoon on and off. Helped for colds and to clear throat. We children loved it. (Delores Mathies, born 1926; Green Bay, Wisconsin, 2000)

PORK

I was raised by my grandmother through much of my childhood and I remember many of her remedies. To cure a sore throat, she would take a soft strip of cloth and sew a piece of salt pork to it. She would then bind it to your neck overnight and in the morning there would be blisters all over your neck, but the blisters would pull all the soreness out. I don't know how it did it, but somehow it would just pull out all the soreness and I felt just fine. (Stella Kirby, born 1894, Decorah, Iowa; reported by Kari Hermeier, 1983)

POTATO

I knew a man [Melvin Haugen] who came on a number of occasions to various functions with a piece of potato in his pocket. Now what he did was to slice that potato down the middle so as to give a great area of exposure, and he turned the meat side, the exposed interior portion of the potato, toward his body and put it in his shirt pocket. He thought this would help to alleviate arthritis symptoms. (S. S. Urberg, born 1932, learned of this superstition as a pastor between 1959 and 1963 in Hannaford, North Dakota; reported by Ingrid Urberg, 1983)

POULTICES

Our grandmother used a poultice made of home-baked bread and milk. She would warm the milk and make a "paste" and put that on the sore and tie with clean rags; she never used gauze or tape, always clean white rags to hold it in place. We believe she added flax to the mixture. Not ground or anything, just plain flax seed. She would also make a poultice of lard, kerosene, and flax, but in what proportions I don't remember. She would use this on infectious sores and also on boils.

We remember her heating a bottle with a small opening, and after the poultice had brought the boil to a head, she would heat the bottle in hot water and place it over the boil to draw out the contents. (Grant Peterson, born 1938; Brookings, South Dakota, 2000)

If you got an infection, you'd dip a piece of bread in milk, slap that on the wound and believe it or not, it would pull out a sliver. This was known as a poultice. (Joe Moen, born 1916; Kindred, South Dakota, 2000)

Whenever we had an infected finger or boil, we made a hot poultice of bread and milk and applied it to the affected area. It worked. (Verna Ellefson, born 1905, Windom, Minnesota; reported by Mark Hostager, 1983)

I had a boil and Mother made a bread and milk poultice and placed it over the boil. (Shirley Olson Sorensen, born 1928; Edina, Minnesota)

SPIRITS

We drank whiskey and sugar in warm water for menstrual cramps. I've heard the theory that this may have led women to alcoholism—but who knows? (Norma Gaffron, born 1931; New Brighton, Minnesota, 2000)

On the second shelf of the pantry cupboard, just above eye level, there stood a large bottle of brandy. It was not regarded as a beverage, but as a medicine. When my father got caught out in the cold autumn rain during fall plowing or corn husking, coming into the house soaked to the skin, the brandy bottle came down. A little glass was enough to "drive out the chill," hopefully preventing a cold or something much worse! During warm summer months, the level of liquid in the brandy bottle stayed exactly the same for the entire season. When the chill winds of autumn and winter blew and the season of colds and "flu" got under way, the visits to the brandy bottle became more and more frequent.

I remember the standard remedy for a serious chest cold or chills and fever. Two extra quilts were added to your bed. Then the potion was mixed: the juice of a half lemon, a generous amount of brandy; then the mug was filled with boiling hot water. A little sugar and a sprinkling of nutmeg smoothed out the flavor. It was best drunk when already dressed in flannel pajamas. The warm coziness set in almost immediately, and the sweat began to ooze out of your pores. Invariably you felt much better in the morning. (Judeen Johnson, born 1925; Brookings, South Dakota, 2000)

SULFUR

To disinfect or fumigate a room that has been occupied by a patient with consumption or tuberculosis: close up the room well, stuff any cracks around windows or doors with bits of cloth. Then place sulfur or brimstone in a tub elevated off the floor on pieces of 2 x 4's. Set fire to the sulfur and leave the room quickly. Keep closed for many days. This was done in my husband's old farm home near Willow Lake, South Dakota, in 1914, after his mother's mother passed away. (Ada Tollefsen, born 1910, Windom, Minnesota; reported by Mark Hostager, 1983)

In the springtime we were each given sulfur and molasses. This was said to "clear out the winter" and all its harmful effects on a person. It didn't harm us, but I'm not sure if it did us any good either. (Stella Kirby, born 1894, Decorah, Iowa; reported by Kari Hermeier, 1983)

TURPENTINE

Little Helga had a hollow cough. There was a trembling movement under her chin every time she took a breath. She sat in her high chair as usual today for breakfast, but this empty cough persisted. Toward noon she seemed to be worse and we again fetched the doctor. He said then that she had "croup" and gave her strong doses of turpentine in milk. He said that she had not more than one chance in ten of recovering; but this we would not believe. The doctor was there until 9 o'clock, Mama and I sat up with her all night. It was so painful for us to see how much she suffered. And so patient and gentle as she was to take the repulsive medicine. We laid cold compresses on her throat and forehead.

Later in the morning we realized that she had little prospect of recover-

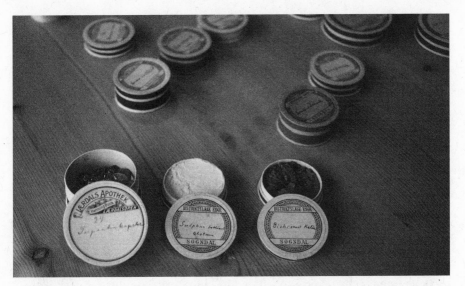

Turpentine and sulfur packaged by an apothecary shop in Lærdal, Norway (*Photo by Stokker*)

ing. We again sent a message for the doctor, who gave her a dose of emetic powder, except she threw it up. Then he gave her an emetic which was supposed to be stronger, but without results. Her stomach had truly become so insensitive from all the turpentine that the emetic had no effect on her. About 7 o'clock she had a strong struggle with death, but she lived until almost 12 on Saturday the 26th of September. (1896 diary entry by Torjus Sondre Reishus, McIntosh, Minnesota; translated by Don Berg, reported by Reishus's granddaughter, Kek Robien, Gurnee, Illinois, 2005)

Ailments

Burns

When I was five years old, I was always in the tool shed. My dad was making something and had the hot anvil there for use on some piece he was welding. Dad asked me for the hammer, which was on the shelf across from the anvil. I guess I took a short cut and came straight across to pick up the hammer and stepped on the red hot anvil he had just taken out of the forge. All the skin from the bottom of my foot was left on the anvil. I screamed and screamed at the top of my voice. Neighbors a quarter-mile away heard the screams and came in a hurry to see what had happened. Martha Urheim ran down our basement to get potatoes. She took a knife and sliced them on my foot. They took the pain away and also helped to heal. For 6 months, I had my foot up while new skin grew on. It did not get infected and healed well. In those days we did not go to doctors. This is a true story and I remember the pain when I stepped on that hot anvil like it was yesterday. (Mrs. E. R. Mitchell, born 1916; Brookings, South Dakota, 2000)

COLDS

For a sore throat and cold, Mom would slice up onions and put them in a handkerchief on my chest. I slept with it only once, never again. Turpentine was also frequently rubbed on the chest for colds. This seemed to help. (Alice Hostager, born ca. 1920, Kenyon, Minnesota; reported by Mark Hostager, 1983)

A home remedy for a cough or sore throat was to rub your neck with camphor oil and fasten a man's woolen sock around your neck. (Ella Grunewald, born 1916; Fergus Falls, Minnesota, 2001)

This is for a sore throat. You wrap a black wool sock around your throat before you go to bed. A warm one from your foot works best. (Ester Hegg, born 1913, Decorah, Iowa; reported by Mark Hostager, 1983)

Rx for bad cold and coughs: Concentrated pine oil ½ oz., good whiskey 2 oz., Mix and shake well. Dose: teaspoonful to tablespoonful every 4 hours. (Notebook kept by Christ Leyse, who emigrated to South Dakota in 1865; reported by his daughter, Eldoris Leyse Hustad, Granite Falls, Minnesota, 2000)

For a chest cold Mom rubbed my chest with goose grease and would place wool or flannel over it. (Ester Hegg, born 1913; reported by Mark Hostager, 1983)

Heated goose oil with a little turpentine mixed in was often rubbed on the chest and back for a cold. (Ada Tollefson, born 1910, Windom, Minnesota; reported by Mark Hostager, 1983)

DIPHTHERIA

Snesrud medicine for sore throats and preventing diphtheria: Mr. Snesrud was an elderly gentleman who seemed to this child to be something of a hermit. But he developed a salt-like product distributed in a bottle with a glass tube used as an applicator. The tube was pressed into the salt-like crystals until about ¼ inch of the tube was filled. The tube was then placed quite far back in the mouth of the patient and the "salt" was blown into the throat. The bottle of "salt" and glass tube were packaged in a small pale green cardboard carton with Mr. Snesrud's name on it and a picture of what I believe was intended to resemble diphtheria germs as seen under a microscope. My mother was our family's contact person for this remedy. She left Norway—the Aremark/Ørje area—when she was 3 years old together with her parents and an older brother, and came to Minnesota. I don't know whether Mr. Snesrud brought any of his ideas from Norway or came up with his "formula" over here. (Orville Bakka, raised in 1920s Minnesota; Rancho Bernardo, California)

PNEUMONIA

When my cousin Gwen Kvilhaug was about 6 months old, she had pneumonia. The doctor said she would die. My grandma—Hilda Mathilda Peterson—asked if she might try her "onion pack." She fried up onions in lard, put them in some type of bag, and then kept the warm onion packs on the little girl. Within a short period of time, the fever broke, the lungs cleared, and Gwen was completely healed. (Grant Peterson, born 1938; Brookings, South Dakota, 2000)

A cure for pneumonia is to put fried onions in camphor and put the mixture in cheese cloth. Then put the cheese cloth on the chest of the sick person. Eldred Christen, born 1918 in Decorah, Iowa, saw this work on a little boy with pneumonia. She really believes this works, but says that people today just laugh at her when she brings it up. (Reported by Suzanne Josephson, 1983)

When people get pneumonia you should take a clean white cloth, fry some onions, place them in the cloth and fasten it shut with a pin. Then you should place the cloth on the chest of the person who has pneumonia. Now if the onions turn black, then the poison that caused the pneumonia has been drawn out of the body. As soon as the onions turn black, you put on fresh applications until they don't turn black any more and then you have drawn out all the evil that caused the pneumonia. However, if on the first application nothing happens and the onions don't turn dark, the person either doesn't have pneumonia or the onion poultice won't do the trick or help the person. They will most likely die. (S. S. Urberg, born 1932, observed this in Hannaford, North Dakota; reported by Ingrid Urberg, 1983)

WARTS

My mother Alida Simonsdatter Veseth, born 1900 in Norway, used to tell us kids that as a child on a small farm on the island of Østerøy off the coast of Bergen, whenever they wanted to get rid of warts they would count the number of warts and cut that many notches in a piece of wood that would then be buried. She always claimed that the warts would disappear. Apparently we were not all that impressed for I don't ever recall that I did this to get rid of the warts that I had. (Ole Veseth; Tucson, Arizona, 2000)

Rub a piece of salt pork on each wart. Take a piece of woolen thread and tie one knot for each wart. Bury the thread and if no one digs it up, the warts will disappear. But if someone does dig up the thread, the warts will remain. (Mrs. Martin Solnordal, born 1904; reported to Sharon Symington, University of California, Berkeley, 1969)

Take a clean, glazed ceramic plate and a sheet of bond paper. Shape the paper into a cone and fasten it with a common pin. Stand the cone on the plate. Light the top of the cone and let it burn down. Blow away the ashes. A yellow residue remains on the plate. Apply this as a salve to the wart. In a week or so, the wart will be gone. This worked on my brother when he had warts. (John Christiansen; Decorah, Iowa, 1999)[5]

My grandmother had a "sure cure" for warts. Just bury a string in the back yard—or in a Bible and the wart will disappear. It seemed to work. Recently I opened a little Bible—a gift to my father from his Sunday school, Christmas 1924—and I found a little string buried at Genesis 23–24. (Sandra Gaudier; Port St. Lucia, Florida, 2000)

My mother's good friend, Astri Senum, came from Lista, Norway. Tante Astri and her family had a summer home next to our summer home in the Pocono Mountains of Pennsylvania. When I was a teenager I developed a wart on my wrist. That summer I told Tante Astri about it. She very solemnly told me that on the night of the full moon I had to rub the wart with bacon fat, and then bury the piece of bacon beneath a rock that had the moon shining on it. I did this, and miracle of miracles, the next morning the wart was gone! I have never had a wart since. (Ingrid Olssen Feingold; Glen Head, New York, 2000)

My grandmother lived on Karmøy near the city of Haugesund. Once when I had an outbreak of small warts all over one hand, Mom said, "Let's try your grandmother's cure." It was simple: take an onion, cut it in the middle, salt both sides and then tie it together with twine and place on a saucer. What dripped from the onion, a combination of salt and onion juice, was applied to the hand in question. This application caused a tingling sensation and two days later, those warts disappeared. (Hilda Thompson Quickstad, in Peterson, Minnesota, ca. 1900; Norwegian American Historical Association [P1317], 1982)

Conclusion

A few folk remedies have lived on in memory, but by the 1940s, most families stopped passing down this information to the next generation. "I have attempted to *pry* some other home remedies from friends," writes Claire Kristensen (born in Brooklyn, 1933), "but I realize that I was fortunate in having a mother who communicated. Others haven't so much to report."[6]

Had this book been written seventy-five years ago, it could have contained much more specific information about the remedies and rituals used by nineteenth-century Norwegians on both sides of the Atlantic. The present effort only suggests the massive medical lore they once possessed.

Yet, some of the questions this study raises seem more relevant than ever before: How does a society provide health care to those who can't afford to pay for it? To what extent is health care the individual's own responsibility? Should the patient's social class determine the quality of the basic health care received? Could an intermediate level of health care be instituted to make services more readily available to the poor? How does faith—whether in the religious sense or in the health care provider—relate to recovery? Should medical education include alternative notions and methods of healing? What is it like to be ill as an immigrant in a new land? How do beliefs and experiences from the homeland influence an immigrant's use and perception of medical care in the new land?

In addition to the issues, some of the remedies pertinent to nineteenth-century Norwegians have also returned: interest in medicinal herbs, the belief that a glass of red wine promotes health, and some mothers' preference for childbirth assisted by a midwife at home. Doctors are finding new uses for leeches and bloodletting, and nutritionists are recommending increased levels of Vitamin D.

Self-care and home-based first aid continue to play a role in our health care, too, though not to the extent it did for nineteenth-century Norwegians,

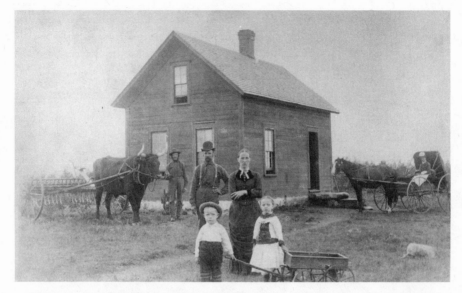

The young I. Ellefson family at home in Hendricks, western Minnesota, about 1880

who applied the remedies that everyone knew "as well as they knew Luther's catechism." They expanded their repertoire by talking to neighbors, relatives, and friends and by reading the doctor books. When home remedies failed, they consulted an impressive array of self-trained specialists and occasionally a professional doctor.

Perhaps the most striking and persistent elements of Norwegian folk medicine are spiritual. The folk religion of the almue—a unique blending of orthodox Lutheranism with pre-Christian and Catholic elements—provided a meaningful framework for the remedies and rituals they employed. Added to these systematic beliefs was the patient's faith in the folk healers themselves, whose memory in many cases survives more indelibly than the specific remedies they used. People long recalled the calming reassurance, penetrating gaze, and powerful personality of healers like Mor Frøisland and Anne Brandfjeld and how, when they were children, they had feared Marit Tofteli and Mrs. Shoemaker Riley as witches.

Norwegian folk healers themselves, meanwhile, risked their personal well-being and reputations to battle disease and, often, government authorities as well. The healers, like their patients, lived in a world where, from the precarious moment of birth, danger lurked in the challenging climate, rugged landscape, and treacherous huldrefolk. Seeking solace in the alcohol that flowed freely during the extended celebrations of weddings, Midsummer's Eve, and other milestones of the life cycle and agricultural year, they also found comfort in the structure of ritual and the insights of tradition, not least the belief that certain individuals could stop excessive bleeding, deliver babies that refused to leave the womb, and treat diseases inflicted by unseen forces.

Only a shadow remains of the rich tapestry of remedies and rituals that helped nineteenth-century Norwegians through their lives. Knowing even a little about their beliefs aids our understanding of the resources they garnered to endure their difficult circumstances.

Notes

Chapter 1. Healing the People

Epigraph: Quoted in *Hordaland og Bergen i manns minne. Dagleliv ved hundreårsskiftet* (Oslo: Det Norske Samlaget, 1974), 156.

1. Facts and figures quoted here and in the next several paragraphs rely on Odd S. Lovoll, *The Promise of America: A History of the Norwegian-American People* (Minneapolis: University of Minnesota Press, 1984), 8–9, and Odd S. Lovoll, *The Promise Fulfilled: A Portrait of Norwegian Americans Today* (Minneapolis: University of Minnesota Press, 1998), 8–11.

2. The notion that certain folk remedies began as human imitations of animal practices dates back at least to Pliny the Elder (23–79 AD), who, in his popular *Natural History*, reported seeing a deer soothe a wound by licking it after chewing leaves of sage (Caius Plinius, *Naturalis Historia*, K. Maghoff, ed. [Lipsïæ, 1875]).

More recently the Norwegian folk healer Hans Kadden (1807–97), seeing a sparrow that had applied a "dough" containing pine sap to its injured foot, analyzed the dough and duplicated it as an ointment for his patients, writes A. S. Hvidbergskår in *Kvaksalvere og folkemedisin på Agder* (Oslo: Universitetsforlaget, 1968), 53.

3. Magical medicine regarded sickness as the harm inflicted by hidden spirits who hit, pinched, blew upon, or threw projectiles at their victims. Present-day Norwegian names for such afflictions as lumbago (*hekseskudd*, witch shot) and hives (*alveblåst*, elves' breath) reflect this once widespread belief.

Curing illness by means of magical charms enjoyed great vogue among the ancient Egyptians, Babylonians, Persians, and Hebrews. They contributed material to the formulas that attained enormous popularity and wide circulation in medieval Europe, as evidenced by catalogs of the prestigious libraries in London, Oxford, Paris, and Berlin that contain numerous manuscripts of magical incantations dating to the eleventh through the sixteenth centuries. Originally in Latin (and sometimes in Greek or Hebrew), these formulas were translated early into vernacular languages and collected in compendia, variously known as leach books, grimoirs, or the Sixth and Seventh Books of Moses.

4. Injald Reichborn-Kjennerud, *Våre folkemedisinske Lægeurter*, published as a supplement to *Maal og Minne* (1922), 6; Harpestreng, *Gamle danske urtebøger, stenbøger og kogebøger*, Marius Kristensen, ed. (Copenhagen, 1908).

5. Erwin Ackerknecht, *Therapeutics: From the Primitives to the 20th Century*

(New York: Macmillan, 1973), 124. About the doctrine of signatures, see Per Holck, *Norsk folkemedisin. Kloke koner, urtekurer og magi* (Oslo: Cappelen, 1996), 23–24.

6. Otto Lindemark, *Medisiner før og nå* (Oslo: Cappelen, 1967), 34–35. C. E. Mangor describes the use of tartar emetic (*viinsten*) in his *Lande-apothek, til landmænds nytte* (Copenhagen: J. H. Schubothe, 1835 [1767]), 126–27.

7. Ira Rutkow, *Bleeding Blue and Gray: Civil War Surgery and the Evolution of American Medicine* (New York: Random House, 2005), 53.

8. Unless otherwise indicated, facts and figures on Norwegian medical history here and in the paragraph below rely on Olav Bø, *Folkemedisin og lærd medisin. Norsk medisinsk kvardag på 1800-talet* (Oslo: Det Norske Samlaget, 1986), 22.

9. The district doctor is quoted in Øystein Lappegard, M.D., *Det var so laga. Om helse og utvikling i Øvre Hallingdal fyrst på 1900-tallet* (Ål: self-published, 1997), 85. Eilert Sundt commented on peasant conditions that challenged cleanliness in *Om renligheds-stellet i Norge. Til oplysning om flid og fremskridt i landet* (Christiania: J. C. Abelsted, 1869).

10. Sherwin B. Nuland, *The Doctor's Plague: Germs, Childbed Fever, and the Strange Story of Ignàc Semmelweis* (New York: Norton, 2003). Norwegian writer Jens Bjørneboe portrayed this dramatic struggle in his play *Semmelweis* (Oslo: Gyldendal, 1986).

11. *Sogn og Fjordane i manns minne. Dagleglid ved hundreårsskiftet* (Oslo: Det Norske Samlaget, 1974), 178.

12. The letter from Johanne Svenningsdatter Sogne, sent from Winnebago County, Ill., to Tvederstrand in Aust Agder, Norway, on July 16, 1854, is quoted in Orm Øverland and Steinar Kjærhiem, eds., *Fra Amerika til Norge. Norske utvandrerbrev*, Vol. I (Oslo: Solum, 1992), 318. The letter from E. T. Rogne to his family, preserved by Elmer Rogne of Minneapolis, Minn., was provided by relative Marlin Heise, St. Paul, Minn. Ragna's letter, from the article "Amerikabreve fra en tjenestepike, Ragna," is on the website of Norway's Nasjonalbibliotek at http://nabo.nb.no/trip?_b=EMITEKST&urn.

13. Knut Gjerset and Ludvig Hektoen, "Health Conditions and the Practice of Medicine among the Early Norwegian Settlers, 1825–65," *Studies and Records*, Vol. I (Northfield, Minn.: Norwegian-American Historical Association, 1926), 32–33. Notable exceptions are Ann Legreid and Rasmus Sunde, who have both dealt with immigrant health issues.

14. Ole Munch Ræder, *America in the Forties: The Letters of Ole Munch Ræder*, Gunner J. Malmin, trans. and ed. (Minneapolis: University of Minnesota Press, 1924), 66.

15. Mandt's story is in C. A. Clausen, *A Chronicler of Immigrant Life: Svein Nilsson's Articles in Billed-Magazin, 1868–70* (Northfield, Minn.: Norwegian-American Historical Association, 1982), 114–17.

16. Quotations here and three paragraphs below are from Ole Løkensgaard, "På Lake Prairie i sekstiaarene," *Hallingen*, Mar. 1921, 884–85.

17. Ester Hegg's comment was collected by Mark Hostager, a student in the author's 1983 folklore class at Luther College, Decorah, Iowa. The observations about the Viking's use of milk are from Aage Bjertnæs, *Groblad, meitamark og krut. Kjerringråd og folkelig behandling i 1000 år* (Oslo: Gyldendal, 1997), 152.

18. Traditionally *makkemjøl* was thought to have magical associations to the sacred power of trees, says Reichborn-Kjennerud, *Lægeurter*, 8, 25. Its use in more recent times is discussed in Alf Mostue, *Slik var hverdagen. Arbeidsfolk forteller fra husmannskår, anleggstid og kriseår* (Notodden: Historielaget, n.d.), 27.

19. Writing in the prestigious British medical journal, *The Lancet*, Jorge Chirife and Leon Herszage concluded in 1982 that "sugar may be considered as a non-specific 'universal' anti-microbial agent, in the sense that pathogens known to be present cannot grow in a sugar solution of high concentration" (J. Chirife and L. Herszage, "Sugar for infected wounds," *The Lancet*, July 17, 1982, 2 [8290]: 157). Hjalmar Lie's experience is from *Østfold og Vestfold i manns minne. Dagleglic ved hundreårsskiftet* (Oslo: Det Norske Samlaget, 1975), 161–62.

20. Ole Løkensgaard, "Nybyggerhistorier," *Hallingen*, Apr. 1918, 147.

21. Other examples of Indians and Norwegian Americans exchanging health care assistance include: Olav-Iver and Johanne Berg (Norwegian Americans stopping at an Indian camp to get aid for frozen feet), in "Pioneers—An account of covered wagon days," by Mathilde Berg Brevstad (born 1862), trans. by Agnes Grevstad Lee, *Studies and Records* 27 (Northfield: Norwegian-American Historical Association, 1977); Nina Maathieu (Indians and Norwegian Americans helping each other through childbirth) in "Our Prairie Home" (typed manuscript at Norwegian-American Historical Association), 36–37; and Hilda Wisness and Levard Quarve, ed. (immigrants helping an Indian family with child care), *Viking: Early Settlement Days 1886–1936* (Viking, N. D.: self-published, 1936), 29–30.

Examples of contact between the Norwegian immigrants and American Indians conducive to the exchange of medical information are found in: J. T. Odegard, *Erindringer I. Lom, Long Lake, Fargo, Minneapolis* (Oslo: self-published, 1930), 9–10; "Six Mile Grove," *Telesoga*, Sept. 1919, 9–10; and H. G. Stub, "Fra fars og mors liv," *Symra. En aarbog for norske paa begge sider af havet*, 1907: 36.

Like Norwegians, American Indians tended to view serious illness as the result of offending one of the many spirits who inhabited the world around them or malevolent actions by other humans. Discovery of who caused the illness was an essential task of the healer. See Virgil J. Vogel, *American Indian Medicine* (Norman: University of Oklahoma Press, 1970), 13–35.

22. Kirby's account was collected by Kari Hermeier, student in the author's 1983 Luther College folklore class. Doris Barnaal (Vesterheim Museum, Decorah,

Iowa) extensively interviewed Stella Kirby in January 1982, and the museum's transcript includes this incident. The pneumonia cure Kirby mentions was common but apparently seemed miraculous each time it worked. See additional examples in Chapter 10.

23. Erwin Ackerknecht, *A Short History of Medicine* (Baltimore: Johns Hopkins University Press, 1982), 223–24. Information about the proprietary schools is from Rutkow, *Bleeding,* 49–52.

24. Caja Munch, *The Strange American Way: The Letters of Caja Munch from Wiota, Wisconsin, 1855–59* (Carbondale: Southern Illinois University Press, 1970), 35 and 75; Ackerknecht, *Therapeutics,* 120. In her letter of Jan. 22, 1856, Caja Munch comments, "We regret we did not bring a larger supply of [medicines] because doctors as well as medicines [here] are only rubbish. A Norwegian doctor would be very welcome here, but his life would be a constant journey, as people live so far apart (35). To the letter dated Feb. 23, 1857, she adds: "This is how medical service is in the country and in the small miserable towns around here where the most prominent article is liquor; in the larger cities there is certainly a little better service available, although it is in a bad way even there" (75). In this letter, too, she notes, "We are often short of medicines; to be sure, you can buy some that are called by the same names here, but one certainly had better not take most of them, for they are not trustworthy" (75).

25. Rutkow, *Bleeding,* 56.

26. Here and nine paragraphs below, Severin Almklov, "En biografi og nogle erindringer," *Nord-Norge* 61 (1931): 8–11. Except as otherwise indicated, this section is based on Almklov's memoir.

27. Kjell Åsen, *Nissedal Bygdesoge. Kultursoga, frå dei eldste tider til år 1900* (Nissedal: Bygdesogenemd, 1986), 352.

28. The Almklovs had six children of their own, five of whom survived infancy; several of his descendents later pursued careers in medicine. The small frame drugstore was damaged by fire in 1905 and replaced by a cement block building, which remained in the family for eighty-nine years (*Griggs County History, 1879–1976* [Dallas: Taylor Publishing, 1976], 56).

Except as otherwise indicated, the information and quotations here and below are from Erlys Haerter, Williston, N. D., letter to the author, Dec. 6, 2002.

29. "Flickertail Pharmacist's Early Study of Skin Diseases Brings Profit to His Store," *Northwestern Druggist,* Sept. 1928.

30. In 1888, Almklov bought both the drugstore and the coffin stock from his predecessor (Dr. George F. Newell) and, like him, stored and displayed the coffins above the drugstore. *Cooperstown, North Dakota, 1882–1982* (Cooperstown: Centennial committee, 1982).

Chapter 2. Folk Healers and Folk Cures

Epigraph: Oluf Turtumøygard, "Gamle helseråder og åtgjerder: Anne Marie Djupedalen i Heidalen fortel," Årbok for Gudbrandsdalen 1969: 202.

1. Except as otherwise noted, the entire account of Mor Sæther's life is based on Karl Haugholt, "Mor Sæther," St. Halvard, 1958: 270–87. The Anatomy Department was originally located in the building still standing at Rådhusgate 19.

2. Erik Henning Edvardsen, Ibsens Christiania (Oslo: Damm, 2003), 16.

3. The quack law is quoted by Hvidbergskår, Kvaksalvere, 69.

4. Unless otherwise indicated, the details of the court cases against Mor Sæther derive from Bø, Folkemedisin, 44–60; the quotations here are at 45–46, and the document (below) signed by the Eidsvoll poverty commission is at 50.

5. Details quoted from the 1842 trial here and below are from Haugholt, "Mor Sæther," 279–81.

6. Madam Sæther, "The queen of all kvaksalvere, the consoler of all sick fools, the medical oracle of the entire nation, the darling of the highest authorities, and the disgrace of our health policy," the doctor further charges, "is making fools of them all" (quoted in Haugholt, "Mor Sæther," 282).

7. During the 1842 trial, thirty prominent citizens of Christiania submitted a statement declaring that they had "known Anne Johannesdatter Sæther for a period of several years" and felt she had "benefited a great number of her fellow human beings through the use she has made of what appears to be a natural ability to cure certain, especially external, illnesses such as lameness and rheumatism." It would therefore "wound our natural sense of justice, if after a life of mostly useful sacrifices for her fellow citizens' well-being she were to be sentenced to punishment in jail" (quoted in Haugholt, "Mor Sæther," 276).

8. The document is quoted in Bø, Folkemedisin, 57.

9. Aloe ferox was obtained by evaporating the bitter yellow latex found in the leaves of the African aloe plant. Its medicinal properties are discussed in Lindemark, Medisiner før og nå, 22; John Crellin and Jane Philpott, Herbal Medicine Past and Present, Vol. II. A Reference Guide to Medicinal Plants (Durham: Duke University Press, 1990, 46–48); and David G. Spoerke, Jr., Herbal Medicines (Santa Barbara, Cal.: Woodbridge Press, 1980), 21. Norwegian herbals do not usually include it.

10. On valerian, see Varro E. Tyler, Lynn R. Brady and James E. Robbers, Pharmacognosy (Philadelphia: Lea and Febiger, 1981), 499–500; Spoerke, Herbal Medicines, 172–73; Francesco Bianchini and Francesco Corbetta, Health Plants of the World: Atlas of Medicinal Plants (New York: Newsweek Books, 1977), 108; Crellin, Herbal Medicine II, 434–36.

11. On hops, see Tyler et al., Pharmacognosy, 486–87; R. A. LeStrange, A History of Herbal Plants (New York: Arco, 1977), 139; Spoerke, Herbal Medicines, 88–89.

About the Norwegian use of hops, Reichborn-Kjennerud wrote in 1922 that people in Hardanger put it into pillows to remedy insomnia (*Lægeurter,* 48), and Holck says that Norwegian apothecaries still sell blossoms of hops as a sedative (*Folkemedisin* 160–61).

12. On the production and medicinal uses of turpentine, see Tyler et al., *Pharmacognosy,* 153–55; Bianchini and Corbetta, *Health Plants,* 203; and, for the Norwegian uses, Lappegard, *Det var so laga,* 113.

13. Unless otherwise indicated, details of Wergeland's life are from H. Lassen, *Henrik Wergeland og hans Samtid* (Christiania: Malling, 1866).

14. For his commitment to their cause, Wergeland continues to hold a special place in the hearts of Scandinavian Jews. In 1849, Danish and Swedish Jews raised the elaborate memorial that still stands on his grave in Oslo's Vår Frelsers Gravlund (Our Savior's Cemetery).

15. Here and below, H. Lassen, ed., *Breve fra Wergeland* (Christiania: Malling, 1867), 164–67.

16. Per Holck, "Henrik Wergelands sykdom og død. Et 150-årsminne," *Tidsskrift for den Norske Lægeforening* 115 (1995): 3734–37. Fifty years before Wilhelm Conrad Roentgen discovered the x-ray in 1896, writes Holck, the stethoscope (invented by French clinician Rene Theophile Laennel, 1781–1826) provided the most useful diagnostic tool for doctors Andreas Christian Conradi (1809–68) and John Andreas Lie (1799–1882), who treated Wergeland from January 1845 until his death seven months later.

17. H. Lassen, *Breve,* 166–67; Holck, "Wergelands sykdom," 3735.

18. Holck, "Wergelands sykdom," 3734.

19. Details here and in the paragraph below are from Wilhelm Lassen and Chr. Brinchmann, "Lidt om Wergelands sidste Levemaaneder," *Edda,* 1918, 98–110.

20. Details of the doctors' treatments are in Holck, "Wergelands sykdom," 3736. Aware that the doctors' impatience with him equaled his own irritation with them, Wergeland wrote (in the formal Latin used in the Rikshospital daily journal) the following parody of his doctors' entry upon his departure: "Thank goodness he is gone! The Institution is glad to be rid of such an unruly and untreatable patient. Insane, superstitious, deaf to common sense, tortured by pain, he complained about everything from the ventilation to the sweet laughter of innocent children" (H. Lassen, *Wergeland og hans samtid,* 215).

21. H. Lassen, *Wergeland og hans samtid,* 216; and Holck, *Norsk folkemedisin,* 181.

22. Haugholt, "Mor Sæther," 284. Haugholt does not date the letter, which must have been sent after the May 13 letter telling of his improvement under Mor Sæther's care.

23. Bø, *Folkemedisin,* 51. Mor Sæther's use of baldrian drops is established in Bø, *Folkemedisin,* 49, 55. In Møre, they mixed valerian with tar and smeared it on

the livestock to protect them from the huldrefolk (Reichborn-Kjennerud, *Lægeur-ter*, 92–93).

24. The Skien newspaper is quoted in Haugholt, "Mor Sæther," 285–86. Long after her death, Mor Sæther remained a controversial figure.

25. The quotations here and on the tombstone mentioned below are from "Mor Sæther," *Nylænde*, Mar. 1, 1908, 70–72. Dr. DeBesch reported that on her deathbed Mor Sæther told him about the remedies she had used in her practice, "especially aloe, sulfur, valerian, several aromatic oils and some common Norwegian plants."

26. Most self-trained healers lacked the powerful spokesmen Mor Sæther enjoyed and fared considerably worse. Ole Olsen Huset in Nedre Telemark, for example, was sued in 1833, 1837, and 1843, and actually served the six-month sentence at hard labor stipulated by the quack law. In 1846, with his future in Norway ruined, Huset emigrated to America (Bø, *Folkemedisin*, 64–79).

27. Some sources give Anne Brandfjeld's birthplace as Vartdal in Sunnmøre (as do Haakon B. Nielson, *Byoriginaler* [Oslo: Cappelen 1966], 18, and Holck, *Norsk Folkemedisin*, 192), and a great deal of other mistaken information has been published about her, as well. This account is based on a lecture ("Anne Brannfjell, *signekonenes dronning* [Queen of the folkhealers]") that Berit Øiseth Bakken delivered on Jan. 21, 1999, to clear up the confusion, but I have retained the more traditional spelling of the healer's name. Bakken's lecture is available at http://home .online.no/~blfblf/Annabrann.htm.

28. At the time there were several small farms on the large Ekeberg estate, then outside of the city limits. Brandfjeld was the southernmost subdivision.

29. T. Kiellend-Torkildsen made a drawing of the street that is reprinted in Haakon B. Nielson's *Byoriginaler*, 21. Until the 1960s the area escaped urban renewal and still resembled a street in a small Norwegian town.

30. "Anne Brandfjeld," *Urd*, Jan. 14, 1905, 22.

31. Juniper's anti-inflammatory effects have been demonstrated (Crellin, *Herbal Medicine II*, 144–45), but modern herbalists advise against taking juniper internally (Spoerke, *Herbal Medications*, 102). About the Norwegian use of juniper, see Mangor, *Lande-apothek*, 35, and Reichborn-Kjennerud, *Lægeurter*, 20.

32. Martin Tidemansen (born 1892 at Hoff in Vestfold) describes the process employed for making juniper oil: "We filled a big iron cauldron with dry juniper wood, then we turned the cauldron upside down on a flat stone that slanted to one side to allow the oil to run off. Then we smeared clay between the lip of the cauldron and the stone, leaving just a small opening for the oil to run out. Then we lit a wood fire on top of the up-turned cauldron and soon the juniper oil would be running out onto the flat stone. It was pitch black. My father used it as a salve and said that it soothed his rheumatism. He also gave it to others who said it helped" (*Østfold og Vestfold i manns minne*, 163).

In south Norway, Torijus Lien (born 1775 in Hægbostad, Agder) became well-known for making a salve from juniper berries and sweet cream that soothed rheumatism, eczema, and other pains and rashes (Hvidbergskår, *Kvaksalvere*, 33).

33. Nielson, *Byoriginaler*, 23–24.

34. The sign is located near the northernmost cabin built by *Sanitetsforeningen* (a volunteer public-health organization) near the Ekebergsletta playing field.

35. Flatabø worked as a teacher in Kvam, Hardanger, and attained enormous popularity as an author in the late 1800s and early 1900s. He is virtually forgotten today.

36. Passages from the novel and its preface are quoted from Odd Nordland, "The Street of the Wise Women," *Arv. Yearbook of Scandinavian Folklore* 18–19 (1962–63): 105–16.

37. This scene was originally attributed to Mor Sæther by her niece (born 1841) in the Mar. 1, 1908, issue of *Nylænde*, 71. Little concrete information remains about the individual folk healers, and their stories often borrow details from each other.

38. The section on Valborg Valand builds primarily on the information found in Hvidbergskår, *Kvaksalvere og folkemedisin på Agder*; Bjørn Slettan, *Holum: Gardshistorie* (Mandal: Mandal Kommune, 1977); and a personal visit in 2005 assisted by Kari Grønningsæter of Kristiansand. In addition to Holmen in Søgne, where Valborg's childhood home once stood, we visited the yellow house at Valand where she lived her adult life, as well as the churchyard at Holum where she is buried. We met local historian Bjørn Slettan and several of Valborg's descendents (sons and a granddaughter of Else Valand, referred to below), who have preserved the recipe for her salve.

39. Hanson's story here and Skeie's in the paragraph below are at Hvidbergskaar, *Kvaksalvere*, 66 and 63.

40. A much-used doctor book gave these instructions for making *Blyvand*: Dissolve lead extract in a tablespoon of French cognac or Aquavit. Once it has dissolved, shake the mixture with a half-quart of pure spring water (C. E. Mangor, *Lande-apothek, til landemænds nytte* [Kjøbenhavn: J. H. Schubothe, 1835], 24. The 1899 *Merck Manual* (Ready pocket reference for practicing physicians) similarly recommends "lead water" for bruises; *Merck's Manual of the Materia Medica* (New York: Merck and Col, 1899), 97.

41. On yarrow's medicinal preperties, see Ann McIntryre, *Folk Remedies for Common Ailments* (Toronto: Key Porter Books, 1994), 72, and Crellin, *Herbal Medicine II*, 462–65. On its Norwegian use, see Reichborn-Kjennerud, *Lægeurter*, 92–93, and Holck, *Norsk folkemedisin*, 174.

42. On tormentil red, see Holck, *Norsk folkemedisin*, 177.

43. On tormentil's medicinal properties, see Spoerke, *Herbal Medications*, 172,

194; Bianchini and Corbetta, *Health Plants*, 62, 194; and on its Norwegian use, Reichborn-Kjennerud, *Lægeurter*, 61–62.

44. About the Norwegian use of dock, see Holck, *Norsk folkemedisin*, 62, and Reichborn-Kjennerud, *Lægeurter*, 50.

45. Modern herbalists credit "rumicin" (chrysophanic acid) as the active ingredient in several of the herbs known as "dock" that makes them useful in treating chronic skin diseases among patients suffering from scrofula; see W. T. Fernie, M.D., *Herbal Simples Approved for Modern Uses of Cure* (Bristol: Jon Wright [1895], 1914), 146; Tyler, *Pharmacognosy*, 66–67; McIntyre, *Folk Remedies*, 69; and M. Grieve, *A Modern Herbal in Two Volumes*, Vol. I, 258–60.

Valborg's choice of vinegar (*eddik*) may derive from Mangor, who calls it "such a superb solvent with so many uses that I would not think well of a housewife who did not constantly use it in her home" (Mangor, *Lande-apothek*, 132).

46. Here and below, see Hvidbergskår, *Kvaksalvere*, 64, 66–67, and (below) 79. According to Valborg's neighbor, Oskar Torkelsen Valand, Valborg also used leeches, which he collected for her.

47. Long known for its beneficial effects, Riga Balsam remains a popular tourist item in Latvia and is named for its capital city.

48. On the medicinal use of tobacco in Scandinavia, see Holck, *Norsk folkemedisin*, 178; Mangor, *Lande-apothek*, 121; and Reichborn-Kjennerud, *Lægeurter*, 84–85.

49. T. J. Ritter, M. D., The *People's Home Medical Book*, constituted one third of *The People's Home Library. A library of three practical books* (Cleveland, Ohio: R. C. Barnum, 1915).

50. Bø, *Folkemedisin*, discusses Valborg's legal trials on 102–9 and the ensuing Storting debate on 133–42; quotations below are at 133–34 and 141–42.

51. Ueland was the father of the prominent Minneapolis judge Andreas Ueland (born 1835), who was the husband and father of well-known women's rights advocates Clara and Brenda Ueland.

52. *Folketidene* was published in Mandal from July 5, 1865, to Dec. 31, 1879, with Jaabæk as editor. Here and below, Jaabæk is quoted from Bø, *Folkemedisin*, 142.

53. The almue stood firmly behind this woman, "who has soothed so many pains and with a loving heart and open hand given help where it was needed," declared *Fædrelandsvennen* on June 7, 1886. Sentiment in rural areas rapidly grew against the law that seemed to oppose people trying to improve life in their communities while receiving little or nothing in return. Some district doctors helped folk healers by ignoring their legal obligation to report the activities of these individuals to the authorities.

Most of the local health commissions created in 1860 to improve hygienic conditions opposed changing the quack law, a decision Jaabæk felt represented the will not of the people but of the district doctors, who, as the commissions' self-elected presidents, dominated them (Bø, *Folkemedisin*, 141–42).

54. Hvidbergskår, *Kvaksalvere,* 74.

55. The newspaper reports about Valborg are quoted in Bø, *Folkemedisin*, 107; about Valborg's wealth, see Hvidbergskår, *Kvaksalvere*, 76–77.

56. Else Valand, "Valborg Valand," *Vår arv* (Holum Historielag) 4[1985]:5; and Hvidbergskår, *Kvaksalvere*, 78.

57. The story of Ivar Ringestad below is from A. M. Mohn, "Et Kapittel af de norske indvarndrernes historie," *Samband* 1914: 326–31 (Apr.), 379–82 (May), 426–30 (June), and 487–92 (July).

58. The brother of Anne Ringestad, Nils Olsen Brandt (born 1824 in Vestre Slidre) graduated from the University of Christiania in 1849, was ordained as a Lutheran minister in 1851, emigrated to America the same year, and became the first Norwegian pastor to visit settlements west of the Mississippi River. He served as a professor at Luther College from 1865 to 1882, was one of six Norwegian pastors who organized the Norwegian Synod in 1853, and served as its vice president from 1857 to 1871, writes G. J. Lomen, *Geneologies of the Lomen [Ringstad], Brandt, and Joys Families* (Northfield: Mohn, 1929), 47.

59. Mohn gives Anne's birth year as 1812, but Lomen's genealogy says 1810. She was a descendant in the fourth generation of Johan Fredrik Brandt, who immigrated to Norway from Copenhagen in 1730 (and is said to be the person who first brought potatoes to Valdres). Her first husband was Sheriff Johannes Andersen of Toten, a resident of Løken, Vestre Slidre. Anne had seven children by her first marriage and three by her second to Ivar Ringestad, the brother of Jørgen G. Lomen. Anne died in Decorah in 1884 (Lomen, *Geneologies*, 47).

Anne had a son born in 1850 near Janesville, Wisc., just as she and Ivar set out on the trek for Decorah, Iowa, by ox team and covered wagon. Their daughter, Anna Elisabeth Ringstad, born in Madison Township in 1852, later married Professor Th. N. Mohn, the first president of St. Olaf College (1874–99). As a bride of twenty-three, she went to Northfield to take up the work of building the school (Lomen, *Geneologies*, 53–54). While the Loman genealogy spells the name "Ringstad," I have retained the spelling used in Mohn's account.

60. Though Anne Mohn gives Ivar's birth date as 1813, his obituary in the Sept. 13, 1892, *Decorah Posten* says 1812, as does the obituary in the Sept. 15, 1892, Decorah *Republican*, which states that Ivar "was buried in the Lutheran cemetery, beside his wife." Don Berg provided the obituaries and noted the discrepancy.

61. The interview of Oline Dahl Skrove (Sept. 2, 1937) is at Otter Tail County Historical Society, Fergus Falls, Minn., where files also contain a similar interview about Olava given by Mrs. Julius Johnson on February 8, 1939. Olava's descendent, LeRoy Larson of Rochester, Minn., alerted the author to her story in May 2002.

62. "Lest we forget," by Viola Johnson Behrends and a "Memoir" written in the 1940s by Mrs. Oliver A. Rustad (translated from the Norwegian by Duffy O. Rustad) also contain details of Olava's story. They are both at www.webfamilytree. com/mn_otter.htm.

63. Rustad, "Memoir," 7.

64. The account of Anne Ludvikke Løberg is based on letters received from her granddaughter, Carla Waal, Columbia, Missouri, Feb. 3, 2003, and Feb. 26, 2006. Carla also loaned me the family copy of Raspail's book, no longer easily found. Background information about her grandfather comes from Øyvind Gulliksen and Carla R. Waal, "Peder Kristoffersen Waal: En utvandrer fra Notodden," *Notodden Historielag Årskrift* 1986: 66–77.

65. Ackerknecht, *Therapeutics*, 120, and Erwin Ackerknecht, A *Short History of Medicine* (Baltimore: Johns Hopkins, 1982), 226.

66. Ackerknecht, *Therapeutics*, 120–21. In 1865 Lister pioneered antiseptic surgery, which Ackerknecht terms "the greatest single advance in modern medicine." Pasteur had disovered in 1864 that microscopic organisms are responsible for putrefaction, but his sterilization techniques were unsuitable for surgical use. Lister experimented further and in 1865 succeeded by using carbolic acid.

Chapter 3. The Pastor as Doctor

Epigraph: Prost Henrik Seip, "Åseral prestegård," in Elisabeth Christie, *Prestegårdsliv. Minner fra norske prestegårder I* (Oslo: Gyldendal, 1966), 81–82.

1. A formative version of this chapter appeared in Todd W. Nichol, ed., *Crossings: Norwegian-American Lutheranism as a Transatlantic Tradition* (Northfield: Norwegian-American Historical Association, 2003), 119–38.

2. Details about the early history of medicine in Norway are from Per Holck, "The Very Beginning. Folk medicine, doctors and medical services," in *The Shaping of a Profession: Physicians in Norway Past and Present*, Øyvind Larsen and Bent Olav Olsen, eds. (Canton, Mass.: Science History Publications USA, 1996), 32.

The Age of Enlightenment advanced the idea that improving the people's standard of health constituted an integral part of the clergy's task. The international nature of these views is documented by George Herbert (1593–1653), who sets out as one of the responsibilities of the parson's wife, the "curing and healing of all wounds and sores with her own hands which skill either she brought with her or he takes care she shall learn it by some neighbor" (68).

About the pastor in his circuit, Herbert says, "If curing poor people, he supplies them with receipts [remedies] and instructs them further in that skill showing them how acceptable such works are to God and wishing them ever to do the cures with their own hands and not to put them over to servants" (75); see George

Herbert, *The Country Parson and the Temple*, John W. Wall, Jr., ed. (New York: Paulist Press, 1981).

3. Peder Harboe Hertzberg also wrote a book describing the healing mineral spring at Finnås Prestegård, published by the academic society of Trondheim (Bø, *Folkemedisin*, 26).

4. O. Olafsen, "Provst Niels Hertzberg som Læge," *Hardanger* 1918: 19–20. When Hertzberg's parishioners initially resisted the procedure, he vaccinated his family members and relatives to convince them it was harmless. The epidemic passed over those who had been vaccinated, and opinions soon changed.

5. Holck, "The Very Beginning," 32. Dr. Møller from Arendal, who served as physician for the first Norwegian national assembly in Eidsvoll in 1814, cited this attitude among the parishioners to explain why a doctor could not make a living, even as the only physician in a community of 30,000 or 40,000 people. As late as 1880, a doctor from Nordfjord recorded that only two out of 117 people who had died in his district had been attended by a doctor during their last illness (Holck, "The Very Beginning," 36).

6. Details here and in the next paragraph quoting Hertzberg rely on Bø, *Folkemedisin*, 30.

7. Munch, *Strange American Way*, 107.

8. Joseph M. Shaw, *Bernt Julius Muus: Founder of St. Olaf College* (Northfield, Minn.: Norwegian-American Historical Association, 1999), 374, n 8. The same source reports that Mrs. Muus practiced bloodletting among the Indian families she visited.

9. Mrs. Assur H. Groth, a girl of nineteen when she made the journey with Claussen in the spring of 1853, is quoted in Hektoen and Gjerset, "Health Conditions," 11. Mrs. R. O. Brandt tells her story in "Some Social Aspects of Prairie Pioneering: The Reminiscences of a Pioneer Pastor's Wife," *Studies and Records VII* (Northfield, Minn.: Norwegian-American Historical Association, 1933), 6–7.

10. Elisabeth Koren, *The Diary of Elisabeth Koren, 1853–55*. Translated and edited by David T. Nelson (Northfield, Minn.: Norwegian-American Historical Association, 1955), 144.

11. During their first three nights in Iowa, the Korens stayed with the family of Nils Katterud. The one-room cabin where the Korens spent the next two and a half months—living with Erik Egge (1826–1905), his wife, Helene (1824–1902), and her two children from a previous marriage, aged four and six—is now at Vesterheim Museum in Decorah (Peder H. Nelson, "Et nybyggerhjem," *Årbok for Hadeland* 1982: 30–34).

12. Caja Munch's letter dated Feb. 23, 1857, revealed how "frightening" it was to be "so absolutely devoid of a physician's aid" but noted that "*Mangor's Country Pharmacy* stands us in good stead." Since the pioneer pastors and their families came from strikingly similar backgrounds in Norway and kept close contact in the New

Land, it is highly likely that Elisabeth Koren also used Mangor's *Lande-apothek*. Both she and Caja probably had the 1835 edition, now the only version found in the United States; the only known copy is at the Kierkegaard Library at St. Olaf College in Northfield, Minn.

13. Diary citations here and in the next paragraph are at Koren, *Diary*, 240, 244–45, and 253.

14. Frederic Hoffmann (1660–1742), a professor of medicine at Halle and a well-known chemist, explained disease as disturbances in the "hydraulics of nerve juices" and felt that his drops constituted one of only twelve medications necessary to treat them all (Ackerknecht, *Therapeutics*, 79). "Huslægen" constitutes ninety-two pages of *Husvennen* (The home campanion) (La Crosse, Wisc.: *Fædrelandet og Emigrantens Trykkeri*, [1882]), quote at 50. The other half is devoted to housekeeping and cooking. *Lægebog for hvermand* was published as a separate volume (Chicago: J. T. Relling & Co., 1879), quote at 175. Both volumes arrived as premiums to subscribers of Norwegian American newspapers (and are discussed in Chapter Five).

15. Here and below, Koren, *Diary*, 267 and 262; Mangor, *Lande-apothek*, 566–67. Eye ailments occur frequently throughout the diary. On Monday, January 23 (the day before Mrs. Dysje's first visit), Elisabeth tells of setting out at eight o'clock in the morning, wading through deep snowdrifts, and swallowing her fear of relentlessly barking dogs, all in order to go to the Katterud's for an "eyestone" (a small, smooth, lens-shaped object commonly used to remove foreign substances from a person's eye) to treat Helen's daughter (Koren, *Diary*, 141).

16. Neglected eye infections generally disappear but can result in the far more serious condition known as granular conjunctivitis, advised D. W. Hand, M.D., *Report of Diseases of Minnesota and the Northwest* (St. Paul: Daly and Hofer, 1876).

17. Koren, *Diary*, 295.

18. H. Chr. Mamen, "Prestens bibliotek," *Prestegårdsliv II. Minner fra norske prestegårder* (Oslo: Gyldendal, 1967), 158–75. For an analysis of Black Book Minister legend motifs, see the following articles by Kathleen Stokker: "Between Sin and Salvation: The Human Condition in Legends of the Black Book Minister," *Scandinavian Studies* 67 (1995): 91–108; "ML 3005—'The Would-Be Ghost': Why Be He a Ghost? Lutheran Views of Confession and Salvation in Legends of the Black Book Minister," *Arv: Scandinavian Yearbook of Folklore* 47 (1991): 143–52; and "To Catch a Thief: Binding and Losing and the Black Book Minister," *Scandinavian Studies: Nordic Narrative Folklore* 61 (1989): 353–74.

19. Bø, *Folkemedisin*, 26.

20. Hans Eivind Næss, *Trolldomsprosessene i Norge på 1500–1600-tallet* (Oslo: Universitetsforlaget, 1982); Mamen, "Prestens bibliotek," 168. Though magical incantations go back to ancient times, the witch trials seem to have revived their currency in popular culture.

21. Pastor Schive's story is from Joh. T. Storaker, *Sagn og gaader* (NFL #47) (Oslo: Norsk Folkeminnelag, 1941), 15.

22. Information about Pastor Ruge comes from J. T. Ødegard, *Erindringer,* 29–31.

23. Dagmar Blix, *Og draugen skreik. Tradisjon frå Lofoten* (NFL #93) (Oslo: Norsk Folkeminnelag, 1965), 23.

24. Kirsti Magelssen, "Der mitt hjarta er fest [Prestefolk i Gildeskål, 1897–1906: Nils Stockfleth Magelssen]," *Prestegårdsliv II. Minner fra norske prestegårder* (Oslo: Gyldendal, 1967), 24.

25. Of Hans Haaga, Holand writes: "In the early years, Coon Valley had no medical help. The nearest doctor lived 150 miles away. People resorted to family remedies . . . and 'homemade doctors.' Hans Haaga from Haagadalen was one of these. . . . People maintained that he had the Black Book and could understand it. Although many were of the opinion that this mystical knowledge was very risky business, others gave him even greater respect." Hjamar Rued Holand, *Coon Prairie: An Historical Report of the Norwegian Evangelical Luther Congregation at Coon Prairie Written on the Occasion of its 75th Anniversary in 1927,* Oivind Hovde, trans. (Decorah, Iowa, 1977), 49–50.

"It is said of Peder Enger," writes O. S. Johnson, "that he knew more than the Lord's Prayer. . . . People thought he must be in possession of the Black Book, which could cure this or that ill, but since Peder Enger only did well towards his fellow beings, he could not have had the devil in his service" (O. S. Johnson, *Nybyggerhistorie fra Spring Grove* (Minneapolis: self-published, 1920), 227.

The one Norwegian American source that does mention the black book in connection with the clergy is Peer Strømme's 1893 novel, *Halvor.* About one character (Jens Knudsen) it is said that "he firmly believed that pastors had the 'Black Book' in their possession, and could do whatever they chose, and that there was nothing under the sun they did not know" (Peer Strømme, *Halvor: A Story of Pioneer Youth,* Inga B. Norstog and David T. Nelson, trans. [Decorah, Iowa: Luther College, 1960], 37). On the previous page, however, Jens Knudsen is described as "dreadfully ill-informed."

Although Thor Helgeson did include an account of the black-book minister in the legends he recorded from his neighbors in Waupaca, Wisc., the account describes a black-book minister in Norway, Malcolm Rosholt: *From the Indian Land: First Hand Account of Central Wisconsin's Pioneer Life* (based on Rosholt's translations of *Fra Indianernes lande,* compiled by Thor Helgeson) (Iola, Wisc.: Krause Publications, 1985).

26. The letter continues: "Anyone can understand how much easier it is for a troubled soul to confess to an open and mild man. I can testify from personal experience that it is very difficult for a person troubled by sin to open his heart to a pastor [in Norway]. He is regarded as a haunting spirit, if not worse. People scare children by saying that the pastor will come and take them away." The letter, originally published in *Agder,* Feb. 21, 1879, is reprinted in Frederick Hale, *Their Own Saga: Letters from*

the Norwegian Global Migration (Minneapolis: University of Minnesota Press, 1986), 128–29.

Caja Munch, on the other hand, expresses her preference for the privileges of her class. "These silly peasants for the most part cannot comprehend at all that we are a step above them and have more requirements. No, they regard themselves maybe fully as high and always say *du* [the form of address used among equals] and many such things, which sometimes really are highly ridiculous. For example, many will simply call me Caja" (Munch, *Strange American Way*, 30). Caja and her husband soon returned to Norway to stay.

27. A. Sophie Bøe, "The Story of Father's Life," unpublished manuscript in Luther Seminary archives, St. Paul, III. Bøe's inclination toward medicine, she notes, had already surfaced during his student days at Augustana Seminary in 1866, when he volunteered to quarantine himself for a month as the caregiver for five fellow students with smallpox.

28. Mitchell's words are quoted in Gunter B. Risse, "From Horse and Buggy to Automobile and Telephone: Medical Practice in Wisconsin, 1848–1930," *Wisconsin Medicine: Historical Perspectives*, Ronald L. Numbers and Judith Walzer Neavitt, eds. (Madison: University of Wisconsin Press, 1981), 27.

29. The *Wisconsin State Board of Health Seventh Annual Report* is quoted in Dale Treleven, "One Hundred Years of Health and Healing in Rural Wisconsin," *Wisconsin Medicine*, Numbers and Leavitt, eds., 138.

30. Laurence M. Larson, *The Log Book of a Young Immigrant* (Northfield, Minn.: Norwegian-American Historical Association, 1939), 72. The importance of personality in healing is also attested by Leroy Davis in reminiscences of the 1870s diphtheria epidemic: "The physicians' big job was to keep up the courage of the parents and cheer up his patients and perhaps incidentally, but most importantly of all, to keep up his own courage" (Leroy Davis, "Reminiscences," 79, typed manuscript, Minnesota Historical Society, St. Paul).

Chapter 4. The Black Book

Epigraph: "Svarteboka," *Skilling Magazin* 1859, 218. A preliminary version of this chapter appears in *The Nordic Storyteller: A Festschrift to Niels Ingwersen*, edited by Tom DuBois and Susan Brantly, University of Wisconsin Press (forthcoming).

1. Carl M. Roan, "The Immigrant Wagon: A Trustworthy Narrative of Pioneer Events," 177, typed manuscript, 1946, Minnesota Historical Society.

2. Rasmus Nyerup, *Almindelig Morskabslæsning i Danmark og Norge igjennem Aarhundreder* (Copenhagen: Andreas Seidelins Forlag, 1816), 195.

3. Storaker, *Sagn og gaader*, 24; Edvard Langset, *Segner-gåter-folketru frå Nordmør* (NFL #61) (Oslo: Norsk Folkeminnelag, 1948), 110; and Knut Hermundstad,

Kvorne Tider. Gamal Valdres Kultur VII (NFL #86) (Oslo: Universitetsforlaget, 1961), 93.

4. In 1996, Aud Ross Solberg, curator of the Heibergske Samlinger in Kaupanger, Norway, arranged interviews with thirteen elderly residents in Balestrand, Vik, Sogndal, Kaupanger, Fjærland, and Fortun about the home remedies that had been used in their families. "I can't recall that there were any who had seen this Black Book at any rate," continued the quoted informant, "but they sure talked about it a lot."

5. Ottar Evensen, "Svartebøkene fra Rustad," *Årbok for Elverum* 1994: 90–134. According to a tradition quoted by Johannes Storaker, the black books in circulation are copies of one original manuscript: "Most people have heard of the Black Book, but here in this community not many people own one. And if they did, it was usually just a copy. The Black Book itself is printed in red letters and written by a man of God by the name of Cyprianus in the city of Wittenberg. It may not be obtained from anyone but the devil himself" (Storaker, *Sagn og gaader*, 20).

6. Here and several paragraphs below, letter to the author from Mary Rustad, Elverum, May 1, 2003. Like those found at Rustad, "black books" can range from coherent booklets carefully written in ornate script to random items hastily scribbled on the backs of discarded documents or the leftover pages of outdated ledgers.

The Rustad black books were probably written sometime at the end of the 1700s and based on excerpts of earlier texts. A Rustad ancestor, possibly Tollev Helgesson Kilde (born 1772), might have written these formulas, which primarily consist of white magic (calling on good powers for help in sickness and other trouble), though there are also hints of black magic (prayers that appeal to darker powers). Per Sande deciphered the gothic writing and Per Holck translated the old-style language to modern Norwegian, which Mary Rustad then translated into English. The books had apparently been a well-kept secret for many years because the find also came as a surprise to Nils Rustad's father. Mass media in Norway ran several articles about the Rustad find, including *Allers* on May 11, 1999, and *Aftenposten* on May 16, 1999. Mary's translation of the Rustad black books was published as Mary S. Rustad, *The Black Books of Elverum* (Lakeville, Minn.: Galde Press, 1999).

7. Ottar Evensen, "The Black Books from Rustad in Norway," in Rustad, *Elverum*, xxxiv. A traditional account expressing the same fear of finding a black book is in Lars M. Fjellstad, *Haugfolk og trollskap. Folkeminne frå Eidskog II* (NFL #74) (Oslo: Norsk Folkeminnelag, 1954), 20.

8. Hans Eyvind Næss, *Med bål og brann. Trolldomsprosesser i Norge* (Oslo: Universitetsforlaget, 1984), 16, 39. Næss says that of the 860 men and women accused as witches whose names were known, 350 were executed for trolldom in Norway. From these figures, Næss estimates that, in all, about 1,750 individuals were accused and about 20 percent of them were executed.

9. Details of Nypan's trial unless otherwise stated derive from Næss, *Med bål og brann*, 41. Casting out disease by similar means occurs in the Bible in Matthew 8:22 ("That evening they brought to him many who were possessed with demons and he cast out the spirits with a word, and healed all who were sick"). The Bible also contains an example of disease being transferred into a herd of swine.

10. *Den kloge kones bog* (1886), reprinted with a commentary by Birgitte Rørbye (Copenhagen: Jul Strandbergs Forlag, 1975), 111.

11. *Hexevæsen og Troldskab i Norge. Meddelt til Læsning for Menigmand* (Christiania: Bentzens, 1865), 14 and 21.

12. Here and below, Næss, *Med bål og brann*, 39, 53. The Bible and other Christian texts were routinely used to drive out evil spirits during Norway's Catholic period, when priests also read annual benedictions to bless farm fields, houses, ships, and roads.

13. Lieutenant Colonel Hoff, in his description of Berg parish in Smålenene, observed that the almue seldom consulted doctors because "their forefathers knew best how each type of illness could best be healed and had handed down the best cures" (quoted in N. A. Quisling, *Overtroiske kure og folkemedisin i Norge* [Kristiania: Aschehoug, 1918], 62).

14. Anton Christian Bang, "Gjengangere fra Hedenskabet og Katholicismen blandt vort Folk efter Reformationen," *Theologisk Tidsskrift for den evangeliske lutherske Kirke i Norge Ny række* 10 (1885): 187. They "no longer regarded the Catholic remnants [the sacred words] contained as expressions of Christian piety," he continues. Bang attributes the almue's use of these formulas, as does the author, to people's "constant feeling of helplessness," "eternal fear of magic," and "ever-present fear of deviltry" (218). But while these same dangers had lurked no less threateningly before the Reformation, people's perception of danger apparently increased dramatically in its wake. Missing the old protections of pilgrimage, prayer, and penance, whereby they could appeal directly to the deity, they did as custom decreed in other areas of life: they looked back to the means used by their forefathers and consequently continued to rely on the protective power of ritual healing that had been part of Catholic doctrine.

15. Bang, "Gjengangere," 187 and 211. "It can be a consolation that although the entire population believed in the reality [of this magic], surely only a relatively small number actually practiced these arts in their worst form—although the Catholicized, epic-legendary formulas were certainly known and used by a larger majority" (218).

16. Arne Bugge Amundsen, "Kilde og kirke. En fromhetshistorisk undersøkelse av legekilden ved Trømberg kirke," *Ung Teologi* 1 (1981): 20–40.

17. Landstad quoted in Jens M. Alm, ed., *Bygd og by i Norge–Vest Oppland og Valdres* (Oslo: Gyldendal, 1982), 409. About devotional churches, see Anne Eriksen,

"Lovekirker i Norge etter reformasjonen," M. A. thesis, Dept. of Folklore, University of Oslo, 1986. About the Vatnås church, Andreas Mørch reports, for example: "It was common belief among people that if they had an illness and then promised to give a present to the church, they would get well. In this way the church received many gifts in the old days" (Mørch, *Frå gamle dagar*, 84).

18. Ystad's account of the St. Olav spring is in *Trøndelag i manns minne* (Oslo: Det Norske Samlaget, 1969), 128.

19. Olav Haraldsson (King Olav II) had continued in 1015 the work of converting Norway to Christianity, begun by Olav Tryggvasson (King Olav I, 995–1000), and he also used force to achieve this goal. Working with Bishop Grimkjell, Olav II presided over the assembly at Moster in 1024 that adopted Christianity as Norway's official religion. Just four years later, however, enraged peasants and Viking chieftains drove Olav II out of the country. His attempt to return to power was permanently blocked two years later on July 29, 1030, at the Battle of Stiklestad (Olav Bø, *Heilag-Olav i norsk folketradisjon* [Oslo, 1955].

For popularized accounts of St. Olav's life and legend, see Kathleen Stokker: "In the Footsteps of Olav, Norway's Super Saint," *The Norseman*, Nov. 1988; "Wishing Wells and Sacred Springs: Treasure Troves of Norwegian Culture," *Viking Magazine*, Apr. 1991; and "The Miracles of St. Olav: Secrets of a medieval altar," *Viking Magazine*, July and Aug. 1992.

20. Andreas Mørch, *Frå gamle dagar. Folkeminne frå Sigdal og Eggedal* (NFL #27) (Oslo: Norsk Folkeminnelag, 1932), 83–84.

21. Major A. F. Mockler-Ferryman, *In the Northman's Land: Travel, sport and folklore in the Hardanger fjord and fjeld* (London: Sampson Low, Marston & Company, 1896), quotations here and below at 154.

22. Here and below, Ørnulf Hodne, *Mystiske steder i Norge* (Oslo: Cappelen, 2000), 193–98. It is unclear what if any action the Oslo bishop took with regard to the pilgrimages, but for two hundred years more, people continued to descend upon Røldal from all directions. Nearby place-names such as Krossli and Krossluten identify resting places along their route.

23. Lorentz Dietrichson, 1892, in *De norske stavkirker. Studier over deres system, oprindelse og historiske udvikling*, quoted in Peder Anker, *Stavkirkene. Deres egenart og historie* (Oslo: Cappelen, 1997), 185, on which the additional information on stavechurches relies.

24. Andreas Faye, *Norske Folke-Sagn* (NFL #63) (Oslo: Norske Folkeminnelag, 1948 [(Christiania, 1844)]).

25. Olav's shrine consisted of three different casings; the innermost of wood was housed in a slightly larger one of silver that was encased by jewel-encrusted gold. It is the silver casing that probably resembled the style of the Vatnås reliquary (which has been at Copenhagen's National Museum since 1748), while the St. Olav shrine

was lost at sea on its way to Copenhagen to be melted down for the royal coffers. Rolf Erikson, *Nævra-Erikson: A Sigdal Family* (Madison, Wisc: self-published by Michael Freidel, 1996), contains a photo of the reliquary.

26. Pastor Bernhoft is quoted in Ørnulf Hodne, *Mystiske steder,* 191–92.

27. This custom, forbidden by the Law of Gulating, is further discussed in Kathleen Stokker, *Keeping Christmas. Yuletide Traditions in Norway and the New Land* (St. Paul: Minnesota Historical Society, 2000), 7–8, 106, 308 n 53 and 309 n 9.

28. Sigurd Nergaard, *Hulder og trollskap. Folkeminne fraa Østerdalen IV* (NFL #11) (Oslo: Norsk Folkeminnelag, 1927), 48.

29. Evensen, "Svartebøkene," 131–32.

30. Here and below, Reidar Svare, *Frå gamal tid—Tru og tradisjon. Vefsn Bygdebok II* (Mosjøen: Vefsn Bygdeboknemd, 1973), 319–20. A story printed in the 1901 *Décorah Posten* makes the same point about the black book losing its mystical image.

31. Holstad is quoted in *Møre og Romsdal i manns minne* (Oslo: Det Norske Samlaget, 1969), 109.

32. Ystad's account here and below is from *Trøndelag i manns minne,* 123–26; the formula is at 126.

33. Information on Ole Toftelien here and below relies on Per Kollstad, "Ei Svartbok frå Dovre," *Årbok for Gudbrandsdalen* 1959, 58–61. Johan Meyer, *Fortids kunst i Norges bygder: Dovre* (Oslo: Nasjonalforlaget, 1978), plate VI, shows Toftelien's rosemaled room from the Lindsø farm as painted in 1850 (and drawn by Meyer in 1911).

Tofte, one of the oldest farms in Dovre and by far the largest, is located, like the best farms in the area, midway up the east side of the valley and is mentioned in the medieval Saga of Harald Hårfagre, who "had a chapel built there where none had stood before" (Gunnar Kaas and Arnfinn Engen, *Bygdefok for Dovre (2). Gaardar, hus, folk* [Dovre: Dovre Kommune, 2003–04]).

34. Velle Espeland (Department of Folklore, University of Oslo) provided a photocopy of Toftelien's black book in Oct. 2000.

35. Meyer, *Fortidskunst,* 11–12. In 1837, Ola Hansson from Åkerjordet and his wife, Eli Samuelsdatter, took over Toftelien, a cotter's place owned by the Tofte royal estate. The 1865 census shows Ola Toftelien as a cotter with land, 56.9 years old; Eli Samuelsdatter, his wife, 57.9 years old; and their daughter, Marit Olsdatter 22 years old. Ola Toftelien and Eli left for America in 1869. Marit, born Nov. 16, 1844, had gone to Trondheim in 1866, but returned and emigrated with her parents (Kaas and Engen, *Bygdebok for Dovre 2,* 368–69).

36. This and other oral traditions about Ole Toftelien are quoted in Velle Espeland, *Svartbok frå Gudbrandsdalen* (NFL #110) (Oslo: Universitetsforlaget, 1974), 63–67.

37. The story of Ola Sætrum's cow is quoted in Kaas and Engen, *Bygdebok,* 269.

38. The turnip story is quoted in Espeland, *Svartbok*, 67, and I heard it again while visiting Dovre in August 2005.

39. Toftelien sold his black book to Peder E. Tallerås, the father of Gunnar Rudi, who eventually inherited it. Rudi described it as a "book of 'white magic,'" used for healing and other beneficial purposes, though he speculated that "Toftelien probably used 'black magic' too." Rudi's grandson, Gunnar Rudie, who lived and worked as a curator in Oslo, had by the 1970s inherited Toftelien's black book and deposited a photocopy of it in the Archives of the University of Oslo Folklore Department, where it is catalogued as *NFS, Svartebok from Dovre* (Espeland, *Svartbok*, 66).

40. Stimulated by his grandmother's stories, Doug Becken wrote about Old Man Tufteli's suitcase and Mati's black book (below) for a class at Mankato State University in 1986. (I have abbreviated these accounts.) The suitcase story resembles one told to me at Toftelien in 2005 about a trunk hidden on the farm that, if moved, would bring misfortune. Rev. Sarah Oelberg, pastor at Nora Church, 1991–2003, sent me Becken's story on Aug. 20, 2003.

41. Letter to the author from Forrest Brown, May 7, 2003. In this letter Brown suggested contacting Sarah Oelberg, who had mentioned hearing parishioners tell of a local folk healer who some had suspected of witchcraft. Thanks to Brown and Oelberg, the stories of Ole Toftelien and Old Man Tufteli finally came together.

42. "The village had no library, but Nora Church had one and made its books available to the public," writes Nina Draxten in *Kristofer Janson in America* (Boston: Twayne, 1976), 331.

43. A full list of Toftelien's books is available at the Norwegian-American Historical Association.

44. Before the hospital opened, states the book written to mark Hanska's centennial, the rule for treating serious illness and delivering babies was that "brave and skilled women would come to the rescue through storm and night." Among those named is "Marit Toftelien (home medicine and healing)." *Hanska: A Century of Tradition, 1901–2001* (Hanska: Centennial Committee, 2001), 203.

45. According to Lorraine Becken (letter sent July 17, 2004), Pastor Whalen drowned when he accidently fell into in an outdoor cistern (commonly used to collect rainwater for household use).

46. L. Pio, ed., *Cyprianus* (Copenhagen: Immanual Ree, 1870), foreword, n.p. The Norwegian-American Historical Association "Svartebok" file (P374) contains three additional black books: 1) *Svarteboka*, published in Fredrikstad, Norway, in 1859 and consisting of eighteen formulas found in the 1830s under the altar cloth of North Norway's Vesteraalen church (also published in *Skilling Magazin*, 1859); 2) *Det sorte kabinet i Stockholm* (the black cabinet in Stockholm), probably published by John Anderson in Chicago; and 3) *Den Sorte Bog* (The black book), trans-

lated from French and subtitled "How to achieve your goal," and apparently intended to help immigrants adjust to middle-class life by addressing matters of hygiene, clothing, and social deportment. The last one shows how the term "black book" eventually came to connote "powerful" information of all kinds.

47. The tradition from Eidskog quoted here and in the next paragraph is from Fjellstad, *Haugfolk og trollskap*, 20.

48. Tormod Skatvedt, *Sigdal og Eggedal V. Bygdehistorie* (Eggedal: Historielag, 1965), 880.

49. Birgir Osland, *A Long Pull from Stavanger: The Reminiscences of a Norwegian Immigrant* (Northfield: Norwegian-American Historical Association, 1945), 16. The other best sellers he identified as "the Bible, Norwegian hymnbooks, *Troens Harpe* [Harp of faith], *Gjest Baardsen* [Story of a master thief], and *Farming med Hoved og Hænder* [Farming with head and hands]"—titles that reflect the mixture of pious Christianity, magic, and everyday pragmatism that characterized the nineteenth-century Norwegian almue.

As the term "black book" eventually came to connote "essential knowledge," black books for learning magic tricks, card games, and other social skills were advertised in the Norwegian American press. A 1901 article in the *Decorah Posten* debunked the mysticism of the black book and showed that individuals reputed to "know more than the Lord's Prayer" actually depended on keen powers of observation and psychological insight rather than supernatural wizardry.

50. Someone has written by hand on the first page of one of the Rustad black books, for example, "A copy of the actual Black Arts Book written at the University of Wittenberg in the year 1529 and thereafter found at the castle in Copenhagen in the year 1591 in a white marble casket, written on parchment."

Though *Oldtidens Sortebog* names no publisher, Osland's comments strongly suggest John Anderson. Anderson once told the immigrant historian Hjalmar Holand that he "didn't want the Norwegian American clergy in his hair" (Hjalmar Holand, *My First Eighty Years* [New York: Twayne, 1957], 169), reason enough to disavow any involvement with the black book.

Velle Espeland identified the precise precedent of the Chicago black book, which Professor John Christianson originally called to my attention.

51. The key had to be memorized, says Thormod Skatvedt; "it was like taking an oath" (*Sigdal og Eggedal V*, 870).

52. From the foreword to the black book published in the 1890s by Helge Shultz, quoted in Asbjørn Sæbø, "Svarteboka," *Romsdal Sogelag Aarskrift* 1966: 33–34.

53. For a more detailed analysis, see Kathleen Stokker, "Narratives of Magic and Healing: *Oldtidens Sortebog* in Norway and the New Land," *Scandinavian Studies* 73 (Fall 2001): 399–416.

54. "Sympathetic magic" was one of the many concepts of medieval magic that

Heinrich Cornelius (1486–1535), better known as Agrippa von Nettesheim, systematized and explained in his highly influential treatise on the occult, *De Occulta Philosophia*. Agrippa's book became a standard reference for astrologists, alchemists, and magicians of his day, causing a unified set of concepts and procedures to infuse all manner of European books of magic for centuries to come (Velle Espeland, "Å mane djevelen [Conjuring the devil]," unpublished manuscript used with permission, letter to the author from Espeland, Sept. 12, 1996).

Agrippa systematized the three classical categories of medications as animal, vegetable, and mineral. Thus arranged, the *materia medica* of *Oldtidens Sortebog* are: 1) chemical (camphor, lead subacetate, naphtha, salt peter, alcohol); 2) plant (calmus root, plantain, juniper oil, garlic, anise, pine knots); and 3) animal (urine, collodium, and tallow). All are standard folk remedies that were once used in conventional medicine, as well.

55. Therapies based on excrement were preserved not least in the writings of Galen (ca. 130–200 AD). A Greek physician in the court of the Roman emperor Marcus Aurelius, Galen described the principles of classical medicine so effectively that they remained in use well into the 1700s. He devoted considerable space to therapies based on excrement (Weiser-Aall, *Svangerskap*, 124).

56. Letters to the author from Philip B. Olsen, Honolulu, Hawaii, Mar. 10, 1996, and June 6, 2000.

57. Håvard Skirbekk, "Svartboka, 'Ein kleiner Sibrianus,'" *Årbok for Glåmdalen* 1973: 83. The clandestine aura surrounding the black book had not entirely disappeared, as Velle Espeland (born 1945) learned in 1966 while clerking at a general store in his hometown of Sør-Fron in Gudbrandsdal. One day an older man came into the store to get insecticide for the wasps' nests in his farm outbuildings. "Things were different in the old days when old Marianne Ånekerlykkjun was still around," the man said. "She had the black book and knew how to enchant the wasps so they wouldn't sting. No one needed to buy insecticide then." Espeland wanted to hear what else this man knew about the black book, "but when the man noticed my interest, he just wanted to pay for the insecticide and leave. The black book is not something to chat about idly over the counter of a country store."

Later, as Espeland was gathering material for his *Svartbok* (published 1974), several individuals told him that they didn't "believe in such things, but there are those who do, so it's best forgotten" (Espeland, *Svartbok*, 9).

58. The Torvald and Ole Thompson story written by Harry Thompson is from Gladys Thompson Boril, "Thomas Anderssen Perlesteinbakken Family History" (Tower, Minn.: self-published, 1999), 45.

59. The beliefs about witchcraft noted here and in the paragraph below come from Bente Alver, *Heksetro og trolldom. Et studie i norsk heksevesen* (Oslo: Universitetsforlaget, 1971), 192–209.

60. The words of Hilda Kongsberg (born 1899 in Rolsvøy) document further the ambivalent attitude toward black-book formulas: "Father was often bothered by water on the knee, and went to a woman who healed it. There were two women at Hauge who could do that. Father once got hold of a verse they used. It contained some religious words, but still we thought it was an abomination" (*Østvold og Vestvold i manns minne*, 162).

Chapter 5. Doctor Books

Epigraph: Albert Lea *Tribune*, Sept. 12, 1996, p. 10.

1. Munch, *Strange American Way*, 65 and 75.

2. E-mail to the author from Muriel's sister, Jeanette Mortinson, Albert Lea, Minn., Oct. 20, 2003; T. J. Ritter, "People's Home Medical Book," in *People's Home Library: A Library of Three Practical Books* (Cleveland, Ohio: R. C. Barnum, 1915).

3. Mary Rued, who grew up in north Minneapolis during the 1950s, wrote that "the book [*Twentieth Century Cook Book and Practical Housekeeping* (Chicago: J. B. Smiley, 1905)] belonged to my grandmother, Stella Sage Johnson, and then to my mom, Rosella Johnson Rued. We don't have a family Bible as some families do, but this book has 16 blank pages for memoranda so Grandma's has recipes, one being 'modified milk for babies' and a note: 'Brandy and Indian Turnip Root and rock candy good for coughs,' along with the family birth and death information" (Letter to the author from Mary Rued Martin, Minneapolis, June 24, 2006). Though not technically a doctor book, this one, with its section of "Medical Hints," shows the standard inclusion of such information in cooking and housekeeping manuals, as well as how such a book, passed from one generation to the next, could attain surprising significance.

4. Termed by medical historian Erwin Ackerknecht (*Therapeutics*, 34) "one of the most influential works in all medical history," Dioscorides divided his work into five books: 1) spices, oils, ointments, trees; 2) animal parts and products—honey, fat (goose grease), cereals, blood, excrement, urine, vegetables (mustard, pepper); 3) roots, juices, herbs, and seeds; 4) remaining herbs and roots; 5) wines and metals, mineral water, vinegar (Robert T. Gunther, *The Greek Herbal of Dioscorides* [New York: Hafner, 1959]).

5. "The modern science of pharmacology can be traced back to the efforts of Dioscorides to systematize knowledge of the materials of medicine," writes Frank J. Anderson in his *Illustrated History of the Herbals* (New York: Columbia, 1977), 7.

6. Henrik Harpestreng, *Gamle danske urtebøger, stenbøger og kogebøger*, Marius Kristensen, ed. (Copenhagen, 1908). The University of Wisconsin, Madison, owns a copy of Harpestreng's *Liber Herbarum*. Excerpts are also available at "Plants in the cloister garden at Esrum" (Denmark), www.esrum.dk/kloster/klosterhavens_

planter.htm. Surviving manuscripts of Harpestreng are in Danish, Swedish, and Icelandic, but the original was probably written in Latin, then translated into local languages (Reichborn-Kjennerud, "En oversikt over og karakteristik av de gamle nordiske legebøker," *Tidsskrift for praktisk medisin*, ny række 44 [1924]: 384). "The only medicinal plant that has come onto the world market from Norway, *kvann* must have been among our oldest medicinal herbs, known at the end of Middle Ages as an export article from Norway for medicinal use," writes Reichborn-Kjennerud, *Lægeurter*, 6: 73–74.

7. The saga was written by Snorri Sturluson (ca. 1179–1241).

8. For further information on kvann, see Reichborn-Kjennerud, *Lægeurter*, 6, 73–74.

9. The information on kvann here and below is based on Anne Marte Borgen, *Urtehagen på Knatten* (Oslo: Gyldendal, 1973), 42–43, except as otherwise noted.

10. This description of scurvy, written by the author of a book about North Norway, is quoted in Schnitler's "Description of Nordland," Sept. 7, 1744 (UB manuskript nr. 253).

11. Munthe's book of remedies is described in O. Olafsen, "Folkemedisin efter en gammel lægebok for folket," *Hardanger* 1924: 30–36.

12. Non-Scandinavian sources do not usually recognize angelica's Norwegian background. "Little is known of the herb's early history," writes LeStrange in his *History of Herbal Plants*, "other than that when it was introduced to the warmer countries of Europe it was found to flower on May 8 [the day of the archangel Michael], and therefore got its Latin name" (23–24). Used in many rituals chiefly as a preventative against witches and their spells, angelica was introduced to England by the 1550s, where, as in other countries, it soon naturalized. Becoming a very common garden plant, it was widely regarded as the "antidote" to the plague and incorporated in many useless and superstitious cures (LeStrange, *History of Herbal Plants*, 23–24).

13. General information about the doctor books here and below relies on I. Reichborn-Kjennerud, "En oversigt over og karakteristik av de gamle nordiske læge-bøker," *Tidsskrift for den Norske Lægeforening*, ny række 44 (1924): 381–87, 424–29, 461–67. Pedersen's books (discussed at 425) were never reprinted as doctor books, but a facsimile edition exists (Poul Hauberg, *Christiern Pedersens Lægebog Malmø 1533* [Copenhagen: Levin and Munksgaard, 1933]).

14. Smid's name sometimes appears as Smith. His book about the preparation of medicines from herbs was essentially a translation of Hieronymus Bock, *Krautterbuch*, which first appeared in Strassburg in 1539 and was reissued in 1546. He names as his sources Hippocrates (460–377 BC), Galen (129–199), and Dioscorides (1 AD), as well as the Persian, Avicenna (930–1037), and the Arab, Rhases (d. 923), each of whom had written an encyclopedia of remedies (Reichborn-Kjennerud,

"Gamle nordiske lægebøker," 425). Copies of Smid are at the University of Minnesota, University of Chicago, and Luther College in Decorah, Iowa.

15. Reichborn-Kjennerud, "Gamle nordiske lægebøker," 426. Quoted in the foreword to the 1870 edition of Smid, Professor Kristian Torkelsen Morsing explained that "not many doctors of medicine could make a living here both because of little income and disregard for the doctor's art—which is greater in these kingdoms than in any other place." Quotations and information about Smid here and in the paragraphs below are from Anna-Elisabeth Bræde, *Henrik Smith's Lægebog I–VI* (Copenhagen: Rosenkilde og Bagger, 1976), 3–37, especially 16–17 and 20–21.

16. As late as 1923, a doctor in Ålborg, Denmark, published a translation of Smid stating in the foreword that it could still be of use to those unable to afford consulting a doctor. Smid's book, says Bræde, "represents a part of the history of the Norwegian people in which we can see their daily anxiety and fear of illnesses that they could not understand, much less cure." When Smid's books appeared, she adds, they represented the best official medicine of their time (Bræde, *Henrik Smith's Lægebog*, 21).

17. James O. Berdahl, "The Berdahl Family" (Sioux Falls, S.D.: unpublished manuscript at St. Olaf College library, n.d.), 43.

18. The Age of Enlightenment performed an enormous service for folklore when the clergy were required to write descriptions of their parishes, including the popular customs. Two examples noted later are J. N. Wilse's *Beskrivelse over Spydeberg Præstegjæld* (1779) and H. J. Wille's *Beskrivelse over Sillijord* (1786). Hans Strøm's *Beskrivelse over Fogderiet Søndmør I and II* (Copenhagen, 1762–66) is his best-known work.

Bjørn Davidsen has performed an enormous service in transcribing Strøm's *Kort Underviisning* and making it available online through Norway's Association for the Deaf and Blind, http://home.online.no/~fndbred/hstrom1.htm. Citations here refer to that transcription.

19. As befits such a learned clergyman, Hans Strøm was said to have the black book (Storaker, *Sagn og gaader*, 23). Citations here and below, Hans Strøm, *Kort Underviisning*, 3–4 and 21.

20. Citations here and below, Strøm, *Kort Underviisning*, 26 and 6–7.

21. C. E. Mangor was born in 1739, became a physician in 1764, practiced in Viborg, and was the city physician of Copenhagen. Citations are from the 1835 edition of C. E. Mangor, *Lande-apothek*, preface, n.p. (a reissue of the 1826 edition). While the second edition (1791) significantly expanded upon the first (1767), all editions after 1803 are essentially identical.

The 1803 edition appeared two years after Mangor's death, supplemented by Doctor J. C. Tode (1736–1806), who added updating remarks at the end of each article and in parentheses. J. C. W. Wendt (1778–1838) intended to revise this edition in

1826 but, to meet the "abiding interest in the volume," decided to issue it unchanged. Wendt, who had a degree in surgery and significant medical experience and was a well-known scholarly author, acknowledged in the preface that although certain doctors "believe that such books do harm, by encouraging kvaksalveri, it is also true that even the best things in life can be misused." The seventh (and last) edition of Mangor's *Lande-apothek* appeared in 1863 (Birgitte Rørbye, *Kloge folk og skidtfolk. Kvaksalveriets epoke i Danmark* [Copenhagen: Politikens Forlag, 1976], 219).

22. Mangor, *Lande-apothek*, 132. "What is said about the elderberry's necessity on every farm," adds Tode, "is the greatest truth [and] can't be recommended too strongly" (49). Modern herbals share this enthusiasm for elderberry; see Fernie, *Herb Simples*, 3; Bianchini and Corbetta, *Health Plants*, 214; and Crellin, *Herbal Medicine II*, 199–201.

Elderberry also appears in the Old Norse *Edda* and in Harpestreng. According to Reichborn-Kjennerud, the tree often served as a sacred *tun-tre*—the tree that farm residents traditionally regarded as the seat of their ancestors' spirits and a protector of their own health and good fortune (*Lægeurter*, 89–90).

23. "Huslægen" in *Husvennen* (La Crosse, Wisc.: Færdrelandet og Emigrantens Trykkeri, 1882), 19 (quotation below about treating wounds and cleanliness at 45).

24. *Lægebog for hvermand* (Chicago: J. T. Relling & Co., 1879), on camphor (169), Spanish fly (185), rigabalsam (182), poultices (180), turpentine (186–87), tar (187), and wounds (86).

25. Frederik Mohn, *Før Doktoren kommer. Letvindt lægehjelp og sundhedspleie* (Decorah, Iowa: Decorah Postens Damptrykkeri, 1892), 28. The international research referred to below ranged from the Frenchman Louis Pasteur's initial discovery of bacteria and its practical application in the sterile technique developed by the Scotsman Joseph Lister, to the ability to identify the individual bacteria as the cause of specific diseases. This officially began with the German Robert Koch's identification of the TB bacillus, but had preliminary input from Norway's Armaer Hansen, who isolated the leprosy bacillus in 1873 (but could not prove it caused the disease).

26. Matthias Johnson, *Det sunde og syge menneske* (Decorah: self-published, 1892), quotations here and below at ix–xiv.

27. Channing's lecture is quoted in Lamar Riley Murphy, *Enter the Physician: The Transformation of Domestic Medicine, 1760–1860* (Tuscaloosa: University of Alabama Press, 1991), 112. Additional information on the changing nature of doctor books comes from John B. Blake, "From Buchan to Fishbein: The Literature of Domestic Medicine," *Medicine without Doctors*, Guenter B. Riise, Ronald L. Numbers, and Judith Walzer Leavitt, eds. (New York: Science History Publications, 1977), 11–30.

28. Ritter, *Home Medical Book*, i–ii. "Only the very best [home remedies] have

been saved for this work and after having had over 30 years of experience as a practicing physician, I can pronounce them absolutely safe and reliable," says Ritter, who concludes, "Truly this is the People's Book for it was not only written for the people, but the people themselves helped get it up."

29. E-mail to the author from Lynn Sove Maxson, Chicago, Feb. 26, 2002.

30. Paul "Bud" Hanson, "Heritage Bits: Home Remedies," Albert Lea *Tribune*, Sept. 12, 1996, 10.

31. Letters to the author from Crystal C. H. Lokken, Berkeley, Cal., Sept. 17, 1999, and from Norma Bondeson Gaffron, New Brighton, Minn., Apr. 15, 2000.

Chapter 6. Birthing Children

Epigraph: Borghild Melbye, *Borghild: A History of Pioneer Days in Eastern Clay County* (Hawley, Minn.: The Hawley Herald, 1977), 38.

1. The adage is quoted in Lily Weiser-Aall, *Svangerskap og fødsel i nyere norsk tradisjon* (Oslo: Norsk Folkemuseum, 1968), 113. Norwegian health authorities today recommend that all births take place at a hospital with a professional midwife present and where an obstetrician, anesthetist, and children's doctor can be quickly summoned if necessary, writes Øyvind Lappegaard, M.D., from Ål in Hallingdal. Childbirth shifted into hospitals at different times throughout Norway. Home births remained common in Hallingdal until the Ål hospital was completed in 1968 (Lappegaard, *Det var so laga*, 54–56).

2. Roan writing about childbirth, here and below, from "Immigrant Wagon," 57–59 (quote at 59). Hope is quoted in *Hordaland og Bergen i manns minne* (Oslo: Det Norske Samlaget, 1974), 151.

3. Ida Blom quotes this statistic in her *"Den haarde Dyst": Fødseler og Fødselshjelp gjennom 150 år* (Oslo: Cappelen, 1988), 10.

4. Helen Olson Halvorsen and Lorraine Fletcher, "19th Century Midwife: Some Recollections," *Oregon Historical Quarterly* 70 (Mar. 1969): 44.

5. Quotations here and below from Carl Roan, *Home, Church and Sex* (New York: I. Washburn, 1930), 117–19. "Those pioneer women froze, they sweltered, they hungered, they worked a man's labor, they slept little, they spared themselves not," writes Roan (119). "They bore and raised children in large numbers and made sacrifices in order that their children might have an opportunity to participate in benefits that would come from the development of the national resources that lay before them" (117–18).

6. Valborg Skåret, "Frå småkårsfolks historie. Fødselshjelp, barnedåp, tro, overtro," *Trysil Årbok*, 1985, p. 73 (describing childbirth in the time of her grandmother, Oline Kjærnet, ca. 1850–60). In addition to the fresh fragrance, the spruce branches she mentions were traditionally thought to protect the mother and child

from the hidden powers to which they would remain vulnerable until the child was baptized (Reichborn-Kjennerud, *Lægeurter*, 8).

Though not mentioned by Skåret, Norwegians often used chamomile (*kamillie*) during childbirth to soothe the pain and stop hemorrhage. Scientific studies have since confirmed the anti-inflammatory properties of this herb, primarily due to its volatile oils, especially chamazulene (Mangor, *Lande-apothek*, 63–64, and Tyler, *Pharmacognosy*, 476–77). To stimulate the delivery of the child or the afterbirth, says Reichborn-Kjennerud, some Norwegians used mugwort (*burot*), a use also mentioned by Dioscorides and Harpestreng. The herb has dark-green, sword-shaped leaves and is native to Europe, where it was also used to instigate menstruation (Reichborn-Kjennerud, *Lægeurter*, 94; Grieve, *Modern Herbal*, 556–58).

7. Roan, "Immigrant Wagon," 87.

8. Berdahl, "Berdahl Family," 34, 44.

9. Quoted in Ann Gesme, *Look to the Rock: The Gesme Episode* (Cedar Rapids, Iowa: self-published family history, 1985), 131.

10. Mary King, "Memories of a Prairie Girlhood," typed manuscript, Minnesota Historical Society, 29–30.

11. Berdahl, "Berdahl Family," 34.

12. Bjarne Hodne, *Å leve med døden. Folkelige forestillinger om døden* (Oslo: Aschehoug, 1980), 61.

13. Roan, "Immigrant Wagon," 94.

14. *Østfold og Vestfold i manns minne*, 149.

15. Berkenes is quoted in *Rogaland i manns minne* (Oslo: Det Norske Samlaget, 1970), 165. Vesterheim Museum has many exquisite examples of the *ambar* used to carry porridge to new mothers, and Theodore Kittelsen delightfully captured their use in his 1904 painting, *Grautkjerringer* (Porridge ladies), reproduced in Odd Hølaas, *Th. Kittelsen. Den norske faun* (Oslo: Gyldendal, 1967), 179.

16. *Buskerud og Telemark i manns minne* (Oslo: Det Norske Samlaget, 1971), 104.

17. Erling Ylvisaker, *Eminent Pioneers: Norwegian-American Pioneer Sketches* (Minneapolis: Augsburg, 1934), 97.

18. Roan, "Immigrant Wagon," 94.

19. Michael Krohn, "Om behandlingen av svangre, fødende, og barselqvinder," lecture given Apr. 29, 1861, available at www.uib.no/isf/hist/krohn.htm. The website also contains details of Krohn's social background, other lectures, and annual reports, along with those of his successors. Quotes here and below on p. 4.

20. "Kari" quoted in Ola J. Rise, *Oppdalsboka. Historie og folkeminne I* (Oslo: Tanum, 1947), 243.

21. Lars Skjeldsø, *Frå hverdagslivet i Øvre Gjerstad, 1850–90* (Kristiansand: Gjerstad Historielag, 1979), 63.

22. Rise, *Oppdalsboka*, 243. "The services of the hjelpekone were necessary for

the delivery, of course," writes Valborg Skåret from Trysil, "but her work did not end there. She stayed and helped with child care and housework. . . . Often she would go and take care of the mother and child the first days after the birth, then continue to lend a hand during the first weeks, especially when the family was large and had livestock to care for as well. This work was never paid for; it was a matter of course that they helped each other. 'Today it's my neighbor, tomorrow it may be me,' was the rule" (Skåret, "Småkårsfolk," 75).

23. Krohn, "Om behandling av svangre," 3.

24. The swaddling directions from Østerdal appear in Nergaard, *Hulder og trollskap*, 71.

25. Mostue discusses makkemjøl in *Slik var hverdagen*, 27.

26. Swaddling directions from Voss are quoted from *Hordaland og Bergen i manns minne*, 152–53.

27. Myrvold quoted in *Buskerud og Telemark i manns minne*, 104.

28. Skåret, "Småkårsfolk," 76.

29. Søilen quoted in *Hordaland og Bergen i manns minne*, 152–53.

30. Johannes Gotaas, " Om spæde Børn og om Jordmødre," *Folkevennen* 1859: 292–93.

31. Baastad quoted in *Østfold og Vestfold i manns minne*, 158.

32. Ludvik Hope quoted in *Hordaland og Bergen i manns minne*, 151.

33. Michael Krohn, "Medicinal-Indbretning for året 1856."

34. "On the journey to church with the baptismal child, three strong men walked in front, followed by the one who carried the child; then came the rest of the party," says Ole Fjell (born 1890, Langøy in Hordaland), in *Hordaland og Bergen i manns minne*, 143. About the baptismal clothes as protective, see Inger Lise Christie, *Dåpsdrakter* (Oslo: C. Huitfeldt, 1990), 19.

35. E-mail to the author from Ann Gesme, Cedar Rapids, Iowa, Feb. 24, 2000.

36. Ørnulf Hodne discusses the medicinal properties of baptismal water in *Norsk folketro* (Oslo: Cappelen, 1999), 50.

37. Roan, "Immigrant Wagon," 60.

38. Martin Bjørndal, *Segn og tru. Folkeminne fra Møre* (NFL #64) (Oslo: Norsk Folkeminnelag, 1949), 92–93.

39. Anton Christian Bang, *Norske Hexeformulare og Magiske Opskrifter* (Kristiania: Dybwad, 1901–02), 354.

40. Nina Mathieu, *Our Prairie Home* (New Hope, Minn.: self-published, 1989), 22. Approximately two of every ten infants died in the period between 1750 and 1850, says Sølvi Sogner in *Far sjølv i stua. Trekk fra norsk familiehistorie før og nå* (Oslo: Universitetsforlaget, 1990), 61. Paintings of upper-class families included these children in lighter colors.

41. Hjalmar Holand, *Norwegians in America—The Last Migration: Bits of Saga*

from Pioneer Life, Helmer Blegen, trans. (Sioux Falls, S.D.: Center for Western Studies, Augustana College, 1978), 92; and Holand, *Coon Prairie*, 42–43.

42. Berdahl, "Berdahl Family," 34, 37, 39, 40–44. That Norwegians continued to avoid doctors even after more effective medical care was available, on the other hand, is also a matter of historical record. The Wisconsin State Board of Health singled them out for trusting "too extensively to the preachers' rather than the doctors' directions" (*Wisconsin State Board of Health, Seventh Annual Report, 1882*, 201, quoted in Treleven, "Rural Wisconsin," 138).

43. Holand, *Coon Prairie*, 42–43. Holand also provides statistics showing the number of childrens' deaths in Coon Valley, Wisc., by decade: 1861–70, 11 deaths; 1871–80, 20; 1881–90, 35; 1891–1900, 50 (Holand, *Last Migration*, 92). In his March 1861 lecture on child care, Krohn supplied similarly horrifying statistics from Ytre Nordhordland of the number of children born and the number who died before reaching one year of age—1855: 223 born, 32 died; 1856: 202, 27; 1857: 224, 31; 1858: 211, 29; 1859: 244, 57; and 1860: 233, 31 (Michael Krohn, "Om børnepleien").

Dr. Øyvind Lappegaard shows how those statistics improved later in the century, noting that "during the last 30 years of the 1800s, 16.1% died before the age of one year in Hol, Hallingdal; that number was reduced to 7.6% by 1905" (Lappegaard, *Det var so laga*, 56).

44. Halvorsen and Fletcher, "19th Century Midwife," 45–46.

45. Michael Krohn, "Om børnepleien," Mar. 8, 1861.

46. Valdres midwife quoted in Ørnulf Hodne, "Spedbarnet i norsk folkekultur," *Barn av sin tid. Fra norske barns historie*, Bjarne Hodne and Sølvi Sogner, eds. (Oslo: Universitetsforlaget, 1984), 32.

47. I. Reichborn-Kjennerud, *Elskov og overtro fra Vår gamle trolldoms-medisin* (Oslo: Universitetsforlaget, 1985), 84–86.

48. E-mail to the author from Travis Cleveland, Dorchester, Iowa, Jan. 26, 2000.

49. Quotations from Skåret, here and below, from "Småkårsfolk," 77.

50. Krohn, "Om børnepleien," 2.

51. Martha Myrvold quoted in *Buskerud og Telemark i manns minne*, 104.

52. Mathieu, "Prairie Home," 11.

53. Quotations here and below from Michael Krohn, "Om folkets standpunkt," lecture delivered Mar. 22, 1858, 5; see www.uib.no/isf/hist/krohn.htm.

54. Thomas Collett was the district doctor for Ytre Nordhordaland from 1863 to 1884; his Medisinalberetninger for 1864 are also on the Web at www.uib.no/isf/hist/krohn.htm. Lappegaard writes that as recently as 1895, the jordmor in Hol, Hallingdal, complained of being called in on only ten births (Lappegaard, *Det var so laga*, 56).

Still, Collett could write in his 1869 annual report that "faith in the trained jordmor is increasing and she has in the past year assisted thirty-one births. (But she is poorly paid and applications to increase her salary have been rejected by the Community Council)." The wielders of political power made the life of the trained midwife at least as difficult as did the almue's avoidance of her services.

55. Unless otherwise indicated, information here and below about midwifery relies on Kristina Kjærheim, *Mellom kloke koner og kvitkledde menn. Jordmorvæsenet på 1800-talet* (Oslo: Det Norske Samlaget, 1987).

56. Quoted in Gerd Søraa, *Hent jordmora!* (Oslo: Gyldendal, 1984), 77.

57. The description of delivery is at F. C. Faye, *Lærebog i Fødselsvidenskab* (Kristiania, 1844, 1857, 1872, 1886), 63.

Bloodletting equipment constitutes a significant portion of the midwifery kits owned by Decorah's Vesterheim Museum. One belonged to Marit Engebretson (born 1816 in Fron, Gudbrandsdal), who worked as a midwife around La Crosse, Wisc., during the 1870s and 1880s. She apparently kept up with the latest developments in Norway, for her kit also contains a copy of the 1886 Vogt-revised edition of Faye's classic midwifery textbook.

Faye's book was used by Mrs. M. Seehus, as well. Her copy, also at Vesterheim, contains the following handwritten inscription: "By this book Mrs. M. Seehus practiced as Midwife in Norway and Chicago, Illinois, delivering into the world more than 5,000 children. She is the mother of Pastor Emeritus Knute Seehus, and she educated her two sons—one as pastor and one as doctor of medicine, Martin Seehus of Decorah. This notation made by Pastor Knute Seehus, at the age of 94 yrs and 4 months, living with Herman F. Dale, 505 Leiv Erikson Dr., Decorah, Ia, dated Oct. 10, 1953."

Vesterheim also has the midwifery kit of Julia Olson Lindquist containing twenty-two instruments of various types in a small, well-worn leather satchel. Originally accompanying them, according to the catalog card, were a certificate indicating that she had passed the midwifery exam, a little notebook including the names of 237 "married ladies," a letter of recommendation signed by the parish minister, and the 1886 edition of Faye's text. The owner graduated from midwifery school in Norway on Apr. 29, 1889, and practiced in Merrill, Wisc., from the late 1800s until the 1930s.

58. J. N. Wilse's 1779 *Beskrivelse over Spydeberg Præstegjeld* quoted from Per Holck, *Livets høytider. Skikker og overtro fra vugge til grav* (Oslo: Cappelen, 1995), 23.

59. Holck, *Livets høytider*, 13. Michael Krohn's words are from his 1858 annual report. "Birth is in an upright position, usually kneeling," echoes the journal *Ugeskrift for Medicin og Pharmacie* (Medicine and pharmacy weekly) in its Feb. 6, 1843, issue, quoted in Weiser-Aall, *Svangerskap*, 112.

60. Telemark woman quoted in Weiser-Aall, *Svangerskap*, 112; Halvorsen and Fletcher, "19th Century Midwife," 45.

61. Observer from Sogn og Fjordane quoted in Weiser-Aall, *Svangerskap*, 113.

62. Kjærheim, *Jordmorvæsenet*, 51, and Søraa, *Hent jordmora*, 85.

Doctors warned against having the room too warm and advised that the window be opened. This sharply conflicted with folk custom, which held that births ideally took place in a room without windows to protect mother and child from the huldrefolk and other lurking dangers. Any jordmor who insisted on opening the window would have no credibility among the almue (Søraa, *Hent jordmora*, 59).

The kondisjonerte class, by contrast, used professionally trained midwives and, to the extent possible, continued that practice in America. Thus Caja Munch writes in a letter dated Oct. 28, 1857, about the delivery of Pastor Dietrichson's wife: "She had an excellent and capable certified midwife, who had just arrived from Norway, and it was a pleasure to watch how well and able Mrs. Dietrichson was all the time" (Munch, *Strange American Way*, 124). J. W. C. Dietrichson (1815–83) organized the Koshkonong, Luther Valley, and eight other Norwegian Lutheran congregations in Dane County, Wisc. (Koren, *Diary*, 182 n).

63. Krohn, "Medisinalberetninger fra 1862."

64. The discussion of forceps here and below relies on Søraa, *Hent jordmora*, 109–15. Christoffersen's article (from the *Norsk Magazin for Lægevidenskaben*) is quoted at 114–15.

65. Kjærheim, *Jordmorvæsenet*, 100. The 1844 and 1886 editions of Faye about childbed fever are quoted at 82–83.

66. *Lægebog for hvermand*, 5.

67. Quotations here and in the paragraph below are from Kjærhiem, *Jordmorvæsenet*, 83–84.

68. P. M. Dreijer (1853–1920), "Om dødeligheten på barselseng i Norge," *Norsk Magasin for Lægevidenskaben*, 1907, is quoted in Kjærheim, *Jordmorvæsenet*, 83. The following formula from one of the Rustad black books (Evensen, "Svartebøkene," 94) is known to have been used in childbirth:

Stat stille Blod Flod paa N. N.
lige som Strømmene stille stod
der Jesus med sine 10 Disiple over for,
i 3 Navne Faderen, Sønnen og hellige Ånd.

(Be still the bleeding of N. N. [the mother's name],
like the river ceased its roar
when Jesus and his 10 disciples crossed o'er.
In the name of the Trinity:
The Father, Son and the Holy Spirit.)

The danger of hemorrhage in childbirth—and resourceful ways to treat it— emerge in a more recent incident described to Joan Jurs of Decorah, Iowa, by her mother. During the 1930s a woman began to hemorrhage while giving birth, and when the doctor was unable to get to the house, he advised the women assisting her to pack the birth canal with oats. The bleeding stopped and the woman survived (told to the author by Jurs, March 2005).

69. Kjærheim, *Jordmorvæsenet*, 80. In 1860, seven died per thousand births; by 1899 the number had fallen to 3.2 per thousand births.

70. Krohn, "Om folkets standpunkt," www.uib.no/isf/hist/krohn.htm. Dr. Øyvind Lappegaard similarly charged that the hjelpekoner "killed more infants than they helped [by] hanging the birth mother up by the legs, shaking her, even kicking her in the back to change the child's position" (Lappegaard, *Det var so laga*, 56).

71. Both midwives quoted in Kjærheim, *Jordmorvæsenet*, 87–88.

72. *Nord Norge i manns minne* (Oslo: Det Norske Samlaget, 1973), 11. Even an authority like Professor Edvard Schønberg (1831–1905), a member of the faculty of the Kristiania midwifery school, asserted that being assisted by a self-trained hjelpekone usually presented no extra danger (Kjærheim, *Jordmorvæsenet*, 92).

73. Before midwifery training was even available in Norway, a Royal Decree issued in 1810 had divided the country into official midwife districts. The decree further granted to the officially appointed jordmor (then trained in Copenhagen) a monopoly on assisting childbirth in each district and barred *hjelpekoner* (self-trained birth helpers). Several lawsuits tested the legality of this monopoly; mothers were even brought to court for assisting their daughters, and many others were also sued for delivering friends and neighbors who could arrange no other assistance. In 1838, the court finally struck down the law barring untrained birth assistants, regarding it as inappropriate governmental interference (Kjærheim, *Jordmorvæsenet*, 19).

74. Kjærheim, *Jordmorvæsenet*, 92. Though professional midwives gradually received the almue's acceptance, they had no easy life, "never a single night throughout the year going to bed completely at ease." In addition to the "constant loss of sleep and working amid pain and suffering" were "taxing journeys to be made night and day, in all kinds of weather, whether along the stormy coast, or through long valleys, often high up into the mountains and to places with barely passable roads. Neither permitted nor having the heart to say no, she risks her life in order, if possible, to save others, as she becomes old before her time" (quoted from professional midwives' journal [(*Tidsskrift for Jordmødre*, 1908], in Kjærheim, *Jordmorvæsnet*, 50).

Chapter 7. Rickets Remedies and Lore

Epigraph: "En Signekjerring," originally published in 1845, here from Asbjørnsen og Moe, *Norske folkeeventyr I* (Oslo: Den norske bokklubben, 1982), 277–78.

1. Quotations from Mangor here and below are from the 1835 edition of his *Lande-apothek*, 220–22. The preeminent nineteenth-century physician Sir William

Osler noted, too, that "like scurvy, rickets may be found in the families of the wealthy under perfect hygienic conditions" (William Osler and Thomas McCrae, *The Principles and Practice of Medicine: Designed for the Use of Practitioners and Students of Medicine* [New York: Appleton, 1921], 436). Scientists had learned to associate unhygienic conditions with the lower class, and since bacteria had become the ready explanation for all disease, the presence of rickets among the upper class was hard to explain. Many attributed rickets to "a still unidentified bacillus," as did M. Greve (director of Norway's National Hospital) in his book of popular medicine, *Veileder i Sundhed og Sygdom. Lægebog for norske Hjem* (Kristiania: Cammermeyer, 1904), 164.

2. Lovmø's account here and below is from *Hedmark i manns minne* (Oslo: Den Norske Samlaget, 1972), 128–29.

3. Osler's textbook notes, "Prolonged lactation and suckling of the child during pregnancy are accessory influences in some cases" of rickets, which he observes is "most common in children fed a diet rich in starches," and that "rapidly repeated pregnancies and suckling a child during pregnancy seem important factors in the production of the disease" (Osler and McCrae, *Principles*, 436, 440). All were common circumstances in nineteenth-century Norway.

4. The discussion of vitamins relies on Audrey Davis, "The Rise of the Vitamin-Medicinal as Illustrated by Vitamin D," *Pharmacy in History* 24, no. 2 (1982): 59–72 (quotation at 60).

5. Oluf Turtumøygard, "Gamle helseråder og åtgjerder: Anne Marie Djupedalen i Heidalen fortel," *Årbok for Gudbrandsdalen 1969*, 203. This article does not provide Djupedalen's dates, but they appear in the *Årbok for Gudbrandsdal 1946*, 158. All further references to the "Vågå folkhealer" rely on Turtumøygard, 203.

6. "When a child fails to thrive it should be passed under a coffin," notes Johannes T. Storaker in *Menneskelivet i den norske folketro* (NFL #35) (Oslo: Norsk Folkeminnelag, 1935), 17. He further notes the practice of "stroking the hand of a corpse or its clothes" (17) and advises that "in some illnesses it is good to be touched by a dead man's hand—or to touch a corpse" (15) and that "stubs of candles that had burned on a coffin" were used as medicine (14).

Andreas Mørch gives an example of smøyg being performed in Vatnås church: "Around 1840 a child was passed under the church's altar cloth. It was a child they didn't think would grow into adulthood. One woman stood on each side of the altar and the one sent the child under the cloth and the other received him. The child grew up and became a normal adult" (Mørch, *Frå gamle dagar*, 84).

7. O. S. Johnson, *Nybyggerhistorie*, 227.

8. Wayland D. Hand, "Measuring and Plugging. The magical containment and transfer of disease," *Bulletin of the History of Medicine* 48 (1974): 221.

9. I. Reichborn-Kjennerud, "Åndetruer i norsk trolldomsmedisin," *Syn og segn*,

1925, 398. Other folk healers used the so-called "stone test" to discover the source of a child's disorder. Michael Krohn (1822–97), who found the practice still in use in Ytre Nordhordland, described it in his 1855 annual report: "They take a cauldron of cold water, one stone from the church yard, one from the countryside and one from the sea, heat the stones and put them in cold water, carefully observing which stone gives off the most steam, as this indicates the place from which the illness has come, whether the churchyard [the dead longing for the child to join them], the country-side [evil spirits], or the sea [ghosts of the unburied dead]." Krohn is quoted in Hogne Sandvik, "'Dei Vise forvidle være!' En distriktleges kamp mot overtro og trolldom på 1800-tallet," *Tidsskrift for den Norske Lægeforening* 29 (1993): 3572–73.

The belief in the necessity of destroying hair was long-lived, here collected by Judy Finanger, a student in my 1983 folklore class: "Never throw hair out without burning it," said Ella Knight (born 1906), a Norwegian farmwife from Decorah, Iowa, "because the hidden people that lived near you would then get it and would then have control over you. So my mother and grandmother used to either bury the hair in the ground or burn it."

Mary Cary, also originally of Decorah, provided this example: "Alden Grinna, our neighbor as I was growing up, made an opening in the bathroom wall to put razor blades in (for disposal), carrying on an old Norwegian custom. He said it had originated in Norway for fear that witches would use samples of men's whiskers to make evil potions and cast spells on the hapless individual" (Letter to the author from Mary Cary, La Crosse, Wisc., Feb. 16, 2000).

10. Ragnvald Sveine, "Mor fortalte meg. An outline of Garmo history as told by my mother Ingebjørg Henningsdtr Garmo Svein," Lillehammer, 1960, typed manu-script in the author's possession, 34.

11. "En signekjerring" appears in Asbjørnsen og Moe, *Norske folkeeventyr I* (Oslo: Den norske bokklubben, 1982), 268–80. English translations (below) are based on Marte Hult, *Framing a National Narrative: The Legend Collections of Peter Christen Asbjørnsen* (Detroit: Wayne State University Press, 2002), 122–28.

12. *Bevergjel*, a secretion of the beaver's sex glands, was in great demand during the 1800s. Glands removed as soon as the beaver was shot could be sold for good money to the apothecaries. Having an extremely unpleasant smell, bevergjel was believed to offer protection from serpent attack, and, as reflected in the story, many people also wore it as an amulet against the huldrefolk. Bevergjel was kept in tiny containers, such as a hollow metal button pierced by a sewing needle, as pictured in Skjedsø, *Øvre Gjerstad*, 83.

13. Krohn quoted in Sandvik, "Dei Vise forvidle være," 3572–73.

14. Asbjørnsen's newspaper article quoted in Hult, *National Narrative*, 90.

15. Very few changes were made in content in the three editions of Asbjørnsen's stories. "En Signekjerring" is an exception, says Hult, for it did not end with Gubjør

saying: "Oh, it's your husband who's coming . . . don't be afraid, I will go down past the church yard, then he won't see me." Instead, the original has the husband saying to Marit, "Let me tell you this, if she comes back again, I'm going to have her thrown in jail! And you, woman, will hear a tale of a different color!" (from the notes of folklorist Knut Liestøl, quoted and discussed in Hult, *National Narrative*, 127–29).

Fueling the husband's anger is also the realization that his wife has given pork to Gubjør, a dish they rarely permit themselves even on Sunday. Hult suggests that Asbjørnsen removed this ending from the 1859 and 1870 editions to make a more effective narrative since the husband's entrance is an anticlimax. But the original version more faithfully reflects Asbjørnsen's view that the old folk beliefs had dire consequences.

16. N. A. Quisling, *Studier over Rakitens Væsen og Aarsagsforholde* (Kristiania, 1886), and Edvard Schønberg, "Fra Børnepoliklinikken i det gamle Rikshospital, Rakitt," *Norsk Magasin for Lægevidenskaben* 1887: 740–45.

17. Edvard Schønberg, "Svek," *Norsk Magasin for Lægevidenskaben*, 1892: 1180–216. "*Svek* is not a foggy expression for all kinds of debility," argued Schønberg, "but a well-defined identification of the disease." Schønberg may have given more credit to the almue than they deserved, for through much of the century they used the term loosely to refer to several wasting diseases associated with the huldrefolk. Still, Schønberg observed that parents recognized the disease in their own children more readily than did doctors, who rejected their diagnosis of svekk as pure superstition.

18. Here and several paragraphs below, Inga Bjørnson, "Signekjerringer. Et besøk hos en av dem," *Social Demokraten*, Sept. 14, 1911. Bjørnson visited Mrs. Syvertsen, who lived next door to the house where Anne Brandfjeld had lived.

19. Though the name is now spelled "Frøysland," I have used the more common spelling of the name (though she and some contemporaries used "Frøsland"). Unless otherwise noted, the general information about her comes from David Seierstad and Ingeborg Sæther, "Mor Frøisland," *Gamle minner* (Lena: Totens Trykkeri, 1943), 3–21, referred to below as the "traditional account." Seierstad's experience (below) at 3; Sæther's quotes (below) at 7, 17, 9–10.

20. Erik Åsdokken's account from Gunnar Skrutvold, "Mor Frøisland eller 'Frøisland-kjerringe," *Tidskrift for Valdres Historielag* 8 (1959): 142.

21. Dr. Nils Aal Kolbjørnsen was appointed as doctor for the poor in Nordre and Søndre Land in 1861, writes Svein-Erik Ødegard in "Mor Frøisland—historien bak en legendarisk kvinneskikkelse," *Boka om Land X. Torpa. B* (Gjøvik: Nordre Land Kommune, 2002), 321–45.

On the basis of contemporary documents, Ødegard disputes the "traditional account" of Mor Frøisland recorded by Seierstad and Sæther. He points out that the treatment of Karen's knee was more complicated, the court trial less colorful, and the story (below) that Mor Frøisland treated Dr. Kolbørnsen's daughter unlikely. I have nevertheless chosen to base this account on the version that lived on in tradition, because it shows how much Mor Frøisland's doctoring meant to her contemporaries.

22. The letters are quoted in Ødegard, "Mor Frøisland—historien," 337, 338, 339. That Mor Frøisland solicited some of the many letters herself is seen when she wrote to her former patient Juls Skrutvold on Jan. 23, 1881: "I am accused of carrying out my 'kvaksalveri' for the sake of profit, which I deny. . . . I find it necessary to appeal to individuals familiar with my activity, to request declarations of support concerning patients I have treated." Mor Frøisland had cured Skrutvold of a stomach ailment, and he had subsequently recommended her services to others.

Repeating the instructions she had received, Mor Frøisland stipulated that the declaration "ought to give the nature of the ailment, its extent and duration, if the sick person was treated by a doctor and if so, by whom, and with what result, as well as what the doctor's treatment cost compared to that of my treatment." The declaration must furthermore be attested by "the signatures of two trustworthy men, preferably prominent individuals such as the president of an organization, or a mayor, deputy, dean of ministers, or school teacher" (Skrutvold, "Mor Frøisland," 134–35).

23. Ødegard, "Mor Frøisland—historien," 339. Bø discusses Mor Frøisland's trial in his Folkemedisin, 121–32, and there also describes the medications she used to treat Karen's knee.

24. Ødegard tells the story of Karen's operation and recovery in "Mor Frøisland—historien," 330–31; he discusses the trial's aftermath at 341–42 and the story of the Kolbjørnsens' daughter (below) at 339–40. Sæther's words above and below are at Seierstad and Sæther, "Mor Frøisland," 12–13.

25. Inge Torstensen, "Signekjerringer i storbyen," M.A. thesis for the Department of Folklore at the University of Oslo, Spring 1979, 88–96.

According to the website of the Peter Møller company (one of Norway's largest producers of cod-liver oil), tran had traditionally been made by placing a large container of cod livers in sunlight and allowing the oil to float to the surface as they rotted, producing an upper layer that had a "golden color and mild taste," while the rest was "less so." In 1854 the pharmacist Peter Møller introduced the new method of heating up the cod livers with steam, resulting in golden tran that "tasted fresh." While only about 50 percent of the liver fat was used for medicinal purposes (the rest being employed as lamp oil and fodder), now most cod-liver oil is medicinal (www.petermoller.no/. See also Lindemark, Medisiner, 17–18.)

26. Ruth A. Guy, "The History of Cod Liver Oil as a Remedy," American Journal of Diseases in Children (1923): 112–16; quote at 115. Guy's 1923 article could report

that "recently well controlled experiments both in the rat and in the human infant have demonstrated beyond criticism the efficacy of cod-liver oil in the cure and prevention of rickets, and attention may now be directed to the mechanism which brings about this effect" (116).

Before this discovery, Norwegian American doctors, too, used cod-liver oil as an all-purpose medicine. James Berdahl reports that when his fifth daughter (born in April 1887) was "affected with some serious lung trouble," the doctor "prescribed for her as the only possible remedy to use wine and cod-liver oil. After taking a large quantity of that prescription, she speedily recovered" (Berdahl, "Berdahl family," 42).

27. Greve, *Veileder*, 650. By contrast, a Norwegian American book of popular medicine published in Decorah in 1895 made no mention of cod-liver oil in its otherwise accurate description of the disease (Johnson, *Det sunde og syge*, 231). By 1915, however, Ritter in his *Home Medical Book*, terms cod-liver oil "in doses from ½ to 1 tsp, very advantageous" (440).

Lappegaard reports the district doctor's words in *Det var so laga*, adding that "a varied diet, tran, and a vitamin supplement to all newborns has made rickets unknown for several decades. But a few years ago it showed up again among the community's refugees who with their dark skin have even greater need for sunlight" (31). Since the 1970s refugees from Pakistan and other countries nearer the equator have been settling in Norway.

Nineteenth-century folk healers had the advantage of seeing many more cases of rickets, Dr. Schønberg noted in his 1892 article, since the almue hid this condition "especially from doctors and ministers" ("Svek," 1181).

28. Jessie Johnson (Mrs. C. Wallace Johnson, Alexandria, Minn.), "Reminiscing," typed manuscript, Minnesota Historical Society, 1970–71, part III (The Hanson family), 2–3 (F605.1.J66 A3).

29. Letter to the author from Claire Kristensen, May 9, 2000. Concerning the oil's foul taste, Dr. Guy writes in 1923 that when demand for cod-liver oil became so great around the mid-1800s, substitutes had to be devised and one of these was flavored with decayed herring to give the "characteristic offensive taste and smell" (Guy, "Cod-liver oil," 114).

Since infants were customarily kept indoors when there was frost in the air during the 1800s, babies born in the fall or winter (as are an overwhelming number of Norwegian children) risked never getting outside until spring. In the early 1900s, children's doctors began to counter this custom, urging mothers to let their children enjoy the health benefit of fresh air and sunlight during the winter.

30. An article about "English Disease" in the Sept. 28, 1923, *Decorah Posten* said that "with the right nutrition for both mother and child as well as sun and a little cod-liver oil, it is possible to cure this illness in relatively short time" ("Den engelske Syge," *Decorah-Posten*, Sept. 28, 1923).

31. Letter to the author from Dr. Sarah Oelberg (pastor at the Nora church, 1991–2003), Hanska, Aug. 20, 2003.

32. Marit lived across the street from H. F. Fredericson, the grandfather of Muriel Jeske, who gives this account: " I remember Marit as a small lady who wore dresses that hung down to the ground. She loved flowers and had beautiful flower beds in her yard. I recall people saying she didn't care much for children. I think there were some naughty children who played tricks on her, and the story was that she would chase them with a teakettle of boiling water. It was also said that parents would threaten to take their children to her if they misbehaved, so as a child I feared her.

"One incident I remember is a time when Marit was not feeling well. My grandmother made homemade soup and asked me to take a bowl to her. I was petrified, but in those days, you didn't refuse to do what your grandmother asked, so I went. The house was dark and gloomy inside, as I remember, and she was lying on a cot when I got there. I vividly remember I was scared to death, but as it turned out, she thanked me for bringing her the soup and I realized she was really a very nice, caring old lady" (*Hanska, a Century of Tradition, 1901–2001* [Hanska: Centennial Committee, 2001], 226–28).

33. The Hanska *Herald's* obituary on Aug. 10, 1934, noted that she "passed away Sunday morning [Aug. 5], at 1:30 o'clock, after a short illness, at the age of 89 years, 8 months and 18 days. Funeral services were held last Tuesday afternoon from the Zion church, and interment was made at the Zion Lutheran cemetery, Rev. V. F. Larson officiating."

34. Leif Salomonsen, "Barnet, dets pleie og sykdommer," *Vår helse* (Oslo, 1933), 151–55, and Leif Salomonsen, "Barnet," *Vår helse 2* (Oslo, 1949), 377–79. In 1928 a popular magazine reported: "The time of the klokekoner has past. Though a few are no doubt still to be found here and there, telling fortunes and bleeding patients by means of cupping or leeches, on the whole this class, that during the last century played quite a significant role in the capital city, is now history" ("Kloke koner," *A-Magasinet*, Sept. 13, 1928).

35. Raymond Dalen in "Tran—arktisk vitaminbombe," www.lifekjeden.no/.

Chapter 8. Alcohol as Medicine and Scourge

Epigraph: Erling Bækkestad, "Minne frå eit langt liv," from the local archives at Ål, is quoted in Lappegaard, *Det var so laga,* 77.

1. Eugene Boe, "Pioneers to Eternity," *The Immigrant Experience: The Anguish of Becoming American,* Thomas C. Wheeler, ed. (New York: Dial Press, 1971), 65.

2. Letters to the author from Shirley Olson Sorensen, Edina, Minn., Jan. 11, 1997, and June 7, 1997. Sorensen's grandfather was born in 1857 and married his wife (then nineteen) when he was forty and a widower with five children. She had

emigrated with her parents from Skjåk, Gudbrandsdal, in 1893. In Norway, too, "brennevin played an enormous role as a medicine" (Haugholt, "Mor Sæther," 272).

3. As early as 3000–2000 BC, beer-brewing flourished in Sumerian and Meso-potamian civilization (modern Iraq), with recipes for over twenty varieties of beer re-corded on clay tablets. Information about the history of alcohol is from the Loyola Marymount website: www.imu.edu/headsup/students/history.html.

4. Unless otherwise noted, the information on Norwegian alcohol consump-tion relies on Sverre Brun-Gulbrandsen, "Våre forfedres alkoholforbruk," Alkohol i Norge, Odvar Arner, Ragnar Hauge, and Ole-Jørgen Skog, eds. (Oslo: Universitets-forlaget, 1985), 26–32.

5. The letter is quoted in Stian Vasvik, "Aqua Vita—fra medisin til juledrikk," The Norseman, Nov. 1994: 36–37.

6. The use of beer in Norway dates from the Bronze Age, 500 BC, says Sverre Brun-Gulbrandsen, and it is first documented there by the Greek explorer Pytheas, who in the year 330 traveled to "Ultima Thule" and wrote about the inhabitants brewing beer from grain (26).

Beer was a "drink of the gods," derived from and consecrated to them. One drank to honor Odin, Thor, and the other gods and seek their protection, good crops, and peace. "Everyone should take part in this ritual drinking, at least occasionally, to avoid angering the gods" (27–28).

The earliest Christian law, Gulatingsloven, required landowners to brew beer twice a year to be "consecrated to thanking Christ and the Virgin Mary for a good harvest and peace." Thus, in both pre-Christian and early Christian times, beer had a central position in the relationship between humans and the divine. When the practice changed from honoring the gods to honoring Christ and the Virgin Mary, the tradition of using beer was on the whole preserved (28).

7. Armauer Hansen, Livserindringer og betragtninger (Kristiania: Aschehoug, 1910), 139. Beer that didn't make people drunk reflected badly on the brewer, as did re-fraining from getting drunk on festive occasions. "God help the person who remains unaffected by God's gift," wrote Pastor H. J. Wille in his 1786 Sillejords Beskrivelse, quoting a well-worn saying from Telemark (quoted in Brun-Gulbrandsen, "Alko-holforbruk," 31). Jon Tvinnereim quotes the ale bowl inscription in Grotid i grense-land. Fylkeshistorie for Møre og Romsdal II (Oslo: Det Norske Samlaget, 1992), 151.

8. The official is quoted in Oskar Kristiansen, Edruelighetsforhold i Norge 1814–48 (Oslo: Cammermeyer, 1943), 1.

9. Ellen Schrumpf, "Berus eder!" Norske drikkekulturer i de siste 200 år (Oslo: Unipax, 2003), 20–21.

10. "We recall the widespread joy all around the country that greeted the law of 1816 for free distillation," wrote Bishop J. S. Munch in 1827 (quoted in Schrumpf, Berus eder, 42).

11. The unidentified woman's words appear in "Hvad bestemor fortalte," *Opdalslagets Aarbok*, 1939–41: 44; Ragnar Hauge, "Alkohol i norsk historie," *Norsk Epidemiologi* 6, no. 1 (1996): 18.

12. In response to a particularly devastating string of crop failures, authorities banned the distillation of brennevin in 1756 so that scarce grain resources would go solely to producing bread and porridge instead of alcohol. This restriction remained in effect until 1816, the year that alcohol consumption began to become a problem ("Det historiske grunnlaget for norsk alkoholpolitikk," *SOS-NOU*, 1995: 24).

"Since people believed in the beneficial health effects of brennevin, this drink came to be seen as a daily necessity, not just a festive drink associated with daily rituals and formalities" (Brun-Gulbrandsen, "Alkoholforbruk," 33). Statistics quoted are from Schrumpf, *Berus eder*, 44–45.

13. Schrumpf, *Berus eder*, 42. Statistics quoted here are from "Det historiske grunnlaget," 24.

14. Eilert Sundt, *Om ædruelígheds-tilstanden i Norge*, H. O. Christophersen, et al., eds. (Oslo: Gyldendal, 1976), 51.

15. Åsen, *Nissedal*, 357–58; Christopher Hammer, *Chymisk, Oeconomisk Afhandling om Norske Akeviter, Bær-tinkturer og Bær-Safter* (Chemical, economic treatise on Norwegian aquavits, berry tinctures and berry juices), quoted from Rolf Øvrum, *Akevitt av egen avl. En bok om brennevinskrydring* (Oslo: Damm, 1999), 25–26.

Åsen also tells that the pastor at Nissedal Telemark reported in a letter to the *lensmann* (sheriff) Rasmus Bakke, "Terrible drinking during Sunday services and at weddings." Parishioners came to church drunk and after the services continued drinking "*på kyrkjebakken*" (on the church grounds, where Norwegians traditionally gathered after services to exchange news and greetings, as well as to hear public announcements). Rumor had it that the last time the minister preached at Treungen, parishioners were drinking during the service itself and some were even dancing in the aisles. "I have no choice but to report such behavior," the pastor concluded, urging the lensmann to punish the miscreants. Referring the matter to civil authority, the clergyman apparently objected to the drinking more as a disturbance of the peace than a moral breach, Åsen observes, and not until the temperance movements started taking hold a few years later did drinking become associated with immorality.

Caja Munch writes on Feb. 24, 1857: "Friday I brewed and got a very good beer, although it is a poor substitute for the Bavarian; Munch often wishes for a glass of that." On May 3, 1857, she writes: "We have drawn my wine into bottles; it is exquisite, but I hope to get it even better next year with a little less sugar." On Oct. 28, 1857: "My wine from wild grapes, I believe, will turn out quite good" (Munch, *Strange American Way*, 78, 88, 128).

16. Lars Abraham Bakke, the lensmann of Fyresdal, Telemark, recorded the

transformation of his own attitude toward alcohol in an 1845 diary entry describing an unsettling experience during a wedding at Fjone. "I stood for several minutes and watched the guests, with few exceptions, all inebriated. Men and women, young and old, I watched with rapt attention as they staggered about, wildly gesticulating. I listened to them prattle and roar and swear, and can honestly say their behavior disgraced and dishonored them as members of the human race. On this basis I ground my absolute condemnation of drinking brennevin (except as medicine)," he concluded (Åsen, *Nissedal*, 358).

17. Schrumpf, *Berus eder*, 22, 47, and 48; Brun-Gulbrandsen, "Alkoholforbruket," 32. Similarly, while a government report in 1835 stated that excessive consumption of brennevin should be opposed, it also emphasized that the working class, especially fishermen, needed brennevin. Thus, making it more expensive or unavailable was not the answer (Schrumpf, *Berus eder*, 47).

18. Åsen, *Nissedal*, 352, 358.

19. Aslak Bergland quoted in Carol Hanson Schwinkendorf, *Here Come the Norwegians* (Scottsdale, Ariz.: self-published, 1994), 16. Statistics about temperance are from Schrumpf, *Berus eder*, 48–50. Den norske Forening mod Brændevinsdrik (The Norwegian union against drinking distilled spirits) was established in 1845.

20. P. C. Asbjørnsen, *Fornuftigt Madstel: En tidsmæssig Koge-og Husholdningsbog* (Christiania, 1864), published under the pseudonym "Clemens Bonifacius."

21. Astrid Riddervold, *Drikkeskikker: Nordmennenes drikkevaner gjennom 1000 år* (Oslo: Teknologisk Forlag, 1997), 70.

22. Statistics are from "Det historiske grunnlaget," 24, and Schrumpf, *Berus eder*, 50–52. The Norwegian organization for total abstinence was founded in 1875 with the goal of an alcohol-free Norway. It had broad support and enormous growth, but few members from the upper class.

23. Rasmus Sunde, *Vikjer ved fjorden—Vikjer på prærien. Ein demografisk komparativ studie med utgangspunkt i Vik i Sogn*, 130–31, doctoral dissertation, University of Bergen, 2000.

Caja Munch observed about alcoholism in a letter dated Feb. 23, 1857: "All the liquor that is for sale around here has also caused Munch great vexation, for many are tempted by it . . . and there is unfortunately much drinking among the Norwegians in the congregation. . . . I could possibly say that except two men, they all drink!" (Munch, *Strange American Way*, 76).

24. All details of the Ole Skjækermo story here and below are from Schwinkendorf, *Norwegians*, 25–40.

25. Here and below, Aagot Raaen, *Grass of the Earth: The Story of a Norwegian Immigrant Family in Dakota* (St. Paul: Minnesota Historical Society, [1950] 1994), 40–53, 119–28.

26. Here and below, Aagot Raaen, "Thomas Raaen and Ragnhild Rødningen." The originals are at the Hatton-Eielson Museum, which devotes a room to Aagot's memorabilia—including the red shawl "Mor" pulled over her shoulders when she helped raid the saloon (below). Copies of the papers are also available at the Institute for Regional Studies at North Dakota State University in Fargo.

27. Barbara Handy-Marchello, "Introduction to the Reprint Edition," *Grass of the Earth* (St. Paul: Minnesota Historical Society, 1994), xiv.

28. "He was a man of fine intelligence, talented, well-educated and of unquestioned integrity. He read incessantly books of travel, science, religion, history, and geography and was never without his newspaper, and would go long distances to secure interesting reading materials. He was likewise a keen student of nature. When legal matters were to be transacted, contracts or petitions drawn, he was usually consulted" (quotations here and below from Raaen, "Papers," 8–9).

29. Aagot wrote, "Ragnhild was never able to participate in community affairs or belong to the Ladies Aid. How could she? . . . There was not a home so bare and poverty stricken in Steele County as the Raaen home. Ragnhild and the children during the early years were so poorly dressed that they were hardly covered. One garment (it does not merit the term "dress") was all that each had, and underwear was an unknown thing to them even in the coldest winter weather. As soon as the children were large enough they were sent out to work" (Raaen, "Papers," 10–11).

30. Raaen, *Grass of the Earth*, 121–23. The description of the saloon raid below uses Raaen's words. American temperance movements had begun forming as early as the 1830s, and unlike their counterparts in Norway, they had clerical leadership and used moral suasion from the start.

31. "We had doctors in Cooperstown, but with roads practically impassable at times . . . we were left with our own home medicine and improvised cures," writes Oskar R. Overby, "The Years in Retrospect" (typed manuscript, 1963, at Norwegian-American Historical Association, Northfield, Minn.), 14.

"The newspapers and magazines all carried numerous patent medicine ads to take advantage of the pioneer's isolation and desperation," writes Hiram Drache, noting that the Aug. 20, 1881, issue of the Warren (N. D.) *Sheaf* "carried on one page eleven ads—one for axle grease, another for horse powered threshing machines, another dealing with religion, and eight for patent medicines, all boasting to be the 'genuine wonder drug pain killer'" (*The Challenge of the Prairie: Life and Times of Red River Pioneers* [Fargo: North Dakota Institute for Regional Studies, 1970], 270).

"On the eve of the Civil War in 1859, the proprietary medicine industry had an output valued at 3,500,000," writes James Harvey Young. "By 1904 the sum had multiplied by more than 20 times." "Nostrum literature was piled on the counters of drugstore and country general stores. It was also delivered to the doorstep of the home, sent through mail, and also found in mail order catalogues" (*The Toadstool Millionaires: A Social History of Patent Medicines in America Before Federal Regulation* [Princeton, N.J.: Princeton University Press, 1961], 110, 105).

32. Oskar R. Overby, "Years in Retrospect," 14; Schwinkendorf, *Norwegians*, 177.

33. Details of the Fuglestads' story here and below are from Svanhild Aalgaard, *Though the Mountains Depart* (Minneapolis: self-published, 1977), 41–44.

Elisabeth Koren, too, relied on patent medicines, especially Ayers Cherry Pectoral, which contained alcohol (44 percent) and opium. She writes in a letter to her father on Jan. 28, 1855, from the parsonage into which they had finally settled: "One morning Pastor Clausen drove in. He was on his way home from Iowa City—came this far by stage and got off at Aarthuns in order to go on from there. But he had scarcely got inside before he became so violently ill that a doctor had to be sent for. He looked very sick, but could not be persuaded to stay. He was hurrying home because of his wife; all I could do was give him a little Ayers Cherry Pectoral which is good for a cold; Vilhelm usually takes a small bottle of it with him on his travels (Koren, *Diary*, 355).

The Wiley Act of 1906 required that labels indicate the presence and amount of certain dangerous drugs—alcohol, opiates, chloral hydrate, acetanilde, and others. Manufacturers were forbidden to put on packages any statement, design, or device that was false or misleading.

34. Obstruction can be caused by "external pressure closing the duct, for example, a pregnant uterus," writes Osler in *Principles*, 545–46. All details of Torkelson's story are from Melvin Olaf Torkelson, "Life on the Fraction: The past hundred years." This is an account of early settlers in Smiley Township, Pennington County, Minn. See Torkelson's colorful story at www.service.emory.edu/~marisa/FRAC-TION/fraction.text.html.

35. A copy of the label was kindly sent to me by Milton Sorenson (1917–2002), who remembered the remedy from living with his grandmother on a farm near Toronto, S.D. (letter to the author, June 1, 2000).

36. "Efforts should be made to eliminate the toxins before they produce their degenerative effects by free elimination," writes Osler in *Principles* (551), words that suggest how Kuriko's laxative could have provided effective relief for Torkelson's mother. Ingredients in Kuriko and other patent medicines were reported in Ritter's *People's Medical Book* (1915), but the alcohol content may have been considerably higher before the 1906 law.

37. Nancy Stout, "The Hans Bangen Family History," typed manuscript, Vesterheim Museum, n.p.; *Hostetter Bitters Almanac* quoted in Young, *Toadstool*, 131–32. Doctors also increasingly used alcohol to reduce fever beginning in the 1860s. Erwin Ackerknecht writes of "a new and enormous wave of the therapeutic use of alcohol" whereby "fevers were treated with great quantities of cognac" (Ackerknecht,

Therapeutics, 109). "Only toward the end of the century did this scientifically sanctioned form of alcoholism, often defended by intelligent and honest physicians, retreat" (110). Angostura Bitters ("an aromatic preparation of water, alcohol, gentian," and other vegetable extracts) still advertises its health-promoting effects as an appetite stimulant and flatulence cure.

For some, says Young, taking alcoholic bitters was subterfuge. In 1874 the Women's Christian Temperance Union began its work, and the decade of the 1880s witnessed terrific agitation, some statewide legislation, and the end of liquor sales in many American communities by local option. "For these deprived, one legal and almost respectable resource was open: the steady pursuit of health through high proof bitters" (Young, *Toadstool*, 133).

38. Helleland quoted in *Hordaland og Bergen i manns minne*, 158; and Holstad in *Møre og Romsdal i manns minne*, 109.

39. Margit Samulsen quoted in *Buskerud og Telemark i manns minne*, 116.

40. Frank J. Lipp, *Herbalism* (Boston: Little Brown, 1996), 50–51. Pastor H. J. Wille repeated the Telemark legend in his 1786 description of Seljord parish; it is quoted here from Reichborn-Kjennerud, *Lægeurter*, 67–68.

41. Information about Norwegian use of St. John's wort (*prikkperikum*) relies on Holck, *Norsk folkemedisin*, 172. For information about its general history and effects, see Varro E. Tyler, *The Honest Herbal: A Sensible Guide to the Use of Herbs and Related Remedies* (New York: Pharmaceutical Products Press, 1993), 275–76.

42. *Urtehagen ved Apotekmuseet* (Oslo: Cygnus, en norsk farmasihistorisk skriftserie, May 2001), 27.

43. Here and below, Karen Holtet is quoted in *Østfold og Vestfold i manns minne*, 165–66.

44. Harald Anderson is quoted in *Oslo og Akershus i manns minne* (Oslo: Det Norske Samlaget, 1970), 157. Details of the history of wormwood here and below from Borgen, *Urtehagen*, 55. Mangor describes its traditional use in *Lande-apothek*, 81. Writing in 1922, Reichborn-Kjennerud says that malurt is still cultivated in many places in Norway for medicinal use (*Lægeurter*, 95).

45. Grieve, *Modern Herbal*, 858–60.

46. Wille's use of wormwood is noted in Finn Erhard Johannessen, *Bitre piller og sterke dråper: Norsk apotek gjennom 400 år, 1595–1995* (Oslo: Norsk Farmasihistorisk Museum, 1995), 32. Caja's letter is in Munch, *Strange American Way*, 108.

47. Letters to the author from Ella Grunewald, Fergus Falls, Minn., Feb. 6, 2001, and Marion Oman, Waseca, Minn., Apr. 7, 1997.

48. Holtet, *Østfold og Vestfold i manns minne*, 165–66; letter to the author from Frances Anderson Haase, Staten Island, N.Y., Apr. 25, 2000.

Camphor, a colorless, crystalline, translucent mass with a characteristic mothball odor, is derived from the Asiatic camphor tree by passing steam through the chopped wood. It could be bought in prepared drops or cubes that were to be dissolved in spirits to make camphor drops (Tyler, *Pharmacognosy*, 126–28).

Nineteenth-century Norwegians used camphor drops for many things, and they were a very common home remedy, given in a spoon of water for a cold or dribbled on a cloth placed on the chest for bronchitis and cough. Camphor drops were also dissolved in olive oil for infections and serious illnesses to stimulate heart and circulation (Lappegaard, *Det var so laga*, 113; Mangor, *Lande-apothek*, 81).

49. The informant was among those interviewed in 1996 by Aud Ross Solberg and the author, as noted above.

50. Letter to the author from Olga Edseth, Mt. Horeb, Wisc., Aug. 12, 2000.

51. We "used nothing but oil and brandy and salt," wrote Caja Munch about Else's illness on May 3, 1857 (Munch, *Strange American Way*, 88–89); her extended quotation above about her husband's illness is at 65. Peter A. Munch's comment quoted below is at 257 n 7.

52. Malling published the translation in 1842. Regarding the brochure on salt og brennevin as a greater cause for concern than quack healers themselves, the district doctor of Vestre Nedenes, Henrik Skjeldrup, wrote in his 1842 annual report: "What good are all the laws against kvaksalveri when anyone can write and have printed for sale panaceas for any illness?" (quoted in Sundt, "Gamle medicinal-beretninger," 23).

53. Knut Teigen, *Ligt og uligt. Skisser, humoresker, eventyr og pennebilleder fra livet blandt vestens vikinger* (Minneapolis: Kreidt, 1907), 162–77.

Chapter 9. The Letting and Staunching of Blood

Epigraph: Vadder's letter was sent from Nissedal, Telemark, on July 4, 1862 (quoted in Åsen, *Nissedal*, 474).

1. "Bloodletting," wrote Marshall Hall in *On the Morbid-Curative Effects of Loss of Blood* (1830), "is not only the most powerful and important, but also the most generally used of all our remedies."

Archaeologists have found bloodletting tools dating to Stone Age cultures, write Fields and Kluger, two main sources for the ensuing discussion of bleeding (William S. Fields, "The History of Leeching and Hirudin," *Haemostasis* 21 [1991]: 3; Matthew J. Kluger, "The History of Bloodletting," *Natural History* 87 [Nov. 1978]: 80).

In the 1980s, Canadian doctor Norman Kasting showed that dehydration and hemorrhage stimulate the release of a hormone that does, in fact, lower fever. "Fevers often were dramatically reduced by copious loss of blood," says Kasting, who concludes that bloodletting was introduced as a way of imitating nature. Even a moderate spontaneous loss of blood causes a disproportionate fall in temperature in most fever cases, he says, but the fever-reducing function of bloodletting was replaced in 1899 by the far easier and less risky aspirin (Norman Kasting, "A Rationale for Centuries of Therapeutic Bloodletting: Antipyretic Therapy for Febrile Diseases," *Perspectives in Biology and Medicine* 33 [1990]: 510, 513).

2. Douglas Starr, *Blood: An Epic History of Medicine and Commerce* (New York: Harper Collins, 2002), 19. Starr (7–8) is also the source for the George Washington story below.

3. Facts about blood here and below rely on Audrey Davis and Toby Appel, *Bloodletting Instruments in the National Museum of History and Technology* (Washington, D.C.: Smithsonian Institution Press, 1979), 5–7.

4. Montgomery is quoted in Starr, *Blood*, 23.

5. Flint is quoted in Gilbert Seigworth, "Bloodletting over the Centuries," *New York State Journal of Medicine* 80 (Dec. 1980): 2024.

"During the first five decades of this century, the profession bled too much," wrote preeminent nineteenth-century physician Sir William Osler, "but during the last decades we have certainly bled too little." Feeling certain diseases still had no other or better treatment than bleeding, Osler included the therapy in the 1923 edition of his *Principles and Practice of Medicine* (102).

6. "Phlebotomy, an Ancient Procedure Turning Modern?" *Journal of the American Medical Association* 183 (1963): 279–80; and Charles Lent, "New Medical and Scientific Uses of the Leech," *Nature* 323 (Oct. 9, 1986): 494.

Another article declared in 1983 that regular phlebotomy reduces blood pressure in people suffering from resistant hypertension and suggested that regular blood donations prolong the donor's life by decreasing the risk of heart attack or by stimulating blood and immune functions (G. M. Casale et al., "Does Blood Donation Prolong Life Expectancy?" *Vox Sanguinus* 45 [1983]: 398–99).

7. Kluger, "Bloodletting," 80.

8. Orset's story in *Møre og Romsdal i manns minne*, 109; Rush quoted in Starr, *Blood*, 28.

9. Author interview with Midge Kjome, Decorah, Iowa, Nov. 15, 2003. Venesection employing a slightly larger sneppert was used to treat horses.

10. *Lægebog for hvermand*, 165–66. Norwegians found *årelating* (bloodletting) effective especially to relieve the pain of rheumatism. Nineteenth-century doctors blamed this then-prevalent condition on the punishing physical labor performed by fishermen, foresters, and farmers in relentless cold and damp. "They wade out into frigid, autumnal waters up to the armpits," observed the Telemark district doctor in 1835 (quoted in Åsen, *Nissedal*, 352). "They sit all night in open fishing boats in soaking wet clothes," echoed the Sunnmøre district doctor in 1855 (quoted in Tvinnereim, *Fylkeshistorie II*, 162–63). While the difficult work conditions no doubt sharpened the pain of rheumatism, they did not cause this autoimmune disease, whose actual cause remains unknown.

11. Halvorsen and Fletcher, "19th Century Midwife," 41.

12. J. C. Tode provided this update of Mangor, quoted in Birgitte Rørbye, *Kloge folk*, 219; Fields, "Leeching," 4.

13. Quoted from an exhibit at Sogndal Folkemuseum, Aug. 1999.

14. *Lægebog for hvermand*, 165–66.

15. The popularity of leeching reached its zenith in the first part of the nineteenth century in France with Francois Broussais (1772–1832), a surgeon in Napoleon's army, taking the lead. He attributed every disease to inflammation, i.e., an inordinate collection of blood in one part of the body, and recommended a starvation diet accompanied by heavy leeching (Fields, "Leeching," 4). The details about the prices of leeches derive from Davis and Appel, *Instruments*, 36.

16. Bjerkem quoted in *Trøndelag i manns minne*, 129; Linnerud quoted in *Oslo og Akershus i manns minne*, 38.

17. Holt quoted in *Agder i manns minne*, 214.

18. Søilen quoted in *Hordaland og Bergen i manns minne*, 152.

19. "Uses of Leeches in Plastic and Reconstructive Surgery: A review," *Journal of Reconstructive Microsurgery* 4 (Oct. 1988): 381–86.

20. John Colapinto, "Bloodsuckers. How the Leech Made a Comeback," *New Yorker*, July 25, 2005, p. 72–81 (quotation at 73).

21. Ingeborg Knutsen Fjelly quoted in *Oslo og Akershus i manns minne*, 156.

22. Karen Holtet quoted in *Østfold og Vestfold i manns minne*, 166.

23. Munch, *Strange American Way*, 36.

24. Sandvig's description and the black-book formula were recorded from Maihaugen's exhibit of Sandvig's office, Aug. 2001.

25. Evensen, "Svartebøkene," 97.

26. The finds are described in the 1986 (number 7) issue of Karin Knoph, "Generasjoners kirkegang," *Telemark historie*, 39–47. Herleik Baklid has plausibly argued that these sticks were used in a similar transference ritual to remove warts ("'Dei skar so mange skøre i ein kjeppe': Om pinner med innskårne hakk funnet under kirkegolv," *Heimen* 2004: 179–94).

27. Caption from Maihaugen's exhibit of Sandvig's dental office, Aug. 2001.

28. Hans Bye is quoted in *Oslo og Akershus i manns minne*, 158; and Bjerkem, *Trøndelag i manns minne*, 130.

29. Hans Mohr, "I nær kontakt med bygdens liv," *Prestegårdsliv. Minner fra norske prestegårder II* (Oslo: Gyldendal, 1967), 49.

30. Pastor Høgh's daughter quoted in Åsen, *Nissedal*, 477.

31. Fields, "Leeching," 4–5. Details of nineteenth-century immigrants' use of leeches are from Robert and Michèle Root-Bernstein, *Honey, Mud, Maggots, and Other Medical Marvels: The Science behind Folk Remedies and Old Wives' Tales* (New York: Houghton Mifflin, 1997), 90–91.

32. "Raad og Vink," *Kvinden og hjemmet*, 89. The advice column in another women's magazine (*Kvindens Magazin* [July 1908]) carried a letter from Mrs. A. O. Veien of Route 5, Starbuck, Minn., asking, "Can anyone tell me where I can buy a cupping machine for letting blood?"

33. Fields, "Leeching," 5–7; Colapinto, "Bloodsuckers," 79.

34. Knut Larsen quoted in *Agder i manns minne*, 214.

35. Tarjei Heimdal quoted in Åsen, *Nissedal*, 473.

36. Kasting, "Therapeutic Bloodletting," 513.

37. The history of Arkdale comes from *From Roche-A-Cree to Trinity: The History of Trinity Lutheran Church, Arkdale, Wisconsin, 1853–2003* (Friendship, Wisc.: New Past Press, 2003), 8–9; Olena's story is told in Palma Grahn, "Meet an Old Cupping Lady," in Stoughton's *Syttende Mai Souvenir Edition*, May 1961 (sent to the author by Forrest Brown).

38. Almost a third of the nearly 1,700 formulas in A. C. Bang's classic 1901 compilation of black-book formulas (*Norske Hexeformularer og Magiske Opskrifter*) concern stopping blood. The first formula quoted below is from Bang's collection (#1247d, p. 553), and the second is from Evensen, "Svartebøkene," 95. Despite being firmly anchored in biblical tradition, the second formula's reference to the devil, writes Evenson, has provided fodder to people bent on proving the evil nature of black-book formulas.

39. Berent Skjelbred, "Dei konne lækje sjukdomar då òg," *Årbog for Jæren og Dalene* 1954: 188–89.

40. Letter to the author from Margaret Kray (Elise's daughter), Clara City, Minn., May 19, 2000; Hanna Henriksen Tollaanes quoted in Weiser-Aall, *Svangerskap*, 123.

41. Ludvik Hope quoted in *Hordaland og Bergen i manns minne*, 149; Hvidbergskår, *Kvaksalvere*, 14.

42. Hilda Kongsberg quoted in *Østfold og Vestfold i manns minne*, 162; Tostein Skjelanger quoted in *Hordaland og Bergen i manns minne*, 150.

43. Olav Bø, "Rational Folk Medicine," *Arv: Scandinavian Yearbook of Folklore* 1962: 303. Bø also quotes an unidentified doctor of more recent vintage who calls cobwebs "one of the best hemostatic [blood stopping] means available."

44. Details of the blood-staunching properties of yarrow (*ryllik*), tinder bracket (*kjuke*), and heather (*lyng*) both here and below rely on Holck, *Norsk Folkemedisin*, 165, 168–69, and 174; Pastor Wille's quote (below) at 165.

45. Walter M. Lewis, *Medical Botany: Plants Affecting Man's Health* (New York: John Wiley and Sons, 1977), 340.

46. The following section on blood stopping in North Norway today comes from Linda Vaeng Sæbbe, "Han stenger blodet," *Lørdags Nordlys*, Jan. 8, 1997, p. 36–39.

47. On Sami folk medicine, see Adolf Steen, *Samenes folkemedisin* (Oslo: Universitetsforlaget, 1961). Stewart Holbrook devotes an entire chapter to the Kickapoo

Indian Company and its famous Indian medicine shows. Healy and Bigelow, who patented the labels for "Sagwa" and "Indian Oil" in July 1882, produced "Kickapoo Indian Cough Cure," "Indian Worm Killer," and "Kickapoo Indian Salve" (Stewart Holbrook, *The Golden Age of Quackery* [New York: Macmillan, 1959], 208–15).

48. Kristiansen sees blood-stopping as a more involving religious ritual. A change occurs in people undergoing the process that makes them more receptive to the forces of nature and aware of their place in relation to these forces. Based on the statements of those who have experienced it, Kristiansen concludes that blood-stopping is about mastering these powers (Sæbbe, "Han stenger blodet," 38).

49. Esther Sternberg, M.D., *The Balance Within: The Science Connecting Health and Emotions* (New York: W. H. Freeman, 2000), 7, 12. "Medical science is now at a crossroads of discovery that will finally allow us to piece together the mosaic of the biological basis and physiological effects of sleep, relaxation and even prayer." Sternberg continues, "By understanding these connections in modern times, in the language of molecular and nerve pathways, chemical impulses and hormonal responses, scientists can finally accept such effects as real."

50. Jerome Groopman, M.D., *The Anatomy of Hope: How People Prevail in the Face of Illness* (New York: Random House, 2003), 185 and 175. "The conclusion supported by several research groups," says Dr. Groopman, "is that belief and expectation, cardinal components of hope, can block pain by releasing the brain's endorphins and enkephalins, thereby mimicking the effect of morphine" (170).

51. Davidsen quoted in Groopman, *Hope*, 193.

52. "Recent research shows how catalytic those nerve-chemical changes can be in the course of certain maladies," concludes Kaptchuk, who is quoted in Groopman, *Hope*, 174. Groopman's quote below is at 179.

53. "All of us in the field are just scratching the surface and one day will look back and realize how little we really understood, but that's how science has always been," says Groopman. The so-called "placebo" effect (such as Mor Sæther using the doctor's regimen but achieving greater succeess), though once denigrated and dismissed by scientists, is now seen to have a significant biological effect and to "provide one of the clearest windows into the nexus between the mind and body" (166 and 169). "When confronting suffering and loss in my own life," adds Groopman, "I have found strength and solace in both the insight of tradition and the structure of ritual" (211).

Chapter 10. Remembered Remedies

Epigraph: David Cahoon, Middleton, Wisc., letter to the author, May 19, 2000. The Quisling family, with roots in Telemark, has included several physicians. Four brothers founded the Quisling Clinic in Madison, Wisc., in 1933; one of them is probably the doctor mentioned in the epigraph.

1. Letter to the author from Howard W. Amundsen, Minnetonka, Minn., May 23, 2003.

2. Called by some "the stinking healer," asafetida has a long history and was well established in European medicine by the Middle Ages, recommended by regular physicians as an antispasmodic, stimulant, and expectorant. Its characteristic odor is due to the presence of sulfur compounds, and is apparently the basis of its effectiveness, no other chemical components having been found to explain it (Crellin, *Herbal Medicine II*, 65–66).

Mangor mentions asafetida in his *Lande-apothek*. Calling it by another of its several names, *Dyvelsdræk* (devil's excrement), he says it was taken internally for worms and the discomfort associated with childbirth, and was also spread on the navel or delivered by enema for these same ailments (45). Its more modern usage resembles the way nineteenth-century Norwegians used the equally bad smelling *vendelrot* and *bevergjel* to ward off evil.

Note, too, the similarity between the traditional *føderåd* contract such as Mor Frøisland had with her parents and the way Howard's parents provided for his grandparents.

3. The use of kerosene (a petroleum distillate) probably relates to the medicinal use of turpentine (a pine distillate) that has a long history in Norway (and elsewhere) dating back to the 1600s. Kerosene was regarded as a panacea for colds, diphtheria, sore throat, tonsil troubles, and hoarseness, but it also caused many cases of poisoning in children (Crellin, *Herbal Medicine II*, 338).

4. Carol Gilbertson helpfully provided recipes for Everson's salves:

Grandpa's Black Salve

8 oz. Sweet Oil
4 oz. Red Lead
2 oz. Camphor

Heat the sweet oil, then add red lead. Let boil till it gets black. When partly cooled, add camphor. The camphor should be pulverized with alcohol.

Carol Gilbertson's Aunt Gwen writes: "I do have the salve and have used it. Had the pharmacist in Sturgis make some—had to get the red lead and it stunk up his store for days" (e-mail, June 22, 2006).

Grandpa's Liniment

1 qt. Raw Linseed oil
1 qt. Gum Turpentine

2 oz. Salt Peter

2 oz. Sugar of Lead

3 oz. Sulphuric Acid

Add acid a little at a time for 45 minutes.

(Carol Gilbertson, e-mail to the author, June 30, 2006.)

5. Johs. P. Sorkness (born 1889 in Grue, Hedmark) also tells of *papirolje* being made as Christianson describes and "producing a bad smelling distillate good for warts" (*Hedmark i manns minne*, 125).

6. Letter to the author from Clare Kristensen, Brooklyn, New York, Mar. 31, 2000.

Glossary

NOTE: The Norwegian alphabet has three additional letters following "z": æ, ø, and å.

almue	common folk
blysukker	sugar of lead, lead acetate
blyvann	lead water, lead-acetate solution
brennevin	hard liquor
bytting	changeling
cyprianus	black book
dråper	drops, medicine
fløtegrøt	sweet-cream porridge
gikt	rheumatism
grannelag	social unit of neighboring farms
grautomslag	poultice, literally "porridge wrap"
grep	arthritis, rheumatism
hjelpekone	self-trained birth helper
huldrefolk	hidden people
igler	leeches
jordfaststeiner	earth-fixed stones
jordmor, jordmødre	midwife, midwives
kariole	simple two-wheeled, horse-drawn conveyance
kloke kloner, kloke menn	self-trained healers; wise women and men
kondisjonerte	elite, cultured class
kopping	cupping
kvaksalver	quack, literally "one who cheats with salves"
kvaksalverlov	quack law
legebøker	doctor books
måling	measuring, magical cure
plaster	wound dressing
prest	minister
reive	swaddle

Rikshospital	National Hospital
rømmegrøt	sour-cream porridge
sengemat	bed food, brought to new mother
signekone, signekjerring	folk healer; witch
signeri	supernatural healing
smøyg	passing, magical cure
sortebog	black book
støyping	casting, magical cure
svartebok	black book
svekk	wasting disease, rickets
tran	cod-liver oil
trekkplaster	drawing ointment; attraction, drawing card
trolldom	magic, witchcraft
trollkone, trollkar	female, male magical healer
urter	herbs
valken	wasting disease, rickets
øl	beer
årelating	bloodletting

Bibliography

Aalgaard, Swanhild. *Though the Mountains Depart*. [Minneapolis]: privately printed, 1977.

Ackerknecht, Erwin. *A Short History of Medicine*. Baltimore: Johns Hopkins, [1955], 1982.

———. *Therapeutics: From the Primitives to the 20th Century*. New York: Macmillan, 1973.

Agder i manns minne. Daglegliv ved hundreårsskiftet. Frå Nasjonalforeningens landskonkurranse for eldre (Agder in recent memory. Daily life at the turn of the century. From the national competion for senior citizens). Oslo: Det Norske Samlaget, 1974.

Alm, Jens M., ed. *Bygd og by i Norge—Vest-Oppland og Valdres* (Rural and urban Norway—Vest-Oppland and Valdres). Oslo: Gyldendal, 1982.

Almklov, Severin. "En biografi og nogle erindringer" (A biography and some reminiscences). *Nord-Norge* 61 (1931): 8–11.

Alver, Bente. *Heksetro og trolldom. Et studie i norsk heksevesen* (Belief in witches and magic. A study in Norwegian witchcraft). Oslo: Universitetsforlaget, 1971.

Amundsen, Arne Bugge. "Kilde og kirke. En fromhetshistorisk undersøkelse av legekilden ved Trømberg kirke" (Spring and church. An historical examination of beliefs associated with the healing spring at Trømberg church). *Ung Teologi* 1 (1981): 20–40.

Anderson, Frank J. *An Illustrated History of the Herbals*. New York: Columbia, 1977.

Anker, Peter. *Stavkirkene. Deres egenart og historie* (The stavechurches. Their character and history). Oslo: Cappelen, 1997.

"Anne Brandfjeld." *Urd*, Jan. 14, 1905.

Arner, Oddvar, Ragnar Hauge, and Ole-Jørgen Skog, eds. *Alkohol i Norge* (Alcohol in Norway). Olso: Universitetsforlaget, 1985.

Asbjørnsen, P. Chr. [Clemens Bonifacius, pseudo.]. *Fornuftigt Madstel. En tidsmæssig koge-og husholdningsbog* (Common sense cooking: An up-to-date book of cooking and housekeeping). Christiania, 1864.

———. "En signekjerring." *Norske Folkeeventyr* (Norwegian folk tales), 1: 268–80. Oslo: Den Norske Bokklubben, 1982.

Åsen, Kjell. *Nissedal Bygdesoge. Kultursoga. Frå dei eldste tider til år 1900* (Nissedal local history. Cultural history from the earliest times until 1900). Nissedal: Nissedal Bygdesogenemd, 1986.

Bakken, Berit Øiseth. "Om Anne Brandfjeld: Signekonenes dronning" (About Anne Brandfjeld, queen of the folk healers), lecture, Jan. 21, 1999, transcription at: http://home.online.no/~blfblf/Annabrann.htm.

Baklid, Herleik. "'Dei skar so månge skøre i ein kjeppe': Om pinner med innskårne hakk funnet under kirkegolv" ('They made a number of cuts in a stick.' About sticks with carved incisions found under church floors). Heimen 41 (2004): 179–94.

Bang, Anton Christian. "Gjengangere fra Hedenskabet og Katholicismen blandt vort Folk efter Reformationen" (Ghosts of paganism and Catholicism persisting among our people after the Reformation). Theologisk Tidsskrift for den evangeliske lutherske Kirke i Norge, Ny række, 10 (1885): 161–218.

———. Norske Hexeformularer og Magiske Opskrifter (Norwegian witch formulas and magical incantations). Kristiania: Dybwad, 1901–02.

———. "Svartebogen" (The Black Book). Kirkehistoriske Smaastykker. Kristiania: Cammermeyer, 1890.

Behrends, Viola Johnson. "Lest we forget." Website: www.webfamilytree.com/mn_otter.htm.

———. "Wick (Yttervik)—a family history." [The Dalles, Oregon]: privately printed by Louise Hexum, 1992.

Berdahl, James O. "The Berdahl Family." Sioux Falls, S. D.: typed manuscript, [n.d.], St. Olaf College library, Northfield, Minn.

Bianchini, Francesco, and Francesco Corbetta. Health Plants of the World: Atlas of Medicinal Plants. New York: Newsweek Books, [1975], 1977.

Bjertnæs, Aage. Groblad, meitamark og krut. Kjerringråd og folkelig behandling i 1000 år (Home remedies and folk medicine for 1000 years). Oslo: Gyldendal, 1997.

Bjørndal, Martin. Segn og tru. Folkeminne frå Møre (Norsk Folkeminne Lag [Norwegian Folklore Society publication, hereinafter NFL] #64) (Legends and beliefs. Folklore from Møre). Oslo: Norsk Folkeminnelag, 1949.

Bjørnson, Inga. "Signekjerringer. Et besøk hos en av dem" (Folk healers. A visit with one of them). Social Demokraten, Sept. 14, 1911.

Blake, John B. "From Buchan to Fishbein: The Literature of Domestic Medicine." In Medicine without Doctors, eds. Guenter B. Riise, Ronald L. Numbers, and Judith Walzer Leavitt, 11–30. New York: Science History Publications, 1977.

Blix, Dagmar. Og draugen skreik. Tradisjon frå Lofoten (NFL #93) (And the ghost shrieked. Tradition from Lofoten). Oslo: Norsk Folkeminnelag, 1965.

Blom, Ida. "Den haarde Dyst." Fødsler og fødselshjelp gjennom 150 år ("The hard trial." Birth and midwifery through 150 years). Oslo: Cappelen, 1988.

Bø, Olav. Folkemedisin og lærd medisin. Norsk medisinsk kvardag på 1800-tallet (Folk medicine and learned medicine. Everyday medicine in nineteenth-century Norway). Oslo: Det Norske Samlaget, 1986.

———. *Heilag-Olav i norsk folketradisjon* (St. Olav in Norwegian folk tradition). Oslo, 1955.

———. "Rational Folk-Medicine." *Arv: Scandinavian Yearbook of Folklore*, 1962, 301–11.

Boe, Eugene. "Pioneers to Eternity." In *The Immigrant Experience: The Anguish of Becoming American*, ed. Thomas C. Wheeler, 51–83. New York: Dial Press, 1971.

Bøe, A. Sophie. "The Story of Father's Life." St. Paul: typed manuscript, [n.d.], Luther Seminary Archives, St. Paul.

Borgen, Anne Marte. *Urtehagen på Knattten* (The herb garden at Knatten). Oslo: Gyldendal, 1973.

Boril, Gladys Thompson. "Thomas Anderssen Perlesteinbakken Family History." Tower, Minn.: privately printed, 1999, copy in St. Olaf College library.

Brady, Erika, ed. *Healing Logics: Culture and Medicine in Modern Health Belief Systems*. Logan: Utah State University Press, 2001.

Bræde, Anna-Elisabeth. *Henrik Smith's Lægebog I–VI*. Copenhagen: Rosenkilde og Bagger, 1976.

Brandt, Mrs. R. O. "Some Social Aspects of Prairie Pioneering: The Reminiscences of a Pioneer Pastor's Wife." *Norwegian-American Historical Association Studies and Records* VII (1933): 1–46.

Brun-Gulbrandsen, Sverre. "Våre forfedres alkoholbruk" (Our forefather's use of alcohol). In *Alkohol i Norge*, eds. Odvar Arner, Ragnar Hauge, and Ole-Jørgen Skog. Oslo: Universitetsforlaget, 1985.

Bruun, Erik, and Budde Christensen. *Klassiske legeplanter* (Classical healing plants). Oslo: Aschehoug, 1998.

Buskerud og Telemark i manns minne. Dagleglaiv ved hundreårsskiftet (Buskerud and Telemark in recent memory. Daily life at the turn of the century). Oslo: Det Norske Samlaget, 1971.

Chirife, J., and L. Herszage. "Sugar for Infected Wounds." *Lancet* 8290, July 17, 1982, 157.

Christie, Elisabeth. *Prestegårdsliv. Minner fra norske prestegårder I and II* (Parsonage life. Reminiscences from Norwegian parsonages). Oslo: [Land og Kirke, 1966 and 1967], Gyldendal 1976 and 1977.

Christie, Inger Lise. *Dåpsdrakte*. Oslo: C. Huitfeldt, 1990.

Clausen, C. A. *A Chronicler of Immigrant Life: Svein Nilsson's Articles in Billed-Magazin, 1868–1870*. Northfield, Minn.: Norwegian-American Historical Association, 1982.

Colapinto, John. "Bloodsuckers: How the leech made a comeback." *New Yorker*, July 25, 2005, 72–81.

Cooperstown, North Dakota, 1882–1982. Cooperstown: Centennial Committee, 1982.

Crellin, John, and Jane Philpott. *Herbal Medicine Past and Present, Vol. I: Trying to Give Ease.* Durham: Duke University Press, 1990.

———. *Herbal Medicine Past and Present, Vol. II: A Reference Guide to Medicinal Plants.* Durham: Duke University Press, 1990.

Dalen, Raymond. "Tran—arktisk vitaminbombe." Website: www.lifekjeden.no/.

Davis, Audrey. "The Rise of the Vitamin-Medicinal as Illustrated by Vitamin D." *Pharmacy in History* 24 (1982): 59–72.

Davis, Audrey, and Toby Appel. *Bloodletting Instruments in the National Museum of History and Technology.* Washington, D.C.: Smithsonian Institution Press, 1979.

"Den engelske Syge." *Decorah (Iowa) Posten,* Sept. 28, 1923.

Den kloge kones bog (1886), reprinted with commentary by Birgitte Rørbye. Copenhagen: Jul Strandbergs Forlag, 1975.

"Det historiske grunnlaget for norsk alkoholpolitikk" (The historical basis for the Norwegian policy on alcohol). *SOS-NOU* [Sosial-og Helsedepartementet publication] 1995: 24.

Drache, Hiram M. *The Challenge of the Prairie: Life and Times of Red River Pioneers.* Fargo: North Dakota Institute for Regional Studies, 1970.

Draxten, Nina. *Kristofer Janson in America.* Boston: Twayne, 1976.

Edvardsen, Erik Henning. *Ibsen's Christiania.* Oslo: Damm, 2003.

Eriksen, Anne. "Lovekirker i Norge etter reformasjonen" (Devotional churches after the Reformation). M. A. thesis, Dept. of Folklore, University of Oslo, 1986.

Erikson, Rolf H. *Nævra-Erikson: A Sigdal Family.* Madison, Wisc.: privately printed by Michael Freidel, 1996.

Espeland, Velle. *Svartbok frå Gudbrandsdalen* (NFL #110) (Black Book from Gudbrandsdal). Oslo: Universitetsforlaget, 1974.

Evenson, Ottar. "The Black Books from Rustad in Norway." *The Black Books of Elverum,* ed. Mary S. Rustad, xxxiii–viii. Lakeville, Minn.: Galde Press, 1999.

———. "Svartebøkene fra Rustad" (The Black Books from Rustad). *Årbok for Elverum,* 1994, 90–134.

Faye, Andreas. *Norske Folke-Sagn* (NFL #63) (Norwegian folk legends). Oslo: Norsk Folkeminnelag, [1844], 1948.

Faye, F. C. *Lærebog i Fødselsvidenskaben for jordmødre* (Textbook in obstetrics for midwives). Christiania: Feilberg og Landmark, [1844], 1872.

Fernie, W. T. *Herbal Simples Approved for Modern Uses of Cure.* Bristol: John Wright, [1895], 1914.

Fields, William S. "The History of Leeching and Hirudin." *Haemostasis* 1991 (21): 3–10.

Fjellstad, Lars M. *Haugfolk og trollskap. Folkeminne frå Eidskog II* (NFL #74) (Hidden people and magic. Folklore from Eidskog II). Oslo: Norsk Folkeminnelag, 1954.

"Flickertail Pharmacist's Early Study of Skin Diseases Brings Profit to His Store." *Northwestern Druggist*, Sept. 1928, 22.

Fuglum, P. *Kampen mot alkoholen i Norge, 1816–1904* (The battle against alcohol in Norway, 1816–1904). Oslo: Universitets forlaget, 1972.

Garrison, Dr. Fielding H. "The History of Bloodletting." *New York Medical Journal* 97 (Mar. 1, 1931): 432–37, 498–501.

Gesme, Ann. *Look to the Rock: The Gesme Episode*. Cedar Rapids, Iowa: privately printed, 1985.

Givry, Grillot De. *Witchcraft, Magic and Alchemy*. London: Frederick Publications, 1971.

Gjerset, Knut, and Ludvig Hektoen. "Health Conditions and the Practice of Medicine among the Early Norwegian Settlers, 1825–1865." *Studies and Records* 1 (1926): 1–59.

Gotaas, Johannes. "Om spæde Børn og om Jordmødre" (About infants and midwives). *Folkevennen* 1859, 289–95.

Grahn, Palma. "Meet an Old Cupping Lady." *Syttende Mai Souvenir Edition*. Stoughton, Wisc.: 1961, in Norwegian-American Historical Association Archives, Northfield, Minn.

Grambo, Ronald. *Norske trylleformler* (Norwegian magic formulas). Oslo: Universitetsforlaget, 1979.

Greve, M. *Veileder i Sundhed og Sygdom. Lægebog for norske hjem* (Advisor in health and sickness. Doctor book for Norwegian homes). Kristiania: Cammermeyer, 1904.

Grieve, M. *A Modern Herbal in Two Volumes: The Medicinal, Culinary, Cosmetic and Economic Properties, Cultivation and Folklore of Herbs, Grasses, Fungi, Shrubs, and Trees with Their Modern Scientific Uses*. New York: Dover, [1931], 1971.

Groopman, Dr. Jerome. *The Anatomy of Hope: How People Prevail in the Face of Disease*. New York: Random House, 2003.

Gulliksen, Øyvind T., and Carla Waal. "Peder Kristoffersen Waal. En utvandrer fra Notodden"(An emigrant from Notodden). *Notodden Historielage Årskrift* 1986: 66–77.

Gunn, J. C. *New Domestic Physician or Book of Home Health: A Guide for Families*. Cincinnati: Moore, Wilstace, Keys & Co., 1861.

Gunther, Robert T. *The Greek Herbal of Dioscorides*. New York: Hafner Publishing, 1959.

Guy, Ruth A. "The History of Cod Liver Oil as a Remedy." *American Journal of Diseases in Children* 1923: 112–16.

Hale, Frederick. *Their Own Saga: Letters from the Norwegian Global Migration*. Minneapolis: University of Minnesota Press, 1986.

Halvorsen, Haldor, ed. *Festskrift til Den norske Synodes Jubilæum, 1853–1903*

(Festshrift for the anniversary of the Norwegian Synod). Decorah, Iowa: Den norske Synodes Forlag, 1903.

Halvorsen, Helen Olson, and Lorraine Fletcher. "19th Century Midwife: Some Recollections." *Oregon Historical Quarterly* 70 (March 1969): 39–49.

Hand, D. W. *The Report of Diseases of Minnesota and the Northwest.* St. Paul: Daly and Hofer, 1876.

Hand, Wayland D. "Measuring and Plugging: The Magical Containment and Transfer of Disease." *Bulletin of the History of Medicine* 48 (1974): 221–33. Baltimore: Johns Hopkins University Press.

Handy-Marchello, Barbara. "Introduction to the Reprint Edition." In Aagot Raaen, *Grass of the Earth: The Story of a Norwegian Immigrant Family in Dakota.* St. Paul: Minnesota Historical Society, 1994.

Hansen, Armauer. *Livserindringer og betragtninger* (Life reminiscences and observations). Kristiania: Aschehoug, 1910.

Hanska: A Century of Tradition, 1901–2001. Hanska, Minn.: Centennial Committee, 2001.

Hanson, Paul. "Heritage Bits: Home Remedies." *Albert Lea (Minnesota) Tribune,* Sept. 12, 1996, 10.

Hanson, Ronald, K. *From Roche-A-Cree to Trinity: The History of Trinity Lutheran Church, Arkdale, Wisconsin, 1853–2003.* Friendship, Wisc.: New Past Press, 2002.

Harpestreng, Henrik. *Gamle danske urtebøger, stenbøger og kogebøger* (Old Danish herbals, stonebooks, and cookbooks). Marius Kristensen, ed. Copenhagen, 1908.

Hauberg, Poul. *Christiern Pedersens Lægebog, Malmø 1533.* Facsimile with introduction. Copenhagen: Levin and Munksgaard, 1933.

Hauge, Ragnar. "Alkohol i norsk historie." *Norsk Epidemiologi* 6 (1996): 13–21.

Haugholt, Karl. "Mor Sæther." *St. Halvard,* 1958, 270–87.

Hedmark i manns minne. Dagleglivet ved hundreårsskiftet (Hedmark in recent memory. Daily life at the turn of the century). Oslo: Det Norske Samlaget, 1972.

Herbert, George. *The Country Parson and the Temple,* ed. John W. Wall. New York: Paulist Press, 1981.

Hermundstad, Knut. *Ættararv. Gamal Valdres-kultur* (NFL #65) (Family inheritance. Old Valdres culture). Oslo: Norsk Folkeminnelag, 1950.

———. *Kvorne Tider. Gamal Valdres Kultur VII* (NFL #86) (Times that are gone. Old Valdres culture). Oslo: Universitets Forlaget, 1961.

Hexevæsen og Troldskab i Norge. Meddelt til Læsning for Menigmand (Witchcraft and magic in Norway. Told for the reading of the common man). Christiania: Bentzens, 1865.

Hodne, Bjarne. *Å leve med døden. Folkelige forestillinger om døden* (Living with death. Popular conceptions about death). Oslo: Aschehoug, 1980.

Hodne, Ørnulf. *Mystiske steder i Norge* (Mystical places in Norway). Oslo: Cappelen, 2000.

———. *Norsk Folketro* (Norwegian folk belief). Oslo: Cappelen, 1999.

———. "Spebarnet i norsk folkekultur" (The newborn in Norwegian folk culture). In *Barn av sin tid. Fra norske barns historie*, eds. Bjarne Hodne and Sølvi Sogner, 21–35. Oslo: Universitetsforlaget, 1984.

Høiland, Klaus. *Naturens legende planter. Alt om helseplantenes praktiske bruk og legende virkning* (Nature's healing plants. All about the practical use and healing effect of medicinal plants). Oslo: Hjemmets bokforlag, 1978.

Holand, Hjalmar Rued. *Coon Prairie: An Historical Account of the Norwegian Evangelical Lutheran Congregation in Coon Prairie Written on the Occasion of Its 75th Anniversary in 1927*, trans. Oivind M. Hovde. Decorah, Iowa: [n.p.], 1977.

———. *My First Eighty Years*. New York: Twayne, 1957.

———. *Norwegians in America—The Last Migration: Bits of Saga from Pioneer Life*. Trans. Helmer M. Blegen, ed. Evelyn Ostraat Wierenga. Sioux Falls, S.D.: Center for Western Studies, Augustana College, 1978.

Holbrook, Stewart. *The Golden Age of Quackery*. New York: Macmillan, 1959.

Holck, Per. "Henrik Wergelands sykdom og død. Et 150-årsminne" (Henrik Wergeland's illness and death). *Tidsskrift for den Norske Lægeforening* 115 (1995): 3734–37.

———. *Livets høytider. Skikker og overto fra vugge til grav* (Life's ceremonies. Customs and superstitions from cradle to grave). Oslo: Cappelen, 1995.

———. *Norsk folkemedisin. Kloke koner, urtekurer og magi* (Norwegian folk medicine. Folkhealers, herbal cures, and magic). Oslo: Cappelen, 1996.

———. "The Very Beginning: Folk Medicine, Doctors and Medical Services." *The Shaping of a Profession: Physicians in Norway Past and Present*, eds. Øyvind Larsen and Bent Olav Olsen. Canton, Mass.: Science History Publications USA, 1996.

Hordaland og Bergen i manns minne. Dagleglivet ved hundreårsskiftet. Oslo: Det Norske Samlaget, 1974.

Hult, Marte Hvam. *Framing a National Narrative: The Legend Collections of Peter Christen Asbjørnsen*. Detroit: Wayne State University Press, 2002.

"Huslægen." *Husvennen. Fædrelandet og Emigrantens Præmie for 1883* (The household doctor. The home companion. Subscription premium for 1883). La Crosse, Wisc.: Fædrelandet og Emigrantens Trykkeri, [1882].

"Hvad Bestemor fortalte" (What grandmother told). *Opdalslagets Aarbok*, 1939–1941, 41–44.

Hvidbergskår, A. S. *Kvaksalvere og folkemedisin på Agder* (Quacks and folkmedicine in Agder). Oslo: Universitetsforlaget, 1968.

"Indskrifter paa gamle ølboller" (Inscriptions on old ale bowls). *Samband*, Mar. 1916, 312–14.

Johannessen, Finn Erhard. *Bitre piller og sterke dråper: Norske apotek gjennom 400 år, 1595–1995* (Bitter pills and strong medicine. Norwegian apothecaries through 400 years, 1595–1995). [Oslo]: Norsk Farmasihistorisk Museum [1995?].

Johnson, Jessie Hanson (Mrs. C. Wallace Johnson, Alexandria, Minn.). "Reminiscing," pt. III (Hanson family), 2–3. Typed manuscript, 1970–71, in the Minnesota Historical Society, St. Paul.

Johnson, Matthias. *Det sunde og syge mennekse. En kortfattet, folkefattelig fremstilling af det menneskelige legemes bygning og dets organers forretninger, samt dets sygdomme og deres behandling: med et tillæg om luft, lys, og vand som betingelser for liv og sundhed* (The healthy and sick person. A short, popularized presentation of the human body's construction and the function of its organs, as well as its diseases and their treatments: with a supplement about air, light and water as conditions for life and health). Decorah, Iowa: privately printed, 1892.

Johnson, Nels J. "How 'Doktor Gamla' Cured Ills of the Early Pioneers in the Tumili Township." *Fergus Falls (Minnesota) Daily Journal*, July 15, 1936.

Johnson, O. S. *Nybyggerhistorie fra Spring Grove og Omegn, Minnesota* (Settlement history from Spring Grove and surroundings). Minneapolis: privately printed, 1920.

Kaas, Gunnar, and Arnfinn Engen. *Bygdebok for Dovre (2). Gardar, hus, folk* (Dovre local history (2). Farms, houses, people). Dovre Kommune, 2003–04.

Kasting, Norman. "A Rationale for Centuries of Therapeutic Bloodletting: Antipyretic Therapy for Febrile Diseases." *Perspectives in Biology and Medicine* 33 (1990): 509–16.

King, Mary. "Memories of a Prairie Girlhood." Typed manuscript, 1928, in the Minnesota Historical Society. St. Paul.

Kjærheim, Kristina. *Mellom kloke koner og kvitkledde menn. Jordmorvæsenet på 1800-talet* (Between folk healers and men in white coats. Midwifery in the 1800s). Oslo: Det Norske Samlaget, 1987.

"Kloke koner." *A-Magasinet* (Oslo), Sept. 13, 1928.

Kluger, Matthew J. "The History of Bloodletting." *Natural History* 87 (Nov. 1978): 78–83.

Knoph, Karin. "Generasjoners kirkegang" (Generations of church-going). In *Telemark historie: Tidsskrift for Telemark Historielag* 1986 (7), 39–47.

Kolsrud, Marie Røberg. "Mor Frøisland." *Nylænde*, Kristiania, Oct. 15, 1899.

Kollstad, Per. "Ei svartbok fra Dovre" (A black book from Dovre). *Årbok for Gudbrandsdalen*, 1959.

Koren, Elisabeth. *The Diary of Elisabeth Koren, 1853–1855*. Trans. and ed. David T. Nelson. Northfield, Minn.: Norwegian-American Historial Association, 1955.

Kristiansen, Oskar. *Edruelighetsforhold i Norge, 1814–1848* (Sobriety in Norway, 1814–1855). Oslo: Cammermeyer, 1934.

Krohn, Michael. "Medicinal-Indbretning for året 1856 and 1862 (Annual medical report for 1856 and 1862). Oslo Riksarkivet. University of Bergen's Dept. of Social Medicine (Institutt for samfunnsmedisinske fag): www.uib.no/isf/hist/krohn.htm.

———. "Om behandlingen af svangre, fødende og barselqvinder" (On the treatment of pregnant women and women in childbirth). Lecture, Apr. 29, 1861: www.uib.no/isf/hist/krohn.htm.

———. "Om børnepleien" (On child care). Lecture, Mar. 8, 1861: www.uib.no/isf/hist/krohn.htm.

———. "Om folkets standpunkt" (On the people's point of view). Lecture, Mar. 22, 1858: www.uib.no/isf/hist/krohn.htm.

Lægebog for hvermand. "Nordens" Præmiebog for 1879. (Doctor book for everyone. Norden's subscription premium for 1879). Chicago: J. T. Relling & Co., 1879.

Langset, Edvard. Segner-gåter. Folketru frå Nordmør (NFL #61) (Legends, riddles, folk belief from Nordmøre). Oslo: Norsk Folkeminnelag, 1948.

Lappegard, Øystein. Det var so laga. Om helse og utvikling i Øvre Hallingdal fyrst på 1900-tallet (It was just meant to be. About health and development in upper Hallingdal in the early 20th century). Ål: privately printed, 1997.

Larson, Laurence M. The Log Book of a Young Immigrant. Northfield, Minn.: Norwegian-American Historical Association, 1939.

Lassen, H. Breve fra Henrik Wergeland (Letters from Henrik Wergeland). Christiania: Malling, 1867.

———. Henrik Wergeland og hans samtid (Henrik Wergeland and his times). Christiania: Malling, 1866.

Lassen, Wilhelm, and Chr. Brinchmann. "Lidt om Wergelands sidste Levemaaneder" (A little about the last months of Wergeland's life). Edda [Kristiania] 1918: 98–110.

Le Strange, R. A. History of Herbal Plants. New York: Arco, 1977.

Lent, Charles. "New Medical and Scientific Uses of the Leech." Nature 323 (1986): 494.

Lewis, Walter H. Medical Botany: Plants Affecting Man's Health. New York: John Wiley and Sons, 1977.

Lind J. "Vore gamle urtebøger" (Our old herbals). Farmaceutisk tidende, blad for Dansk farmaceutforening, 1916, 394–99.

Lindemark, Otto. Medisiner før og nå (Medicines then and now). Trans. Johannes Setekleiv. Oslo: Cappelen, 1966.

Lipp, Frank J. Herbalism. Boston: Little, Brown and Company, 1996.

Løkensgaard, Ole. "Nybyggerhistorier I–V." Hallingen, Apr. 1918: 139–50; June 1918: 215–23; Jan. 1919: 319–26; Oct. 1919: 507–17; April 1920: 625–30.

———. "På Lake Prairie i sekstiaarene." Hallingen, Mar. 1921: 883–93.

Lovoll, Odd. *The Promise of America: A History of the Norwegian-American People*. Minneapolis: University of Minnesota Press, 1984.

———. *The Promise Fulfilled: A Portrait of Norwegian Americans Today*. Minneapolis: University of Minnesota Press, 1998.

Magelssen, Kirsti. "Der mitt hjarta er fest." (Where my heart is at home). In *Prestegårdsliv II. Minner fra norske prestegårder*, 7–30. Oslo: Gyldendal, 1977.

Mamen, H. Chr. "Prestens bibliotek" (The pastor's library). In *Prestegårdsliv II. Minner fra norske prestegårder*, 158–75. Oslo: Gyldendal, 1977.

Mangor, Christian Elovius. *Lande-apothek, til landmænds nytte* (The country pharmacy for rural use). Copenhagen: J. H. Schubothe, [1767], 1835.

Matheson, Del. *Reunion East of the Sun*. Eugene, Ore.: privately printed, 1978.

Mathieu, Nina. *Our Prairie Home.*" New Hope, Minn.: privately printed, 1989, in Norwegian-American Historical Association Archives. Northfield, Minn.

McIntryre, Ann. *Folk Remedies for Common Ailments*. Toronto: Key Porter Books, 1994.

Melbostad, Bertemarie. "Norwegian Kopper—Aan Boe." *Spring Grove Herald*, Jan. 18, 1997.

Melbye, Borghild Solwold (Mrs. Henry). *Borghild: A History of Pioneer Days in Eastern Clay County*. Hawley, Minn.: Hawley Herald, 1977.

Merck's 1899 Manual of the Materia Medica: A Ready Reference Pocket Book for the Practicing Physican. New York: Merck & Co., 1899.

Meyer, Johan. *Fortids kunst i Norges bygder. Dovre* (Historical art in Norway's rural communities. Dovre). Oslo: Nasjonalforlaget, 1978.

Mockler-Ferryman, A. F. *In the Northman's Land: Travel, Sport and Folklore in the Hardanger Fjord and Fjeld*. London: Sampson Low, Marston & Company, 1896.

Mohn, A. M. "Et Kapitel af de norske indvandrernes historie" (A chapter of the Norwegian immigrants' history). *Samband*, Apr. 1914: 226–331; May 1914: 379–82; June 1914: 426–30; July 1914: 487–92.

Mohn, Fredrik. *Før doktoren kommer. Letvint lægehjelp og sundhedspleie* (Until the doctor comes. Simple medical assistance and health care). Decorah, Iowa: Decorah Postens Damptrykkeri, 1891.

Mohr, Hans. "I nær kontakt med bygdens liv" (In close contact with rural community life). In *Prestegårdsliv. Minner fra norske prestegårder II*. Oslo: Gyldendal, 1977.

"Mor Sæther." *Nylænde*, Mar. 1, 1908, 69–72.

Mørch, Andreas. *Frå gamle dagar. Folkeminne frå Sigdal og Eggedal* (NFL #27) (From the old days. Folklore from Sigdal and Eggedal). Oslo: Norsk Folkeminnelag, 1932.

Møre og Romsdal i manns minne. Dagleglivet ved hundreårsskiftet (Møre and Romsdal in recent memory. Daily life at the turn of the century). Olso: Det Norske Samlaget, 1969.

Mostue, Alf. *Slik var hverdagen. Arbeidsfolk forteller fra husmannskår, anleggstid og kriseår* (Such was everyday life. Workers tell about cotters, builders of roads, and railways, and times of crisis). Notodden: Historielaget, n.d.

Munch, Caja. *The Strange American Way: The Letters of Caja Munch from Wiota, Wisconsin, 1855–1859*. Carbondale: Southern Illinois University Press, 1970.

Murphy, Lamar Riley. *Enter the Physician: The Transformation of Domestic Medicine, 1760–1860*. Tuscaloosa: University of Alabama Press, 1991.

Næss, Hans Eyvind. *Med bål og brann. Trolldomsprosessene i Norge* (Burning at the stake. Witchtrials in Norway). Oslo: Universitetsforlaget, 1984.

———. *Trolldomsprosessene i Norge på 1500–1600-tallet* (Witchtrials in Norway during the sixteenth and seventeenth centuries). Oslo: Universitetsforlaget, 1982.

Nelson, Peder H. "Et nybyggerhjem" (A pioneer home). *Årbok for Hadeland* 1982, 30–34.

Nergaard, Sigurd. *Hulder og trollskap. Folkeminne fraa Østerdalen IV* (NFL #11) (Hidden folks and magic. Folklore from Østerdal IV). Oslo: Norsk Folkeminnelag, 1927.

———. *Skikk og bruk. Folkeminne fra Østerdalen, V* (NFL #16) (Customs of daily life. Folklore from Østerdal V). Oslo: Norsk Folkeminnelag, 1927.

Nichol, Todd W., ed. *Crossings: Norwegian-American Lutheranism as a Transatlantic Tradition*. Northfield, Minn.: Norwegian-American Historical Association, 2003.

Nielson, Haakon B. *Byoriginaler* (Characters about town). Oslo: Cappelen, 1966.

Nordhagen, Rolf. "De gamle klosterhager" (The old cloister gardens). *Aarsberetning for Foreningen til Norske Fortids Minnesmerkers Bevaring*. 1939. Oslo: Grøndal Boktrykkeri, 1941.

Nordland, Odd. "The Street of 'the Wise Women.'" *Arv* 18–19 (1962–63): 105–16.

Nord-Norge i manns minne. Dagleglivet ved hundreårsskiftet (North Norway in recent memory. Daily life at the turn of the century). Oslo: Det Norske Samlaget, 1973.

Nuland, Sherwin B. *The Doctor's Plague: Germs, Childbed Fever, and the Strange Story of Ignác Semmelweis*. New York: Norton, 2003.

Numbers, Ronald L., and Judith Walzer Leavitt, eds. *Wisconsin Medicine: Historical Perspectives*. Madison: University of Wisconsin Press, 1981.

Nyerup, Rasmus. *Almindelig Morskabslæsning i Danmark og Norge igjennem Aarhundreder* (Reading for the masses in Denmark and Norway through the centuries). København: Andreas Seidelins Forlag, 1816.

Nygaard, Truls. *Norsk Brennevins Leksikon samt brennevinsbrenningens historie i Norge* (Norwegian liquor lexicon and the history of distilling in Norway). Oslo: Cappelen, 1945.

Odegard, J. T. *Erindringer I. Lom, Long Lake, Fargo, Minneapolis* (Reminiscences I). Oslo: privately printed, 1930.

Ødegard, O. K. *Valdrespresta* (The Valdres minister). Kristiania: Det Mallingske Bogtrykkeri, 1917.

Ødegard, Svein-Erik. "Mor Frøisland—historien bak en legendarisk kvinneskikkelse" (Mor Frøisland—the history behind a legendary woman). *Boka om Land,* vol. 10, *Torpa,* B: 321–45. Gjøvik: Nordre Land Kommune, 2002.

Olafsen, O. "Folkemedisin efter en gammel lægebok for folket" (Folkmedicine from an old Doctor Book for the people). *Hardanger* 1924: 30–36.

———. "Provst Niels Hertzberg som Læge" (Dean Niels Hertzberg as a doctor). *Hardanger* 1918: 19–20.

Osland, Birgir. *A Long Pull from Stavanger: The Reminiscences of a Norwegian Immigrant.* Northfield, Minn.: Norwegian-American Historical Association, 1945.

Osler, William, and Thomas McCrae. *The Principles and Practice of Medicine. Designed for the Use of Practitioners and Students of Medicine.* New York: Appleton, 1921.

Oslo og Akershus i manns minne. Dagleglivet ved hundreårsskiftet (Oslo and Akershus in recent memory. Daily life at the turn of the century). Oslo: Det Norske Samlaget, 1970.

Østfold og Vestfold i manns minne. Dagleglivet ved hundreårsskiftet (Østfold and Vestfold in recent memory. Daily life at the turn of the century). Oslo: Det Norske Samlaget, 1975.

Overby, Oscar R. "The Years in Retrospect." Northfield, Minn.: typed manuscript, 1963, in Norwegian-American Historical Association Archives.

Øverland, Orm, and Steinar Kjærheim, eds. *Fra Amerika til Norge: Norske utvandrerbrev,* Vol. 1 (From America to Norway. Norwegian emigrant letters). Oslo: Solum, 1992.

Øvrum, Rolf. *Akevitt av egen avl. En bok om brennevinskrydring (a.k.a. Fra urter til akevitt)* (Akevitt from one's own harvest. A book about flavoring liqueurs). Oslo: Damm, 1999.

People's Home Library: A Library of Three Practical Books. Cleveland, Ohio: R. C. Barnum, 1915.

"Phlebotomy: An Ancient Procedure Turning Modern?" *Journal of the American Medical Association* 183 (1963): 279–80.

Pio, Iørn, ed. *Cyprianus.* København: Immanual Ree's Forlag, 1870.

Porter, Roy. *The Greatest Benefit to Mankind: The Medical History of Humanity.* New York: Norton, 1997.

Quisling, N. A. *Overtroiske kurer og folkemedisin i Norge* (Superstious cures and folk-medicine in Norway). (1918). Oslo: Grenland, 1999.

———. *Studier over Rakitens Væsen og Aarsagsforholde* (Studies of the nature and cause of rickets). Kristiania, 1886.

Raaen, Aagot. *Grass of the Earth: The Story of a Norwegian Immigrant Family in Dakota.* St. Paul: Minnesota Historical Society, (1950) 1994.

———. "Thomas Raaen and Ragnhild Rødningen." Aagot Raaen Papers, 1798–1957. Institute for Regional Studies. North Dakota State University, Fargo, N. D.

Raeder, Ole Munch. *America in the Forties: The Letters of Ole Munch Ræder.* Ed. and trans., Gunner J. Malmin. Minneapolis: Published for the Norwegian-American Historical Association by the University of Minnesota Press, [1924?].

"Ragna, Amerikabreve fra en tjenestepike." National Library, Oslo, website: http://nabo.nb.no/trip?_b=EMITEKST&urn.

Raspail, F. *Huuslægen: Anviisning til selv at tilberede og anvende de vigtigste Lægemidler der tjene til at haelbrede og beskytte mod de hyppigst forekommende Sygdomme* (The house doctor: Directions for preparing and using the most important medications that serve to heal and prevent the most commonly occuring ailments). Copenhagen: Fr. Wøldike, 1863 (4th edition).

Reichborn-Kjennerud, Injald. "Åndetruer i norsk trolldomsmedisin" (Belief in spirits in Norwegian magical medicine). *Syn og segn,* 1925, 398.

———. *Elskov og overtro fra vår gamle troldoms-medisin* (Love and superstition from our traditional magical medicine). Oslo: Universitetsforlaget, [1985?].

———. "En oversigt over og karakteristik av de gamle nordiske lægebøker" (An overview and characterization of the old Scandinavian doctor books). *Tidsskrift for den Norske Lægeforening. Tidsskrift for praktisk medisin, ny række* 44 (1924): 381–87, 424–29, 461–67.

———. *Våre folkemedisinske lægeurter* (The folk medicine of our healing herbs). (Published as a supplement to *Maal og Minne*). Kristiania: Centraltrykkeriet, 1922.

"Return of the Leech: Nature's bloodsuckers are—again—a doc's best friend." *Utne Reader,* May–June 1997, 16.

Riddervold, Astrid. *Drikkeskikker. Nordmennenes drikkevaner gjennom 1000 år* (Drinking customs. One thousand years of Norwegian drinking habits). Oslo: Teknologisk Forlag, 1997.

Rise, Ola J. *Oppdalsboka. Historie og folkeminne I* (Oppdal: history and folklore). Oslo: Tanum, 1947.

Risse, Gunter B. "From Horse and Buggy to Automobile and Telephone: Medical Practice in Wisconsin, 1848–1930." In *Wisconsin Medicine: Historical Perspectives,* eds. Ronald L. Numbers and Judith Walzer Neavitt, 25–45. Madison: University of Wisconsin Press, 1981.

Ritter, T. J. "The People's Home Medical Book." *The People's Home Library. A Library of Three Practical Books.* Cleveland, Ohio: R. C. Barnum, 1915.

Roan, Carl M. *Home, Church and Sex.* New York: I. Washburn, 1930.

———. "The Immigrant Wagon: A Trustworthy Narrative of Pioneer Events." Typed manuscript, 1946, in Minnesota Historical Society, St. Paul.

Rogaland i manns minne. Daglegliv ved hundreårsskiftet. Frå Nasjonalforeningens landskonkurranse for eldre. (Rogaland in recent memory. Daily life at the turn of the century. From the national competition for senior citizens). Oslo: Det Norske Samlaget, 1970.

Root-Bernstein, Robert, and Michèle Root-Bernstein. *Honey, Mud, Maggots, and Other Medical Marvels: The Science behind Folk Remedies and Old Wives' Tales.* New York: Houghton Mifflin, 1997.

Rørbye, Birgitte. *Kloge folk og skidtfolk. Kvaksalveriets epoke i Danmark* (The epoch of quack medicine in Denmark). København: Politikens Forlag, 1976.

Rustad, Mary S., ed. and trans. *The Black Books of Elverum.* Lakeville, Minn.: Galde Press, 1990.

Rustad, Mrs. Oliver A. "Memoir," 1939–1940. Trans. Duffy O. Rustad, Fergus Falls, Minn. Website: www.webfamilytree.com/mn_otter.htm.

Rutkow, Ira M. *Bleeding Blue and Gray: Civil War Surgery and the Evolution of American Medicine.* New York: Random House, 2005.

Sæbbe, Linda Vaeng. "Han stenger blodet" (He stops blood). *Lørdags Nordlys,* Jan. 8, 1997, 36–39.

Sæbø, Asbjørn. "Svarteboka" (The black book). *Romsdal Sogelag Aarsskrift* 1966: 32–39.

Salomonsen, Leif. "Barnet, dets pleie og sykdommer" (The child, its care and illnesses). In *Vår helse* (Our health). Leiv Kreyberg et al., eds., 151–55. Oslo: Nasjonalforlaget, 1933.

———. "Barnet." *Vår helse* 2, 377–79. Oslo: Nasjonalforlaget, 1949.

Sandvik, Hogne. "'Dei Vise forvidle Være!' En distriktleges kamp mot overtro og trolldom på 1800-tallet ("Folk healers delude the world!" A local doctor's struggle against superstition and sorcery in 19th-century Norway). *Tidsskrift for den Norske Lægeforening* 29 (1993): 3572–73.

Schønberg, Edvard. "Fra Børnepoliklinikken i det gamle Rigshospital, 2-Rakit" (From the children's clinic at the old National hospital, 2-Rickets). *Norsk Magasin for Lægevidenskaben* 1887 (48): 740–45.

———. "Svek" (Rickets). *Norsk Magasin for Lægevidenskaben* 1892: 1180–216.

Schrumpf, Ellen. *"Berus eder!" Norske drikkekulturer i de siste 200 år* (Get soused! Norwegian drinking culture during the last 200 years). Oslo: Unipax, 2003.

Schwinkendorf, Carol Hanson. *Here Come the Norwegians.* Scottsdale, Ariz.: privately printed, 1994.

Seierstad, David, and Ingeborg Sæther. "Mor Frøisland." *Gamle minner,* 3–21. Lena: Totens Trykkeri, 1943.

Seigworth, Gilbert R., M.D. "Bloodletting over the Centuries." *New York State Journal of Medicine* 80 (Dec. 1980): 2022–28.

Seip, Prost Henrik. "Åseral prestegård." *Prestegårdsliv. Minner fra norske prestegårder I*, 54-83. Oslo: Gyldendal, 1976.

Selland, S. K. "Folkemedicin." *Hardanger* 1916: 67–68.

Shaw, Joseph M. *Bernt Julius Muus: Founder of St. Olaf College*. Northfield, Minn.: Norwegian-American Historical Association, 1999.

Skåret, Valborg. "Fra småkårsfolks historie. Fødselshjelp, barnedåp, tro, overtro" (From the history of the impoverished. Childbirth, baptism, faith, and superstition). *Trysil årbok* 1985: 72–77.

Skatvedt, Thormod. *Sigdal og Eggedal, Bind V. Bygdehistorie* (Sigdal and Eggedal. Community history). Sigdal og Eggedal: Historielag, 1965.

Skirbekk, Håvard. "Svarboka. 'Ein kleiner Sibrianus'" (The black book. A little Cyprianus). *Årbok for Glåmdalen* 1973: 82–90.

Skjelbred, Berent. "Dei konne lækje sjukdomar då òg" (They could heal illness then, too). *Årbok for Jæren og Dalene* 1954: 188–89.

Skjeldsø, Lars. *Frå hverdagslivet i Øvre Gjerstad, 1850–1890* (From everyday life in Øvre Gjerstad, 1850–1890). Kristiansand: Gjerstad Historielag, 1979.

Skrutvold, Gunnar. "Mor Frøisland eller Frøisland-kjerringe" (Mor Frøisland or the Frøisland woman). *Tidsskrift for Valdres Historielag* 8 (1959): 134–42.

Slettan, Bjørn. *Holum. Gardshistorie* (Holum. Farm history). Mandal: Mandal kommune, 1977.

Sogner, Sølvi. *Far sjølv i stua og familien hans. Trekk fra norsk familiehistorie før og nå* (Norwegian family history now and before). Oslo: Universitetsforlaget, 1990.

Søraa, Gerd. *Hent jordmora!* (Get the midwife!). Oslo: Gyldendal, 1984.

Spoerke, David G., Jr. *Herbal Medications*. Santa Barbara, Cal.: Woodridge Press, 1980.

Starr, Douglas. *Blood: An Epic History of Medicine and Commerce*. New York: Harper Collins, 2002.

Steen, Adolf. "Litt om sjette og sjuende Mosebok" (A little about the 6th and 7th Book of Moses). *Norsk teologisk tidsskrift* 66 (1965): 65–88.

———. *Samenes folkemedisin* (Sami folkmedicine). Oslo: Universitetsforlaget, 1961.

Sternberg, Dr. Esther. *The Balance Within: The Science Connecting Health and Emotions*. New York: W. H. Freeman, 2000.

Stokker, Kathleen. "Between Sin and Salvation: The Human Condition in Legends of the Black Book Minister." *Scandinavian Studies* 67 (1995): 91–108.

———. *Keeping Christmas: Yuletide Traditions in Norway and the New Land*. St. Paul: Minnesota Historical Society Press, 2000.

———. "ML 3005—'The Would-Be Ghost': Why Be He a Ghost? Lutheran Views of Confession and Salvation in Legends of the Black Book Miniser." *Arv: Scandinavian Yearbook of Folklore* 47(1991): 143–52.

———. "'More than the Lord's Prayer': The Black Book Minister on the Prairie." *Crossings: Norwegian-American Lutheranism as a Transatlantic Tradition.* Todd W. Nichol, ed., 119–38. Northfield, Minn.: Norwegian-American Historical Society, 2003.

———. "Narratives of Magic and Healing: *Oldtidens Sortebog* in Norway and the New Land." *Scandinavian Studies* 73 (Fall 2001): 399–416.

———. "To Catch a Thief: Binding and Losing and the Black Book Minister." *Scandinavian Studies: Nordic Narrative Folklore* 61 (1989): 353–74.

Storaker, Joh. T. *Menneskelivet i den norske folketro* (NFL #35) (Human life in Norwegian folk belief). Oslo: Norsk Folkeminnelag, 1935.

———. *Sagn og gaader* (NFL # 47) (Legends and riddles). Oslo: Norsk Folkeminnelag, 1941.

———. *Sygdom og Forgjørelse i den norske Folketro* (NFL #28) (Sickness and healing in Norwegian folk belief). Oslo: Norsk Folkeminnelag, 1932.

Stout, Nancy. "The Hans H. Bangen Family History." Typed manuscript, 1979, Vesterheim Museum, Decorah, Iowa.

Strøm, Hans. *Kort Underviisning om De paa Landet, i Bergens Stift, meest grasserende Sygdomme, og derimod tienende Hjelpe-Midler* (Short instruction on the most common illnesses in rural Bergen parish and their remedies). Trans. Bjørn Davidsen. [1778]. Arendal: 2001. Website: http://home.online.no/~fndbred/hstrom1.htm.

Stuart, Malcolm. *The Encyclopedia of Herbs and Herbalism.* New York: Crescent Books, 1979.

Stubb, H. G. "Fra fars og mors liv" (From father and mother's life). *Symra. En Aarbog for norske paa begge sider af havet* (A yearbook for Norwegians on both sides of the ocean). 1907, 14–42.

Sunde, Rasmus. *Vikjer ved fjorden—Vikjer på prærien. Ein demografisk komparativ studie med utgangspunkt i Vik i Sogn* (People from Vik in Norway and on the prairie. A demographic comparative study based on Vik in Sogn). Ph.D. dissertation, University of Bergen, 2000.

Sundt, Eilert. *Om ædrueligheds-Tilstanden i Norge* (About sobriety in Norway). [Christiania, 1859]. Oslo: Gyldendal, 1976.

———. *Om renligheds-stellet i Norge: til oplysning om flid og fremskridt i landet* (About cleanliness in Norway. For enlightenment about efforts and progress across the land). [1869]. Oslo: Gyldendal, 1975.

Sundt, Halfdan. "Av hvad gamle medicinal-beretninger og andre kilder fortæller om Stavern og Fredriksvern." *Tidsskrift for den norske legeforening* 1927 (1): 19–25.

Svare, Reidar. *Frå Gamal Tid—Tru og tradisjon, Vefsn Bygdebok, Særbind II* (From old times: Belief and tradition in Vefsn). Mosjøen: Vefsn Bygdeboknemd, 1973.

"Svarteboka" (The black book). *Skilling Magazin,* 1859, 218–20.

Sveine, Ragnvald. "'Mor fortalte meg': An outline of Garmo history as told by my mother Ingebjørg Henningsdtr Garmo Svein." Lillehammer, 1960, typed manuscript, author's possession.

Teigen, Knut. *Ligt og uligt. Skitser, humoresker, eventyr og pennebilleder fra livet blandt vestens vikinger* (A little bit of everything. Sketches, humoresques, fairy tales, and drawings from life among the western Vikings). Minneapolis: Kreidt, 1907.

Thomson, William. *Medicines from the Earth: A Guide to Healing Plants.* Revised by Richard Evans Schultes. San Francisco: McGraw Hill, 1978.

Torkelson, Melvin Olaf. "Life on the Fraction: The Past Hundred Years, a tale of Norwegian immigration." Website: http://userwww.service.emory.edu/~marisa/FRACTION/fraction.text.html.

Torstensen, Inge. "Signekjerringer i storbyen" (Folk healers in the big city). Masters degree thesis, Dept. of Folklore, University of Oslo, Spring 1979.

———. "Med bly og tran mot engelsk syke" (With lead and cod-liver oil against rickets). *Byminner* 1986: 3–16.

Treleven, Dale. "One Hundred Years of Health and Healing in Rural Wisconsin." In *Wisconsin Medicine,* eds. Numbers and Leavitt, 133–54. Madison: University of Wisconsin Press, 1981.

Trøndelag i manns minne. Dagleglivet ved hundreårsskiftet (Trøndelag in recent memory. Daily life at the turn of the century). Oslo: Det Norske Samlaget, 1969.

Turtumøygard, Oluf. "Gamle helseråder og åtgjerder: Anne Marie Djupdalen i Heidalen fortel" (Old remedies and cures. Told by Anne Marie Djupdalen from Heidalen). *Årbok for Gudbrandsdalen* 1969: 202–4.

Tvinnereim, Jon. *Grotid i grenseland. Fylkeshistorie for Møre og Romsdal II, 1835–1920* (A time of growth in the border land. Local history of Møre and Romsdal II, 1835–1920). Oslo: Det Norske Samlaget, 1992.

Tyler, Varro E. *Herbs of Choice: The Therapeutic Uses of Phytomedicinals.* New York: Pharmaceutical Products Press, 1994.

———. *The Honest Herbal: A Sensible Guide to the Use of Herbs and Related Remedies.* 3rd edition. New York: Pharmaceutical Products Press, 1993.

Tyler, Varro E., Lynn R. Brady, and James E. Robbers. *Pharmacognosy.* 8th edition. Philadelphia: Lea and Febiger, 1981.

Urtehagen ved Apotekmuseet (The herb garden at the Apothecary Museum). Oslo: Cygnus, en norsk farmasihistorisk skriftserie, May 2001.

"Uses of Leeches in Plastic and Reconstructive Surgery: A review." *Journal of Reconstructive Microsurgery* 4 (Oct. 1988): 381–86.

Valand, Else. "Valborg Valand." *Vår Arv*, Holum Historielag [Our Heritage, published by the Holum Historical Society] 4 (1985): 4–7.

Vasvik, Stian. "Aqua Vita—fra medisin til juledrikk" (Akevit—from medicine to Christmas drink). *The Norseman*, Nov. 1994, 36–37.

Vogel, Virgil J. *American Indian Medicine*. Norman: University of Oklahoma Press, 1970.

Weiser-Aall, Lily. *Svangerskap og fødsel i nyere norsk tradisjon* (Pregnancy and birth in recent Norwegian tradition). Oslo: Norsk Folkemuseum, 1968.

Werner, David, with Carol Thuman and Jane Maxwell. *Where There Is No Doctor: A Village Health Care Handbook*. Berkeley, Cal.: Hesperian Foundation, 1992.

Wisness, Hilda, and Levard Quarve. *Viking: Early Settlement Days, 1886–1936*. Viking, N.D.: privately printed, 1936.

Ylvisaker, Erling. *Eminent Pioneers: Norwegian-American Pioneer Sketches*. Minneapolis: Augsburg, [1934?].

Young, James Harvey. *The Toadstool Millionaires: A Social History of Patent Medicines in America before Federal Regulation*. Princeton, N. J.: Princeton University Press, 1961.

Index

Notes:

Page numbers in *italic* indicate photographs and captions.

Page numbers such as "293n2" indicate information found in end notes (e.g., page 293, note 2).

The letters å, æ, and ø are alphabetized as a, ae, and o, respectively.

A

Aamodt, C. T., 63

Aanen, Andreas Eliasson, 90

Aasen, Ivar, 187

Aasen, Olaug, 189

absinthe, 196

abstinence movement, 183, 184, 192, 284n22

Achilles (Greek warrior), 42–43

Ackerknecht, Erwin, 265n4

acne, treatments for, 55, 59

advertising, and patent medicines, 285n31

Age of Enlightenment, and folklore, 267n18

Agrippa von Nettesheim, 263n54

airborne sickness, treatments for, 78–79, 228–229

alcohol, 177–200; distillation of, 178, *178*; fermentation of, 178; herbal extracts and flavoring, 7, 194–195, 197–200, 286n37; in patent medicines, 191–194; uses of, 10,44, 67, 126. *See also* specific kinds of alcohol

alcoholism: among immigrants, 185–191; behavior attributed to, 182, 283n15; impact on daily life,

185, 186–189; and physical violence, 187

Algaard, Swanhild, 192, 193, 194

Almklov, Leif, 21

Almklov, Severin, 18–22, 190–191, 246n30

Almklov family, 246n28

Almklov's "Itch Specific" salve, 20, *21*

almue. See common classes

aloe (aloe ferox), uses of, 25, 30, 116, 247n9

aloe drops, uses of, 25

ambar (wooden container), 128, 270n15

American Indians: as healers, 223; remedies, 16, 43, 245n21

American Medical Association, 17–18

amputations, 53

Amundsen, Arne Bugge, 84

Amundson, Howard, 227–229

Andersdatter, Anne-Marie. *See* Brandfjeld, Anne

Andersen, Johannes, 252n59

Anderson, Frank J., 265n5

Anderson, Harald, 196

Anderson, John, 99, 263n50

Ånekerlykkjun, Marianne, 264n57

Angostura bitters, uses of, 194, 286n37

Illustration credits

Pages ii, 109, plant drawing from Jens S. Heger, *Herbarium Pharmaceuticum* (1825), reproduced in Erik Bruun og Budde Christensen, *Klassiske legeplanter* (Oslo: H. Aschehoug & Co., 1998); 5, Norwegian Folkmuseum, Oslo; 12, 26, 70, 125, 174, 213, 240, Minnesota Historical Society, St. Paul, Minnesota; 21, courtesy Herbert Peterson, Williston, North Dakota; 36, drawing from *Urd*, 1905; 51, courtesy Louise Hexum, The Dalles, Oregon; 65, 148, 205, 217, Vesterheim Museum, Decorah, Iowa; 77, courtesy Mary Rustad, Nord Rustad, Elverum, Norway; 82, "Hanskrift Samlingen" [collection of handwritten documents], National Library, Oslo (Nasjonalbibliotek); 96, 117, Preus Library, Luther College, Decorah, Iowa; 106, Deichman Library, Oslo; 132, painting by Theodore Kittelson reproduced from Odd Hølaas, *Th. Kittelsen* (Oslo: Gyldendal, 1964); 138, drawing by R. T. Prichett from his *"Gamle Norge"* or *Rambles and Scrambles in Norway* (London: Virtue and Co, 1879); 156, drawing by Theodore Kittlesen, 1887, reproduced in Olav Bø, *Trollmakter og godvette. Overnaturlege vesen I norsk folketru* (Oslo: Det Norske Samlaget, 1987); 161, drawing from N. A. Quisling, *Overtroiske kurer og folkemedisin i Norge* (Superstitious cures and folk medicine in Norway) (Kristiania: Aschehoug, 1918); 165, painting by Adolph Tidemand, *En signekjerring i arbeid* (A folk healer at work), 1848, The National Museum of Fine Arts, Stockholm, Sweden; 178, drawing from Truls Nygaard, *Norsk brennevins leksikon* (Norwegian alcohol lexicon) (Oslo: Cappelen, 1945); 191, courtesy Milton Sorensen, Toronto, South Dakota; 235, Sogn Folkmuseum, Kaupanger.

The text of *Remedies and Rituals* has been set in Adobe Jenson Pro, a typeface designed by Robert Slimbach that captures the essence of Nicolas Jenson, a Renaissance type founder, punchcutter, and printer. Text design and composition by Wendy Holdman, Stanton Publication Services. Printed by Thomson-Shore, Dexter, Michigan.